Computer Access for People with Disabilities

A Human Factors Approach

REHABILITATION SCIENCE IN PRACTICE SERIES

Series Editors

Marcia J. Scherer, Ph.D.

President
Institute for Matching Person and Technology

Professor
Orthopaedics and Rehabilitation
University of Rochester Medical Center

Dave Muller, Ph.D.

Executive
Suffolk New College

Editor-in-Chief
Disability and Rehabilitation

Founding Editor
Aphasiology

Published Titles

Assistive Technology Assessment Handbook, *edited by Stefano Federici and Marcia J. Scherer*

Assistive Technology for Blindness and Low Vision, *Roberto Manduchi and Sri Kurniawan*

Computer Access for People with Disabilities: A Human Factors Approach, *Richard C. Simpson*

Multiple Sclerosis Rehabilitation: From Impairment to Participation, *edited by Marcia Finlayson*

Paediatric Rehabilitation Engineering: From Disability to Possibility, *edited by Tom Chau and Jillian Fairley*

Quality of Life Technology Handbook, *Richard Schultz*

Forthcoming Titles

Ambient Assisted Living, *edited by Nuno M. Garcia, Joel Jose P. C. Rodrigues, Dirk Christian Elias, Miguel Sales Dias*

Computer Systems Experiences of Users with and without Disabilities: An Evaluation Guide for Professionals, *Simone Borsci, Masaaki Kurosu, Stefano Federici, Maria Laura Mele*

Neuroprosthetics: Principles and Applications, *Justin C. Sanchez*

Rehabilitation Goal Setting: Theory, Practice and Evidence, *edited by Richard Siegert and William Levack*

Computer Access for People with Disabilities

A Human Factors Approach

Richard C. Simpson

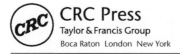

CRC Press
Taylor & Francis Group
Boca Raton London New York

CRC Press is an imprint of the
Taylor & Francis Group, an **informa** business

CRC Press
Taylor & Francis Group
6000 Broken Sound Parkway NW, Suite 300
Boca Raton, FL 33487-2742

First issued in paperback 2019

© 2013 by Taylor & Francis Group, LLC
CRC Press is an imprint of Taylor & Francis Group, an Informa business

No claim to original U.S. Government works

ISBN-13: 978-1-4665-5371-2 (hbk)
ISBN-13: 978-0-367-38042-7 (pbk)

Visit the Taylor & Francis Web site at
http://www.taylorandfrancis.com

and the CRC Press Web site at
http://www.crcpress.com

To my parents, Ted and Mary Ann Simpson, with love.

Contents

Preface

Computer access technology allows people who have trouble using a standard computer keyboard, mouse, or monitor to access the computer. Computer access technology includes relatively inexpensive devices such as trackballs and small-footprint keyboards as well as sophisticated technologies such as automatic speech recognition, eye gaze tracking, and brain–computer interfaces. Computer access technology services are provided by a range of rehabilitation professionals, including rehabilitation engineers, occupational therapists, speech language pathologists, special educators, and vocational rehabilitation counselors.

This book is intended for rehabilitation professionals and special educators who provide computer access services to people with disabilities. The material was originally developed for a course on computer access taught at the master's level to rehabilitation engineers and rehabilitation counselors. My goal was to offer practical guidance on how to provide computer access services along with sufficient background knowledge to allow the reader to interpret the research literature.

Because computer and Internet technology changes so rapidly, I have attempted to avoid references to specific products or operating systems whenever possible. Instead, the book emphasizes fundamental concepts that remain true regardless of which specific operating system or product is being used. The book draws on the literature from rehabilitation engineering and occupational therapy, but also from the human–computer interaction (HCI) literature. As McMillan has observed, most work in computing for people with disabilities is "carried out by professionals in education, rehabilitation and communication disorders, usually in isolation from more theoretical research in the field of HCI" [1].

REFERENCE

1. McMillan, W.W. 1992. Computing for users with special needs and models of computer–human interaction. In *SIGCHI Conference on Human Factors in Computing Systems*. Monterey, CA: ACM Press.

Acknowledgments

I thank the Paralyzed Veterans of America for providing funding to develop the material in this book. I would also like to thank Glen Ashlock, Mary Ellen Bunning, Ray Grott, and Gary Moulton for reading through earlier drafts of the book. Their input was invaluable in improving the final product. I also owe a tremendous amount of thanks to Heidi Koester and Ed LoPresti, with whom I have collaborated on much of my computer access research. Finally, I thank my family and friends for their continuing support.

About the Author

Richard C. Simpson, PhD, received a BS in computer science from Virginia Tech in 1992. At the University of Michigan he earned an MS in bioengineering in 1994, an MS in computer science and engineering in 1995, and a PhD in bioengineering in 1997. Dr. Simpson was certified as an Assistive Technology Professional in 1997. He joined the faculty of the University of Pittsburgh (Pitt) Department of Rehabilitation Science and Technology (RST) in 2000.

1 Introduction

1.1 HOW MANY PEOPLE NEED ALTERNATIVE COMPUTER ACCESS TECHNOLOGY?

It is hard to say exactly how many people need computer access technology. There are lots of different types of disabilities that can affect one's ability to use a computer, and obtaining accurate estimates for how many people have disabilities is difficult. Population-wide demographic data are obtained at different times, from different samples of people, using different definitions of disability [1]. Data are usually obtained from surveys and other "self-reporting" mechanisms, which introduces personal and cultural biases into the data. In addition, people can have combinations of disabilities. Finally, it is hard to account for the fact that people with the same diagnosis can have very different abilities.

1.1.1 COGNITIVE IMPAIRMENT

Individuals with cognitive disabilities comprise the largest single disability group. This is in part because cognition encompasses so many mental skills, processes, and constructs. Subgroups that are typically placed into the overarching category of a cognitive disability include individuals who have learning disabilities (e.g., dyslexia and dysgraphia), attention disorders (e.g., attention-deficit hyperactivity disorder [ADHD]), developmental disabilities (e.g., Down's syndrome, fragile X, autism, and cerebral palsy), and neurological impairments (e.g., Alzheimer's, traumatic brain injury, dementia, and stroke) [2, 3].

In 2004, the UK had 6 million people with dyslexia [4]. In 2002, almost 3 million U.S. students were receiving special education services for a learning disability [5]. Approximately 8% of school-age children in the U.S. are identified as having some form of math disability [6].

A developmental disability is a severe, chronic disability caused by a mental or physical impairment that manifests before 22 years of age. There are almost 4 million individuals in the United States with a developmental disability [7]. An individual is said to have an intellectual disability if he or she has an IQ below 70. There are approximately 7 million people in the United States with an intellectual disability [7]. An estimated 2 million Americans experience a traumatic brain injury every year [8].

1.1.2 SENSORY IMPAIRMENT

Visual impairment includes individuals who are completely blind, individuals who have reduced visual acuity, and individuals with conditions such as color blindness or glaucoma. Visual impairment is often defined in terms of visual acuity, which measures a person's ability to resolve fine spatial detail [9]. Legal blindness is often defined as a corrected visual acuity worse than 20/200 or a visual field of 20° or less [10].

In 2004, the UK had 1.6 million people with visual impairments [4]. Estimates of the prevalence of visual impairment in the United States have ranged from 3.4 million to 13.5 million individuals [1, 11]. The disparity among estimates is often attributed to the inconsistency in the definition of visual impairment used across studies [1]. Approximately 1% of students receiving special education services have a visual impairment [12]. In the United States, 8% of the male population and less than 1% of the female population have some form of color blindness [13].

Between 2 and 3 of every 1,000 children in the United States are born deaf or hard of hearing [14], and approximately 2% of students receiving special education services in the United States have a hearing impairment [12]. Approximately 17% of adults in the United States report some degree of hearing loss [14].

1.1.3 MOTOR IMPAIRMENT

In 2003, 31.7 million working-age Americans had a mild dexterity impairment and 12.0 million had a severe dexterity impairment [15]. Approximately 1% of students receiving special education services have a severe physical disability [12]. An estimated 54,000 to 68,000 people in the United States have incomplete tetraplegia [8]. In 2004, 3.4 million people in the UK had disabilities that interfered with their ability to use a standard computer keyboard, mouse, or monitor [4].

1.1.4 SITUATIONAL/TEMPORARY IMPAIRMENT

In addition to the traditional notion of disability as arising from a medical condition, sometimes the environment or task may induce a situational impairment [16–18] that impacts an individual's ability to use a computer. Examples include performing several tasks at once (multitasking) and working in an environment with loud ambient noise or poor lighting. An individual may also experience a temporary disability, due to something like a sprain or break that requires a cast, side effects from medication, recovery from a medical procedure, or an illness.

1.2   IMPORTANCE OF COMPUTER ACCESS

Computer access technology is critical for enhancing the educational and vocational opportunities of people with disabilities [19, 20]. Computers and the Internet are an important, often unavoidable, aspect of all levels of education, and a computer can be an extremely valuable education tool for students with disabilities [1, 12, 21–34]. Computer use is also required for employment in many fields [1, 22–28, 30–37]. Persons with physical or perceptual impairments are more likely to be employed in professional, administrative, or managerial jobs, which require computer skills, rather than heavy manual labor [3–6]. Employment is a significant predictor of quality of life [8–15], a means to attaining autonomy and independence [16, 17], and an activity that enhances self-esteem and a sense of identity [18]. Employment is strongly linked to feelings of social validity, self-identity, and economic security [28]. Further, employment is a source of personal growth, a place to develop social contacts that lead to a sense of belonging, and a major means of social integration [19]. Positive relationships have been reported between employment and longevity, health status, personal satisfaction, and positive life adjustment following spinal cord injury (SCI) [9, 16, 20–23].

In addition to its importance as an enabler of education and employment, computer access has been shown to contribute to improved health status by providing access to health information and interaction with clinicians and peers [24, 38]. Computer access is also a critical element of community participation and independent living [1, 12, 17, 23, 24, 33, 34, 36, 37, 39, 40]. Access to a computer and the Internet allows individuals with disabilities to perform activities related to

- Government [22, 24, 32]
- Banking [24]
- News and events [22, 24, 35, 37]
- Information [24, 25, 28, 32, 35, 37]
- Shopping [24, 25, 29, 34, 35]

Computer and Internet access has been demonstrated to provide social and psychological benefits to individuals with disabilities [17, 22, 25, 28, 34, 37, 41] and has also been shown to reduce social isolation by eliminating physical barriers, facilitating communication, and providing a forum for the exchange of information [25, 41]. Computer and Internet access allows older adults and people with disabilities to communicate with friends and families [23–26, 28, 33, 34, 36, 37]. Online communities can provide social support and reduce feelings of isolation and loneliness [22, 24, 28, 37]. Computers can be used for leisure time pursuits and entertainment [23, 24, 26, 30, 31, 34, 36, 37]. Individuals with disabilities often appreciate the anonymity of the Internet, where they can be evaluated for the strength of their contributions rather than their physical appearance or disability [26, 27, 42, 43]. The Internet also provides protection against self-consciousness and social anxiety, and active participation can lead to greater levels of self-acceptance and decreased feelings of isolation [28, 29, 44, 45].

1.3   DIGITAL DIVIDE

Individuals with disabilities are much less likely to own or use a computer than their able-bodied peers [15, 25, 28, 46]. While 85% of working-age adults without disabilities use computers, computer usage is 80% among those who have mild impairments and only 63% among individuals who have severe disabilities and are most likely to benefit from the use of computer access technology [15]. Many people with disabilities who do own computers do not take advantage of computer access technology. One study found that only 24% of working-age computer users with severe disabilities use computer access technology [47]. Older adults and people with disabilities often don't know what computer access solutions exist or don't have the expertise necessary to choose and configure the most appropriate computer access solution [1, 23, 27, 28, 48–52].

People with disabilities (particularly individuals outside of a school system or vocational rehabilitation program) do not have regular access to clinicians with computer access expertise [1, 25, 28, 49–51, 53, 54]. Public computers (e.g., computers in libraries) often do not provide any support or instruction [25]. Instead, people with disabilities must rely on themselves, their friends, or their family for support [51, 54]. Many teachers and clinicians don't have training in computer access technology [1, 12, 23, 27, 28, 50, 54–57]. It can also be hard for teachers and clinicians to remain knowledgeable about computer access technology when it isn't their primary focus given the rapid pace of change in the computer industry [50, 58].

Many individuals are reluctant to try and make adjustments to their computer [49, 59–61]. Settings can be confusing or hard to find. Among computer users who do own and use computer access technology, there is ample evidence that it is often not configured correctly. For example, Trewin and Pain reported target acquisition error rates of greater than 10% for 14 of 20 users with physical disabilities, and observed that 55% of the dragging tasks made by these users were unsuccessful [52]. An average of 28% of clicks in this study included a mouse movement, which is a potential source of error, and 40% of multiple click attempts were unsuccessful [52].

Worst of all, approximately a third of computer users who do receive computer access technology wind up abandoning it. A study of 115 individuals with disabilities who received 136 assistive technology devices over 5 years, including computers, communication devices, and adapted software, reported a total abandonment rate of 32.4%. The abandonment rate within the study for computer access and communication devices was 30.8% [62].

1.4 MEASUREMENT

This book emphasizes the importance of quantitative measurement in the computer access assessment process. Measurements rarely tell us anything we can't learn by observation. Instead, their purpose is to summarize our observations in a way that lends itself to description and comparison. Reasons for a clinician to measure a client's performance include

- Document outcomes
- Compare interventions
- Match previous outcomes or literature to new clients
- Create a concise description of a client
- Justify the need for specific interventions

A measurement is a numerical summary of one aspect of the thing being measured. Miles per gallon, time from 0 to 60 miles per hour, and cubic storage space are all measures of specific attributes of a car, but none completely defines the car. Most importantly, which measure is most relevant to you when you're shopping for a car depends on how you intend to use that car. Different performance measures are best suited for different goals. In addition, each performance measure summarizes a unique aspect of a car's performance.

Sometimes, it's not necessary to measure anything. Measurements are most useful for describing things and comparing things. If you want to tell your friend about your car, or you want to compare your car to your friend's car, or maybe compare last year's model to this year's model, it helps to have measurements. On the other hand, if you only have one car to choose from, or you don't have any friends, there's not much point in taking a lot of measurements.

As with cars, there are lots of ways to measure computer access technology, and which measures are relevant depends on what the client wants to do and how the client wants to do it. It's up to the clinician to determine which measures are most relevant to the performance of each client.

1.5 USER MODELING

1.5.1 INTRODUCTION

This book makes use of user modeling techniques to explore several computer access technologies. A *model* is a simplified version of a complex thing that is used to make predictions about how the complex thing will behave under different conditions. As an example, a crash test dummy is a model of a real person used to learn what would happen to a real person in a car crash. A crash test dummy is used by automakers to learn how different people, design decisions, and crash conditions affect the safety of a person in an accident. In this example:

- Different people would be represented by crash test dummies of different weights, heights, and flexibility.
- Different design decisions could include the style of the bumper, the type of seatbelts and airbags, or the construction materials used for the body of the vehicle.
- Different crash conditions could include the speed of the car at impact or the angle and location of the collision.

This information allows automakers to design automobiles that are safe for the greatest number of people under the greatest number of crash conditions.

The user models discussed in this book are often referred to as *models of human information processing*. Models in this category are all similar in that they assume [63]:

1. Humans are composed of interacting subsystems.
2. Humans perform tasks by (1) perceiving observations, (2) deciding on a response to the observations, and (3) acting based on this decision.

Models in this category differ based on what disciplines the models emerged from (psychology, physiology, or sociology) and what aspects of human behavior they incorporate (perceptual, mental, physical, emotional, attentional).

Fitts' law [64, 65] is one of the best-known models used in human–computer interaction (HCI). Fitts' law predicts the time it takes a person to move his or her hand from a starting point to a target based on the size of the target and the distance between the starting point and target. The law states that the time T required to move the hand from a starting point to a target of size S, which is distance D from the hand, is given by

$$T = a + b \log_2 \left(\frac{2D}{S} \right)$$

where a and b are constants that are adjusted for the specific situation being modeled. Examples of how this model is used in HCI include estimating the amount of time it will take a person to move his or her hand from the keyboard to the mouse, or the time required to move the mouse pointer from its current position on the screen to a button at another location on the screen by moving the mouse.

Now consider the task of pressing a switch when a light is switched on. Fitts' law ignores both perceptual activity (identifying when the light is observed) and mental activity (for example, choosing which switch to press from among several choices), and only describes motor activity. Hence, using Fitts' law to model this action would provide an estimate of the time to press the switch, but would ignore the time required to perceive the light or choose which switch to press (out of several possible switches).

The *model human processor* (MHP) [63], on the other hand, is a model of human information processing, derived from psychological data, that represents perceptual, mental, and physical phenomena. The MHP represents a person as a collection of interconnected special-purpose memories and processors. In addition to specifying a *structure* composed of memories, processors, and their interconnections, the MHP also specifies properties of these memories and processors, such as the number of items that can be stored in each memory and the amount of time each processor requires to perform a single action.

The MHP would model the action of pressing a switch in response to a light as follows:

1. The *perceptual processor* observes the light and notifies the cognitive processor.
2. The *cognitive processor* selects the appropriate response and passes this information to the motor processor.
3. The *motor processor* executes the chosen motor command.

The MHP, on its own, is an unwieldy tool for analyzing user interfaces. Instead, the MHP serves as the basis of a family of user modeling methods called GOMS [66], which stands for goals, operators, methods, and selection rules. The members of the GOMS family vary in their assumptions, ranging from very simplified models that provide quick (but less accurate) estimates of user performance to very detailed models that provide labor-intensive (but very accurate) estimates.

A GOMS model uses the components in Table 1.1 to specify the steps used to complete a task. Two key assumptions in all GOMS models are [63]

1. The user will perform the task in the exact same way each time (in other words, each time the user performs the task, the user will follow the same steps, each of which will take the same amount of time).
2. The user will not make any mistakes along the way, nor will the user be interrupted at any point during the task.

TABLE 1.1

Components of the GOMS Framework

Component	Description
Goal	The task the user is trying to accomplish.
Operator	A step performed as part of completing the task. Operators can be perceptual, mental, or physical.
Method	Sequence of operators.
Selection rule	Rule for choosing between potential methods for accomplishing a task or subtask within a task.

Because a GOMS model is based on the MHP, the steps within a task can be associated with the actions of specific processors, which allows quantitative predictions of performance time to be made. Hence, the task of pressing a switch in response to a light would be modeled by the keystroke-level model [67] form of GOMS as:

1. One perceptual processor action to observe the light
2. One cognitive processor action to choose the correct response
3. One physical processor action to move the finger to press the switch

The total time (T_{total}) required for this task would then be calculated as

$$T_{total} = T_p + T_c + T_m$$

where T_p is the time required for a single cycle of the perceptual processor, T_c is the time required for a single cycle of the cognitive processor, and T_m is the time required for a single cycle of the motor (physical) processor.

It's important to understand that models are used to *estimate* behavior, which is much different, and less precise, than *measuring* behavior. To know exactly how a person, or group of people, will perform a specific task with a specific interface, it is necessary to expose the person (or people) to the interface and measure their performance. Models, on the other hand, are used to expose lots of virtual people to an interface to estimate how they would perform. Obviously, the more detailed the model is, the more accurate the estimate will be. On the other hand, the larger the group of people the model is used to represent, the less accurate the estimate will be. In other words, a detailed model tailored to one specific user can be very accurate, but a less detailed model representing many potential users will be less accurate.

However, even if a model is not accurate in an absolute sense, it can still be useful if it is *relatively* accurate. If a clinician wants to compare two interfaces, A and B, it may not be necessary to know precisely how long it would take a user to perform the same task using both interfaces. It may be enough to know that the user will take longer to perform the task using interface A than he or she will take to perform the same task using interface B. In other words, the software designer can use a model to learn that interface B is better *relative to* interface A.

User models are best suited are making relative comparisons between interfaces based on predictions of performance (for example, the number of seconds required to perform a specific task). User models can also be used to identify where errors might occur and to estimate the time required to learn to use an interface. Finally, user models can reduce, but not eliminate, the need to evaluate a user interface with real people. By reducing the amount of testing that must be done with real people, user models can accelerate the process, and reduce the cost, of designing a user interface.

REFERENCES

1. Strobel, W. et al. 2006. Technology for access to text and graphics for people with visual impairments and blindness in vocational settings. *Journal of Vocational Rehabilitation* 24: 87–95.
2. WebAIM. 2007. Cognitive disabilities part 2: Conceptualizing design considerations. Available from http://www.webaim.org/articles/cognitive/conceptualize/ (accessed November 24, 2007).
3. WebAIM. 2010. Cognitive disabilities. Available from http://www.webaim.org/articles/cognitive/ (accessed December 22, 2010).
4. Curran, K., N. Walters, and D. Robinson. 2007. Investigating the problems faced by older adults and people with disabilities in online environments. *Behaviour and Information Technology* 26(6): 447–453.
5. LD Fast Facts. 2009. Available from http://www.greatschools.net/LD/identifying/ld-fast-facts.gs?content=811 (accessed November 2, 2009).
6. Bryant, D.P. 2009. Math disability in children: An overview. Available from http://www.greatschools.net/LD/identifying/math-disability-in-children-an-overview.gs?content=526&page=all (accessed November 2, 2009).
7. Seeman, L. 2002. Inclusion of cognitive disabilities in the web accessibility movement. Presented at Eleventh International World Wide Web Conference (WWW2002), Honolulu, HI.
8. Trewin, S. 2002. Extending keyboard adaptability: An investigation. *Universal Access in the Information Society* 2(1): 44–55.
9. Nunes, F., P.A. Silva, and F. Abrantes. 2010. Human-computer interaction and the older adult: An example using user research and personas. In *PETRA '10: The 3rd International Conference on Pervasive Technologies Related to Assistive Environments*, F. Makedon, I. Maglogiannis, and S. Kapidakis, eds. Samos, Greece: ACM.
10. WebAIM. 2010. Visual disabilities. Available from http://www.webaim.org/articles/visual/ (accessed December 22, 2010).
11. Jacko, J.A. et al. 2003. Older adults and visual impairment: What do exposure times and accuracy tell us about performance gains associated with multimodal feedback? In *SIGCHI Conference on Human Factors in Computing Systems*, G. Cockton and P. Korhonen, eds. Ft. Lauderdale, FL: ACM Press, pp. 33–40.
12. Dugan, J.J., R.B. Cobb, and M. Alwell. 2007. *The effects of technology-based interventions on academic outcomes for youth with disabilities.* Fort Collins: Colorado State University.
13. Meyer, G.W., and D.P. Greenberg. 1988. Color-defective vision and computer graphics displays. *IEEE Computer Graphics and Applications* 8(5): 28–40.
14. Quick Statistics. 2012. Available from http://www.nidcd.nih.gov/health/statistics/Pages/quick.aspx (accessed May 15, 2012).
15. Stevenson, B., and J.L. McQuivey. 2003. The wide range of abilities and its impact on computer technology. A research study commissioned by Microsoft Corporation and conducted by Forrester Research, Cambridge, MA.

16. Newell, A.F., and P. Gregor. 2002. Design for older and disabled people—Where do we go from here? *Universal Access in the Information Society* 2(1): 3–7.
17. Price, K.J., and A. Sears. 2009. The development and evaluation of performance-based functional assessment: A methodology for the measurement of physical capabilities. *ACM Transactions on Accessible Computing* 2(2).
18. Sears, A., and M. Young. 2002. Physical disabilities and computing technologies: An analysis of impairments. In *The human-computer interaction handbook*, J.A. Jacko and A. Sears, eds. Hillsdale, NJ: L. Erlbaum Associates, pp. 482–503.
19. Anson, D.K. 1997. *Alternative computer access: A guide to selection.* 1st ed. Philadelphia: F.A. Davis Company, p. 280.
20. Chen, C.-L. et al. 2006. Enhancement of operational efficiencies for people with high cervical spinal cord injuries using a flexible integrated pointing device apparatus. *Archives of Physical Medicine and Rehabilitation* 87: 866–873.
21. Beigel, A.R. 2000. Assistive technology assessment: More than the device. *Intervention in School and Clinic* 35(4): 237–243.
22. Bowker, N.I. 2010. Understanding barriers to online experience for people with physical and sensory disabilities using discursive social psychology. *Universal Access in the Information Society* 9: 121–136.
23. Burton, M., E.R. Nieuwenhuijsen, and M.J. Epstein. 2008. Computer-related assistive technology: Satisfaction and experiences among users with disabilities. *Assistive Technology* 20(2): 99–106.
24. Czaja, S.J., and C.C. Lee. 2007. The impact of aging on access to technology. *Universal Access in the Information Society* 5(4): 341–349.
25. Fox, L.E. et al. 2009. Public computing options for individuals with cognitive impairments: Survey outcomes. *Disability and Rehabilitation: Assistive Technology* 4(5): 311–320.
26. Fraser, B.A., D.N. Bryen, and C.K. Morano. 1995. Development of a Physical Characteristics Assessment (PCA): A checklist for determining appropriate computer access for individuals with cerebral palsy. *Assistive Technology* 7(1): 26–35.
27. Gallagher, B., N. Connolly, and S. Lyne. 2005. Equal Access to Technology Training (EATT): Improving the computer literacy of people with vision impairments aged over 35. *International Congress Series* 1282: 846–850.
28. Gerber, E. 2003. The benefits of and barriers to computer use for individuals who are visually impaired. *Journal of Visual Impairment and Blindness* 536–550.
29. Kelker, K.A., and R. Holt. 1997. *Family guide to assistive technology.* Billings, MT: Parents, Let's Unite for Kids.
30. Mazer, B., C. Dumont, and C. Vincent. 2003. Validation of the assessment of computer task performance for children. *Technology and Disability* 15(1): 35–43.
31. Ratanasit, D., and M.M. Moore. 2005. Representing graphical user interfaces with sound: A review of approaches. *Journal of Visual Impairment and Blindness* 69–85.
32. Schroeder, P. 1998. *Access to multimedia technology by people with sensory disabilities.* National Council on Disability, Washington, DC.
33. Shih, C.-T., C.-H. Shih, and C.-H. Luo. 2011. Development of a computer assistive input device through a commercial numerical keyboard by position coding technology for people with disabilities. *Disability and Rehabilitation: Assistive Technology* 6(2): 169–175.
34. Williams, M.R., and R.F. Kirsch. 2008. Evaluation of head orientation and neck muscle EMG signals as command inputs to a human–computer interface for individuals with high tetraplegia. *IEEE Transactions on Neural Systems and Rehabilitation Engineering* 16(5): 485–496.
35. Richards, J.T., and V.L. Hanson. 2004. Web accessibility: A broader view. In *13th International Conference on the World Wide Web*, S. Feldman and M. Uretsky, eds. New York: ACM Press, pp. 72–79.

36. Segrist, K.A. 2004. Attitudes of older adults toward a computer training program. *Educational Gerontology* 30(7): 563–571.

37. Taveira, A.D., and S.D. Choi. 2009. Review study of computer input devices and older users. *International Journal of Human-Computer Interaction* 25(5): 455–474.

38. Dobransky, K., and E. Hargittai. 2006. The disability divide in Internet access and use. *Information, Communication and Society* 9(3): 313–334.

39. Bernd, T., D. van der Pijl, and L. de Witte. 2009. Existing models and instruments for the selection of assistive technology in rehabilitation practice. *Scandanavian Journal of Occupational Therapy* 16: 146–158.

40. Jenko, M. et al. 2010. A method for selection of appropriate assistive technology for computer access. *International Journal of Rehabilitation Research* 33(4): 298–305.

41. Drainoni, M. et al. 2004. Patterns of Internet use by persons with spinal cord injuries and relationship to health-related quality of life. *Archives of Physical Medicine and Rehabilitation* 85(11): 1872–1879.

42. Madara, E. 1997. The mutual-aid self-help online revolution. *Social Policy* 27: 20–26.

43. McKenna, K., and G. Seidman. 2005. You, me, and we: Interpersonal processes in electronic groups. In *The social net: Human behavior in cyberspace*, Y. Amichai-Hamburger, ed. Oxford: Oxford University Press, pp. 191–217.

44. McKenna, K., and J. Bargh. 2000. Plan 9 from cyberspace: The implications of the Internet for personality and social psychology. *Personality and Social Psychology Review* 4(1): 57.

45. Morahan-Martin, J., and P. Schumacher. 2003. Loneliness and social use of the Internet. *Computers in Human Behavior* 19(6): 656–671.

46. Vaccaro, M. et al. 2007. Internet use and interest among individuals with traumatic brain injury: A consumer survey. *Disability and Rehabilitation: Assistive Technology* 2(2): 85–95.

47. Stevenson, B., and J.L. McQuivey. 2003. Examining awareness, use, and future potential. Available from http://www.microsoft.com/enable/research/phase2.aspx (accessed 2009).

48. Gregor, P., and A. Dickinson. 2007. Cognitive difficulties and access to information systems: An interaction design perspective. *Universal Access in the Information Society* 5(4): 393–400.

49. Hurst, A. et al. 2008. Automatically detecting pointing performance. In *Proceedings of the 13th International Conference on Intelligent User Interfaces*, S. Staab, ed. Gran Canaria, Spain: ACM, pp. 11–19.

50. Mann, W.C. et al. 2005. Computer use by middle-aged and older adults with disabilities. *Technology and Disability* 17(1): 1–9.

51. Trewin, S., and H. Pain. 1999. A model of keyboard configuration requirements. *Behaviour and Information Technology* 18(1): 27–35.

52. Trewin, S., and H. Pain. 1999. Keyboard and mouse errors due to motor disabilities. *International Journal of Human-Computer Studies* 50(2): 109–144.

53. Bhattacharya, S., A. Basu, and D. Samanta. 2008. Computational modeling of user errors for the design of virtual scanning keyboards. *IEEE Transactions on Neural Systems and Rehabilitation Engineering* 16(4): 400–409.

54. Scherer, M.J. et al. 2007. A framework for modelling the selection of assistive technology devices (ATDs). *Disability and Rehabilitation: Assistive Technology* 2(1): 1–8.

55. Fitzgerald, M.M. et al. 2009. Comparison of three head-controlled mouse emulators in three light conditions. *Augmentative and Alternative Communication* 25(1): 32–41.

56. Gitlin, L., and D. Burg. 1995. Issuing assistive devices to older patients in rehabilitation: An exploratory study. *American Journal of Occupational Therapy* 49(10): 994–1000.

57. Mckenna, M.C., and S. Walpole. 2007. Assistive technology in the reading clinic: Its emerging potential. *Reading Research Quarterly* 42(1): 140–145.

58. Dumont, C., C. Vincent, and B. Mazer. 2002. Development of a standardized instrument to assess computer task performance. *American Journal of Occupational Therapy* 56(1): 60–68.
59. Dillen, H., J.G. Phillips, and J.W. Meehan. 2005. Kinematic analysis of cursor trajectories controlled with a touchpad. *International Journal of Human-Computer Interaction* 19(2): 223–239.
60. Johansen, A.S., and J.P. Hansen. 2006. Augmentative and alternative communication: The future of text on the move. *Universal Access in the Information Society* 5(2): 125–149.
61. Kehoe, A., F. Neff, and I. Pitt. 2009. Use of voice input to enhance cursor control in mainstream gaming applications. *Universal Access in the Information Society* 8(1): 89–96.
62. Riemer-Reiss, M. 2000. Factors Associated with Assistive Technology Discontinuance among Individuals with Disabilities. *Journal of Rehabilitation* 66(3): 44–50.
63. Card, S.K., T.P. Moran, and A.F. Newell. 1983. *The psychology of human-computer interaction*. Hillsdale, NJ: Erlbaum.
64. Fitts, P. 1954. The information capacity of the human motor system in controlling the amplitude of movement. *Journal of Experimental Psychology* 47: 381–391.
65. Fitts, P., and M. Posner. 1967. *Human performance*. Belmont, CA: Brooks-Cole.
66. John, B.E., and D.E. Kieras. 1996. The GOMS family of user interface analysis techniques: Comparison and contrast. *ACM Transactions on Computer-Human Interaction* 3: 320–351.
67. Card, S.K., T.P. Moran, and A. Newell. 1980. The keystroke-level model for user performance time with interactive systems. *Communications of the ACM* 23(7): 396–410.

2 Keyboard-Only Access

2.1 INTRODUCTION

This chapter discusses techniques for using a computer entirely from the keyboard, without any sort of pointing device. Keyboard-only access is important for several different populations of computer users, including [1]

- Individuals who are blind
- Individuals who have low vision that makes it hard to find small objects on the screen
- Users with upper body impairments who have more reliable keyboard access than mouse access
- Users with injuries or temporary disabilities
- Users with poor targeting skills
- Users who want to write robust macros
- People who have difficulty with pointing
- People using an augmentative communication device for computer access

As a general rule, most programs for both Windows® and Macintosh® operating systems let you do the same thing in several different ways, including at least one that only requires the keyboard. For example, there are at least five ways to copy selected text to the clipboard in Word 2010 for Windows [2]:

1. Click the mouse button on the Edit menu, click on the Copy item
2. Alt, E, C
3. Ctrl + C
4. Click the Copy toolbar button
5. Right-click on the selected text to display the context menu, click on the Copy item

Computer users tend to rely on mouse-based methods way too often, because they either do not know about more efficient alternatives or choose not to learn them [2]. There are several advantages to using the keyboard, instead of the mouse [1, 2]. Using the keyboard removes the need for the user to move his or her hands from the keyboard to the mouse. Using the keyboard also eliminates the need to target small items on the screen. Finally, keystrokes are faster than mouse movements. Lane et al. [2] had six able-bodied graduate students perform tasks using the keyboard, toolbar buttons, and menu items. Keyboard shortcuts were much faster than toolbar buttons, and toolbar buttons were much faster than menus [2].

There are also some obstacles to using the keyboard exclusively [1–3]. In particular, it can sometimes be difficult to determine which item on the screen will receive input from the keyboard. In addition, keyboard interfaces can be implemented poorly within an individual application and inconsistently across multiple applications. Finally, some tasks (e.g., drawing) do not lend themselves to keyboard operation.

2.2   INPUT FOCUS

To operate a computer from the keyboard, it is more important to learn a few techniques rather than lots of arbitrary key combinations [1, 3]. To use a computer without the mouse you must be able to perform the following [3]:

1. Identify which item on the screen has input focus.
2. Move input focus to the item on the screen you want to manipulate.
3. Act upon the item that has input focus.

The item with *input focus* is the one item on the screen that receives input from the keyboard. Only one window has input focus at a time, and within the window that has input focus, only one control has focus at a time. If one item gets input focus, another item loses it. Selecting an item with the mouse shifts input focus to that object [1, 3].

2.3   MACROS

A macro is a sequence of commands for performing a task [4]. The principle use of macros is to automate repetitive or fatiguing tasks, but they can also be used to solve accessibility problems [4]. As a general rule, macros that move the mouse pointer tend to be less reliable than keystroke-only macros [4], so it helps to know how to do things by keyboard.

Macro utilities come in different shapes and sizes. Some macro software is built into a single program or suite of programs (Microsoft® Office, for example). Other macro software will run across multiple applications.

Macro utilities also vary in the complexity associated with creating macros. The easiest way to create a macro is to record a series of keyboard and mouse operations, which can then be repeated by the macro utility. While this greatly simplifies the task of creating a macro, the resulting macro is going to be less flexible than a macro that is written in a programming language.

To write a macro:

1. Figure out how to do the task using just the keyboard.
2. List the steps—one step for each keystroke.
3. Write the macro—one command for each step.
4. Develop and test the macro one line at a time.

You can use the following form to organize the information for your macros.

Assumptions

Programs that are running	
Program that has input focus	
Item in active program that has input focus	
Anything else that must be true for the macro to work	

Macro

Step	Keystroke(s)	Macro Command(s)

2.4   MOUSE KEYS

In some circumstances it is impossible to control an application with keyboard short-cuts. In this case mouse keys can be used [5]. Mouse keys allows the user to control the mouse cursor using the number pad on the keyboard. The directions of movement are controlled using the numeric pad keys as shown below. Mouse keys should be considered a last resort, however [1]. Mouse keys are almost always slower than using keystrokes or an actual mouse (Figure 2.1).

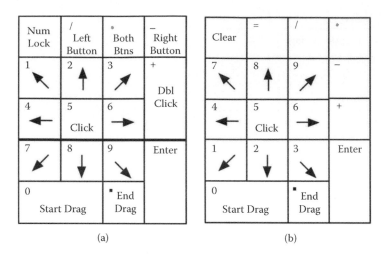

FIGURE 2.1   Mouse keys for (a) Windows 7 and (b) Mac OS X.

2.5   KEYBOARD ACCESS TO WINDOWS 7

2.5.1 DESKTOP

The Windows 7 desktop consists of five regions (Figure 2.2):

- The Desktop folder, which contains the recycle bin, files, folders, and application shortcuts
- The Start menu, which allows the user to launch programs and open folders
- The Task Bar, which shows all open programs and folders and contains quick-launch shortcuts to frequently used programs
- The notification area, which contains icons for background processes
- The Show Desktop button, which minimizes open applications and returns focus to the desktop

The user can move input focus between desktop regions using the F6 key or Tab key. Input focus is moved between items within a region using the up, down, left, and right arrow keys. The item that has input focus can be opened with the space bar or Enter key.

2.5.2 MENUS AND RIBBONS

Most programs in Windows have menus (although some have adopted the "ribbon," instead). There are several ways to access menus and ribbons from the keyboard.

It is possible to navigate through the menu bar using the keyboard. Pressing the Alt key transfers input focus to the menu bar. Input focus can be moved along the menu bar with the left and right arrow keys, and menus can be opened and closed using the up and down arrow keys. Within a menu, input focus is moved between items using the up and down arrow keys, and submenus can be opened and closed using the right arrow key. A menu item is selected using the Enter key (Figure 2.3).

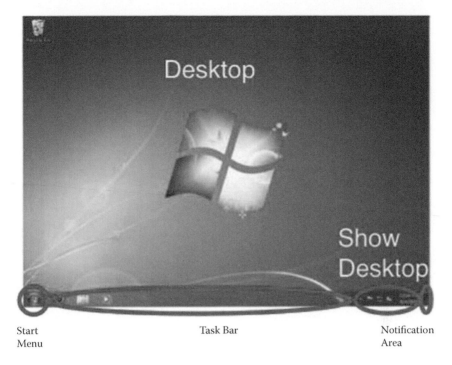

FIGURE 2.2   Components of Windows 7 desktop.

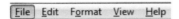

FIGURE 2.3   Menu with input focus.

In addition to using the arrow keys and Enter key to select menu items, a menu item can often be selected using a shortcut key. Most menu names have one letter that is underlined. If you hold the Alt key and press a letter key, then the corresponding menu receives focus. Items within a menu can be selected by pressing underlined letters, too. You may need to press the Alt key for letters to be underlined, but this behavior can be changed (Figures 2.4 and 2.5).

Many commonly used menu items often have direct shortcuts (e.g., Ctrl + C for copy, Ctrl + V for paste). The direct shortcuts are not immediately visible so they have to be remembered. These key combinations are often listed next to their corresponding menu items.

Key tips are available in all applications that have a ribbon. Press Alt to display a letter or number by each ribbon tab or command. After you press a letter or number, you get new key tip letters and numbers to access each command in the location you selected (Figure 2.6).

2.5.3   DIALOG BOXES

Dialog boxes can contain a variety of controls. To cycle input focus between controls, use the Tab key. Pressing the Tab key moves input focus through the controls

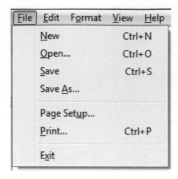

FIGURE 2.4 Menu with shortcut keys and access key combinations.

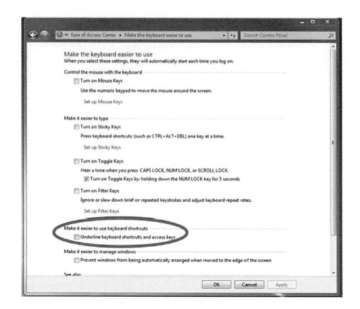

FIGURE 2.5 Underline keyboard shortcuts and access keys.

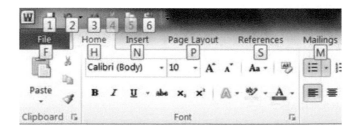

FIGURE 2.6 Key tips on a ribbon.

in the order specified by the software's programmer. Shift + Tab (i.e., holding down the Shift key while pressing the Tab key) moves input focus between controls in the opposite order. It is often possible to move input focus directly to a control with a keyboard shortcut by holding down the Alt key and pressing the key corresponding to the underlined letter in the control's label.

Most dialog boxes have a default button—usually OK or Cancel. If the control with input focus is not a button, the default button is activated when the user presses Enter. If the control with input focus is a button, that button will be activated instead of the default button when the user presses the Enter key. The Escape (Esc) key will nearly always activate the Cancel button.

Dialog boxes use tabs (not to be confused with the Tab key) to group controls within a single dialog box. Ctrl + Tab or Ctrl + PgDown cycles between tabs and Shift + Ctrl + Tab or Ctrl + PgUp cycles through tabs in reverse order (Figure 2.7).

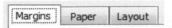

FIGURE 2.7   Tabs on a dialog box.

TABLE 2.1
Controls and Their Appearance with Input Focus

Control	Appearance with Input Focus
Button	Preferences
Check Box	☐ Different odd and even
Drop-Down List	Normal ▼
List Box	First page: Default tray (Tray 2) ▲ Automatically Select Tray 1 Tray 2 Tray 3 (500-Sheet) Tray 3 (1500-Sheet) Tray 4 (500-Sheet) Tray 4 (1500-Sheet) Envelope Feeder ▼
Radio Button	◉ All
Slider	Slow ——————◉—— Fast
Text Field	1-65535

TABLE 2.2

Operating Windows Controls from the Keyboard

Item	Select	Deselect	Activate	Right-Click
Desktop icon	Space bar	Ctrl + space bar	Enter	Shift + F10
Checkbox	Space bar	Space bar		
Radio button	Space bar			
Button			Space bar	
Start menu item	↑ or ↓	↑ or ↓	Enter	Shift + F10
Menu item	↑ or ↓	↑ or ↓	Enter	
Submenu item	↑ or ↓	↑ or ↓	Enter or →	
Combo box	F4 or ↓	F4 or Alt + ↓	Enter	

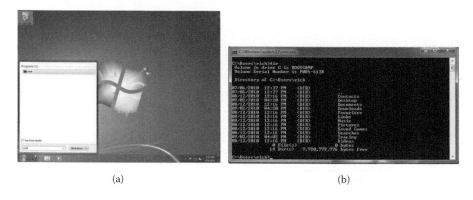

(a)   (b)

FIGURE 2.8   The DOS command line: (a) accessing the DOS command line from the Start menu; (b) the DOS command shell.

2.5.4 Manipulating Files and Folders

There are several options for manipulating files and folders within Windows. These operations include

- Creating, deleting, moving, copying, opening, and closing folders
- Moving, copying, and deleting files
- Launching applications

Although many consider the DOS command line a relic of a different age, it is still alive and well within Windows 7. The command line can be used to manipulate files and folders and launch applications. Because there are no graphical controls, there is no need to worry about where input focus is located. The command line is particularly useful for people who use screen readers (Figure 2.8).

On the other hand, there are some good reasons nearly all computer users have abandoned the command line for graphical user interfaces. A command line imposes a much greater cognitive load on the user. There are no visual prompts for commands

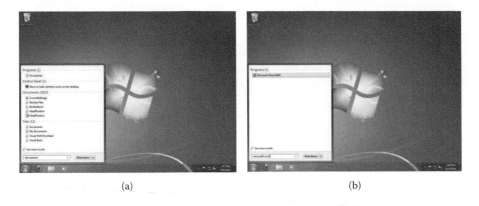

(a)   (b)

FIGURE 2.9   The Start menu can be used to (a) open folders and (b) launch applications.

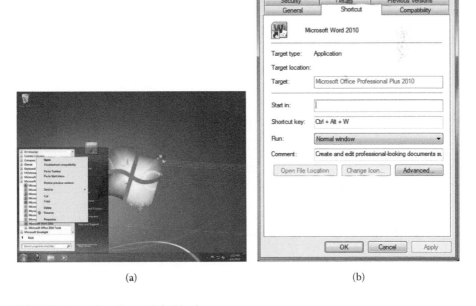

(a)   (b)

FIGURE 2.10   Creating a global hotkey.

(meaning the user must remember them), and the user must maintain an internal representation of the folder structure.

As an alternative to the command line, the Start menu's search field can be used to open folders and launch programs. The search field cannot be used for more advanced operations, however (Figure 2.9).

Windows also allows users to define "global hotkeys" to open a file, folder, or application. Global hotkeys typically take the form Ctrl + Alt + <letter key>. Global hotkeys can be activated at any time in any program and take precedence over any hotkeys defined by the active application (Figure 2.10).

To create a global hotkey:

1. Locate icon of file, folder, or application.
2. Create a Shortcut.
3. Invoke Shortcut's Properties.
4. Go to Shortcut tab.
5. Go to Shortcut key.
6. Press the desired key or key combination.
7. Press Enter.

REFERENCES

1. Cantor, A. 2006. Windows keyboard access FAQ v1.4. Available from http://www. cantoraccess.com/keyaccess/keyaccessfaq.htm.
2. Lane, D.M. et al. 2005. Hidden costs of graphical user interfaces: Failure to make the transition from menus to icon toolbars to keyboard shortcuts. *International Journal of Human-Computer Interaction* 18(2): 133–144.
3. Cantor, A. 2002. *Introduction to keyboard-only access to Windows.* Boulder, CO: Accessing Higher Ground: Assistive Technology in Higher Education. Available from http://www.colorado.edu/ATconference/achandouts2002.html (accessed August 24, 2006).
4. Cantor, A. 2006. Windows macros FAQ v3.0. Available from http://www.cantoraccess. com/macro-docs/macrosfaq.htm.
5. Colven, D. 2006. *Accessing Windows with a keyboard.* Oxford, UK: ACE Centre Advisory Trust.

3 Switches

3.1 INTRODUCTION

A switch is something that opens and closes to control the flow of electrical current. Most switches are open by default and close when activated, but a select few are closed by default and open when activated [1, 2]. A switch typically responds to a single, specific type of input, such as [2]

- Physical pressure
- Air pressure
- Tilt
- Proximity
- Eye blink
- Muscle activity
- Sound

During an assessment for switch access, the clinician's responsibilities are to (1) identify the motor capabilities of the client that are within volitional control, (2) select a switch and an input method that are compatible with the client's motor capabilities, and (3) adapt the environment (e.g., the position of the switch) to maximize the client's performance [3]. During an assessment, the clinician must find the best match between a type of switch and body site. Once a match is made, switch activation becomes a consistent motion and the relationship between the switch site and the consumer's movement remains fixed [3].

3.2 CHARACTERIZING SWITCHES

In this section we discuss the terminology used for describing and comparing switches.

3.2.1 SIZE

Switches come in different sizes. Large switches are advantageous because they allow for larger labels and graphics, and can be activated by larger body parts (e.g., knuckles, toes) [4]. They also provide a larger target for clients with less accuracy. On the other hand, large switches can be more difficult to position and may require greater force to activate (Figure 3.1).

3.2.2 SENSITIVITY

Sensitivity refers to the amount of force or time required to activate a switch [1]. Switches that have high sensitivity respond to very little force or activate immediately after receiving input, and are therefore more likely to be activated inadvertently.

23

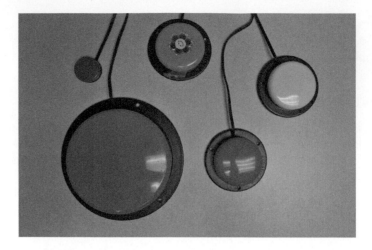

FIGURE 3.1 Push button switches come in many different sizes and colors.

Switches with reduced sensitivity, on the other hand, are less likely to be activated by mistake but require greater force or time to activate.

Choosing the right sensitivity requires balancing between *false positive* errors (the switch activates when it should not) and *false negative* errors (the switch fails to activate when it should). Decreasing sensitivity will reduce false positive errors, but may introduce additional false negative errors. Increasing sensitivity will decrease false negative errors but possibly increase false positive errors.

For example, if a client has tremors that cause him to press a switch several times, instead of just once, then choosing a switch with lower sensitivity can eliminate unwanted switch activations. At the same time, however, choosing a less sensitive switch may also increase the number of instances where the client presses the switch but fails to press hard or long enough, and no switch activation is produced (a false negative error). Similarly, a client with limited strength may need a very sensitive switch, at the expense of additional unintended switch activations (false positive errors).

3.2.3 CONTRAST

Contrast refers to the distinctiveness of the switch in comparison to the background and surrounding switches [1]. Contrast can be

- Visual: Switches can use different colors, labels, or graphics.
- Tactile: Switches can have different surface materials or textures.
- Proprioceptive: Switches can be distinguished by placing them in particular locations.

Increasing the contrast of a switch makes a switch faster and easier to distinguish from other switches. Contrast can be important even if there is only one switch. For example, increasing a switch's contrast from the surface it is mounted on (e.g., a lap tray or table) can be useful for a client with low vision.

3.2.4 FEEDBACK

Feedback describes a switch's response to activation [1]. Feedback can be

- Visual: A switch can change color or light up when activated.
- Kinesthetic: A switch can move when activated.
- Auditory: A switch can generate a click or other sound when activated.

Feedback is important to let users know when they have activated a switch, and to help users figure out whether they have activated the desired switch. Feedback is more important for clients using new input methods, and the need for feedback often dissipates with learning.

3.2.5 FUNCTIONAL TRANSPARENCY

Functional transparency refers to the extent to which a user can determine what a switch actually does when activated [1]. Functional transparency is most directly determined by a switch's label, but can also be influenced by a switch's location, arrangement with other switches, and by convention. For example, switches in a diamond pattern are often assumed to correspond to up, down, left, and right.

Functional transparency is a continuum with items that are *transparent* (the purpose of a switch is obvious) on one end and *opaque* (the purpose cannot be deduced and must be taught) on the other, with the items in between being *translucent* (the purpose isn't obvious but can be deduced). Note that the functional transparency of a switch can vary between people. Something that is transparent to one person may be opaque to another [1].

3.2.6 AFFORDANCE

The *affordances* of an item are the *perceptions* it creates about how it can be used [1, 5]. This is different than how an item can *actually* be used in that an item may imply that it can be used in ways that it can't or may hide functionality it actually has. A switch's affordance is the way in which it is activated. We tend to think of switches as being activated by being pushed and then released, and they *afford* pushing. Some switches, however, are activated by touch and do not actually depress. These switches do not afford pushing, and in fact, some switches can break if pushed too hard.

3.2.7 APPLYING THE VOCABULARY

Consider the following switches (which are only a small sample of the available options) (Figure 3.2):

1. A push button switch measuring 2.5 inches that is activated by pressing anywhere on the top surface. The button provides tactile and auditory feedback.
2. An infrared switch operates by emitting a very low-powered infrared beam. When a surface in front of the beam reflects enough of the light

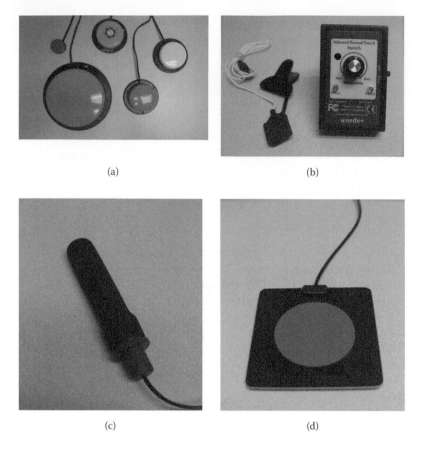

FIGURE 3.2   Switches: (a) push buttons, (b) infrared switch, (c) grasp switch, and (d) plate switch.

back to the receiver, the switch is activated. The surface of virtually any body part can activate the switch by coming close to the sensor or by coming into the field of view of the sensor from the side, thereby reflecting more light. The switch also responds to the difference in reflection between the white of the eye and the closed eyelid or the iris. This enables users who cannot blink to use an infrared switch as an eye movement switch.

3. A grasp switch is activated by squeezing or pinching anywhere on the foam handle.
4. A plate switch is a very thin membrane switch activated with a light touch on the colored circle. Its surface is sealed to prevent moisture damage. No tactile/auditory feedback is provided.
5. A pneumatic switch (often referred to as a "sip and puff" switch) is activated by sipping or puffing on a tube. Each of the two actions activates a different switch.

These switches could be described as follows:

Switch	Size	Sensitivity	Feedback	Functional Transparency
Push button	Varies	Low	Auditory, kinesthetic	Transparent
Infrared switch	N/A	High	None	Opaque
Grasp switch	Large	Low	Kinesthetic	Translucent
Plate switch	Large	High	None	Translucent
Sip and puff	N/A	High	None	Opaque

3.2.8 CHOOSING THE RIGHT SWITCH

To choose the right switch, therapists must understand the factors involved in switch use [3], including reliability, repeatability, timing, and ease of use. The *reliability* of a client's physical actions affects his or her voluntary ability to operate a switch. Reliability can be defined as the consistency with which a consumer completes a motor act to activate a switch. Reliability also implies that a client can make a movement in isolation from other movements. When movement reliability is less than optimal, therapists can respond by changing factors such as switch size, position, and orientation [3].

Movements used for switch pressing should be *volitional* and performed comfortably, without straining or causing uncontrolled movements in other parts of the body. Clinicians should ask clients undergoing a switch assessment to demonstrate movements that have been reliable in the past. Movements that the client has used previously to operate devices may be more reliable than other movements because the client has already incorporated these skills into a reliable movement pattern and has practiced using them [3].

Movements should also be easy to perform. This may seem obvious; however, it is important to remember that, at times, assistive technology providers may request individuals to perform movements that are unnatural. Therefore, movements that come naturally to the end user should be used whenever possible [3, 6, 7]. The client will also need to perform the movement repeatedly over a period of time. To achieve functional outcomes, the client must move reliably not just once or twice, but for as long as the switch is in use. This may last from a few minutes to several hours, depending on the needs of the client and the demands of the activity [3, 6, 7].

Timing must also be critically evaluated when examining switch use. The client must be able to wait until the right time to activate a switch and then be able to activate the switch within a given time window, which takes skill as well as practice [3].

Avoid movements that [8]:

- Are dominated by abnormal reflex patterns
- Cause a significant increase in abnormal tone
- Are abnormal movement patterns such as excessive internal rotation of the arm (i.e., the arm turned inward accompanied by wrist deviation)
- Cause a change in the positioning of the rest of the body

The clinician should also consider the activities and positions the client assumes throughout the day and evening. If the client will be using the switch while in bed and while seated in a wheelchair, or will use the switch for computer access, environmental control, and augmentative communication, then the switch must accommodate these changes [3].

3.3   SWITCH CONFIGURATION OPTIONS

The configuration options described below are not typically built directly into switches themselves. Instead, these configuration options are usually provided by the system the switch is being used to control.

3.3.1   REPEAT DELAY AND RATE

Some switches or switch interfaces allow users to set or adjust the time a switch must be activated before it will start to repeat. Repeating can be turned on for clients who have trouble making rapid consecutive switch activations. Alternatively, repeating can be slowed (or turned off entirely) for clients who find it difficult to release a switch quickly after activating it to avoid errors caused by unwanted repeats [9]. There are two repeat settings [2] (Figure 3.3):

- Repeat delay. The time for which a switch must be activated before the repeat starts.
- Repeat rate. The time between successive repeats once repeating has started.

3.3.2   DEBOUNCE TIME

Debounce time is often used for clients with intention or essential tremors. When a switch activation is accepted, the switch that was pressed is "deactivated" for a specified time. Additional input on the same switch during this time is ignored, but input on other switches is accepted [2, 4, 10]. This means that two different switches can be activated in sequence without any delay, but a delay is required between *two activations of the same switch* (Figure 3.4).

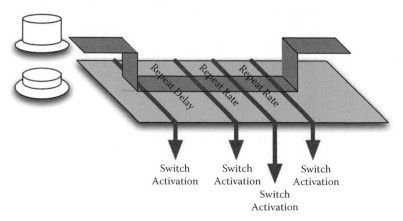

FIGURE 3.3   Repeat keys.

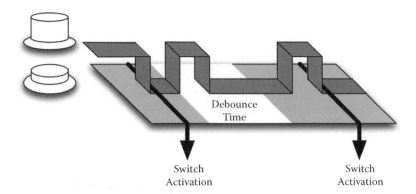

FIGURE 3.4   Debounce time.

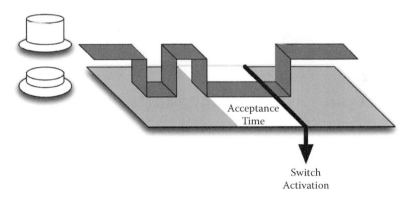

FIGURE 3.5   Acceptance time.

3.3.3   ACCEPTANCE TIME

A switch's *acceptance time* can be changed to increase the time a switch must be activated before the system recognizes the switch activation [2, 10]. Acceptance time is typically increased to ignore unintentional switch presses [2, 11]. Introducing a delay between switch activation and acceptance can be confusing for some clients, particularly if the switch itself has built-in feedback (such as clicking) that signals activation has occurred. If an acceptance time is introduced, look for some way for the system to provide feedback to the client once a switch activation is accepted (Figure 3.5).

3.3.4   MOMENTARY VS. TIMED VS. LATCHED

A switch can be *momentary, timed,* or *latched* [1]. A momentary switch remains closed (or open) as long as it is activated and reverts to its normal state as soon as activation is removed. A timed switch remains closed (or open) for a fixed amount of time after activation and then reverts to its normal state. A latched switch remains closed (or open) until it receives a second input. Some switches have the ability to operate as momentary, timed, or latched. Most switches, however, operate in a single

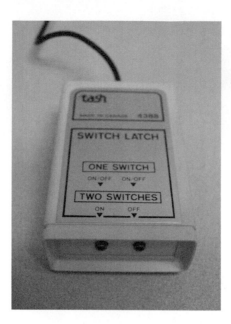

FIGURE 3.6   A switch latch can generate timed or latched switch closures from a momentary switch.

mode. An external "switch latch" can be used, however, to generate timed or latched switch closures from a momentary switch (Figure 3.6).

3.3.5   IN THE CLINIC: CONFIGURING A SWITCH

The following table maps potential problems a client might have with the available configuration options.

Problem	Configuration Option
Client activates switch for too long	Increase repeat delay or eliminate repeat entirely
Client has trouble activating switch multiple times quickly	Decrease repeat delay; use timed or latched switch
Client unintentionally activates the same switch multiple times	Introduce debounce time
Client mistakenly activates switch	Introduce acceptance delay
Client cannot maintain switch activation	Use a switch latch

3.4   SWITCH INTERFACES FOR COMPUTER USE

Most computers do not come with a built-in port or jack for switches. Instead, an external switch interface must be connected to the computer (typically through a USB port). Switch interfaces vary in size, cost, and sophistication.

Switch interfaces also vary in how they interact with the computer's operating system and other software. A switch interface that plugs into the computer's USB port typically appears to the computer to be either a keyboard or a mouse, or both. In

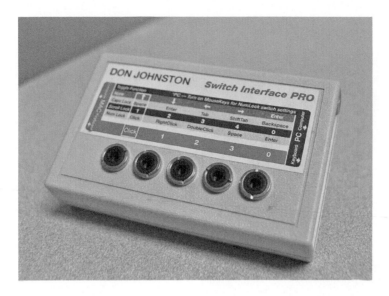

FIGURE 3.7   Switch interfaces for the computer.

response to a switch closure, the switch interface simulates either a key press (e.g., a function key, the Enter key, the space bar) or a mouse click. The more sophisticated switch interfaces allow the user to choose between different key presses or mouse clicks. *What is critical is that the switch interface be able to provide the input that the user's software is expecting* (Figure 3.7).

3.5   SWITCH POSITIONING

Positioning a switch is a critical, but often overlooked, aspect of switch access. Mounts are available that can be attached to a desk or wheelchair to position a switch almost anywhere. Some switch mounts are multijointed arms originally designed to position camera equipment. These mounts are very rigid when tightened and maintain their position when bumped or pushed. They are most appropriate for switches that are going to be pushed hard by the user (e.g., head-operated switches) and switches that rely on precise positioning (e.g., tongue switches). At the other extreme are "gooseneck" switch mounts, which are designed to be positioned (and repositioned) quickly. Goosenecks are appropriate for situations where a switch will need to be moved frequently or when the user will not be applying much force to the switch (Figure 3.8).

A switch user's movements may be limited due to his or her impaired neuromotor system, so the position and orientation of the switch must adapt to the client's abilities as much as possible [3]. The optimal position for a switch relative to the control site is within the individual's range of motion, but not so close that accidental activations occur [3, 8]. Adjust the switch's orientation or angle to ensure that the switch is placed directly in the line of movement, so that the consumer will make contact with the switch each time he or she attempts to activate it [3].

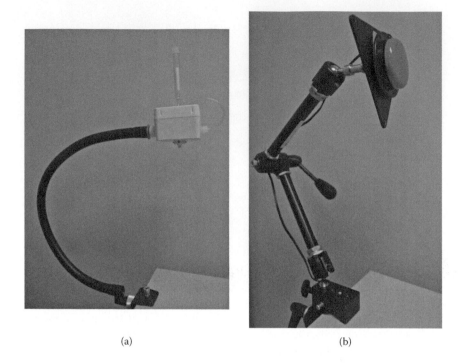

(a)   (b)

FIGURE 3.8   Switch mounts: (a) flexible and (b) rigid.

Safety is also an important consideration. The switch should be attached to a wheelchair or table in a manner that does not endanger the client or others. All wires should be secured to a stable surface to reduce entanglement or the possibility of dislodging the switch. Switches should also be positioned so that body parts, clothing, or jewelry are not entangled [3, 8].

If the switch is going to be mounted on a wheelchair with a tilt-in-space or recline feature, or on a bed with an adjustable frame, make sure the switch is mounted to a component that moves with the client to provide continuous access. Also make sure that the wires connecting the switch to the computer have enough slack to accommodate the full range of motion.

3.6   SCANNING INTERFACES

Scanning is a general term used to describe the process of choosing items from a selection set using one or more switches. Scanning is used by individuals with severe motor disabilities as a method for entering text and data into computers and augmentative communication devices. This need may stem from a variety of medical conditions, such as cerebral palsy, traumatic brain injury, muscular dystrophy, or neuromuscular diseases such as multiple sclerosis and amyotrophic lateral sclerosis, affecting hundreds of thousands of people in the United States.

Scanning involves three essential components: (1) the offer of the item(s) in the selection set to the user, (2) the selection of the item(s) by the user (i.e., conditional activation of the switch to select the target item when offered), and (3) the feedback provided to the user upon selection (switch activation) [12]. Scanning can be accomplished through visual or auditory presentation to the user. Typically items are presented to the individual in a visual array, often accompanied by auditory cues. When individuals have significant visual impairments, they may rely on auditory scanning alone [12].

In most scanning systems, an item is shown to be available for selection (i.e., has *input focus*) through the use of highlighting, typically a flashing or nonflashing light near to, or surrounding, the item (e.g., a red light in the upper left-hand corner near the item, a red box outlining the item, a light highlighting the item) [12]. Items or groups of items are highlighted one at a time. If the selection set is large, only a subset of the items may be displayed at any one time [2].

Although scanning imposes minimal motor demands (i.e., it requires only a single reliable movement to activate a switch), it imposes significant cognitive demands [3, 12]. In order to scan accurately, the client must understand not only what it means when an item is highlighted, but also the relation of the switch to the highlighted item in the selection process. Understanding this relationship is made all the more complex for clients with significant motor impairments because the switch is typically located at a distance from the computer and the actual target items in the selection array, thus obscuring the relationship (e.g., the switch may be mounted beside the user's head 2 feet away from the monitor displaying the target items). Furthermore, the relationship is not a direct one: the switch is used to indicate acceptance of an offered item, not as a means to directly select the target item [12]. Scanning also requires the ability to conceptualize an end product (e.g., a sentence) and the cognitive skill to sequentially construct the elements of that end product.

Scanning, by its nature, also involves a waiting component. The user must wait while items are offered sequentially until the target item is offered, and then must indicate the selection of this target. This waiting component may be especially difficult for young children or individuals with cognitive impairments who may become impatient, fatigued, bored, or distracted. This can have a negative impact on their attention to the task, and thus their overall accuracy of performance [12].

Input methods exist on a continuum. At the slowest end of the spectrum are *scanning input methods*. A very fast user may achieve eight words per minute [13–16], while rates of one word per minute and lower are common [17–19]. In response, product developers have implemented numerous features and configuration options to allow for customization of scanning software, with the goal of increasing text entry rate on an individualized basis. Some of the configuration options available in scanning systems are shown in Table 3.1.

3.6.1 SCANNING MODES

The *scanning mode* refers to the way in which input focus transitions or moves among items or groups of items in the selection set. Clinicians often ignore scanning modes other than automatic scanning, but they should have their clients try the

TABLE 3.1
Configuration Options Found in Commercially Available Scanning Interfaces

Configuration Option	Supported by (%)	Explanation
Scan rate	100%	The amount of time an item is available for selection (i.e., highlighted)
Recovery delay	50%	An additional delay added to the first row or column to provide time for the user to recover from a previous switch activation. Different values may be used for rows and columns in some systems.
Loop count	81%	Determines how many times the system will scan through the columns within a row before resuming between rows.
Reverse scan	19%	The ability to reverse the direction of scanning through a row.
Stop scanning	38%	The ability to stop scanning a row by selecting an item at the beginning or end of each row.
Rescan	19%	The ability to rescan the row by selecting an item at the beginning or end of each row.
Automatic/manual scan initiation	88%	Determines whether the user must press a switch to initiate scanning or if scanning is automatic (and continuous). This setting dictates whether two or three switch presses are required to make a selection.
Switch repeat	50%	Allows user to hold the switch down to register multiple switch activations.
Repeat delay	50%	How long the switch must be held down to register the second activation.
Repeat rate	44%	The length of time between switch activations after the second activation is registered.
Acceptance delay	69%	The length of time a switch must be activated before the activation is registered.
Switch hold escape	6%	The length of time a switch must be held before an exit/escape of the current row or column occurs. Scanning restarts at the top of the matrix.
Character prediction	13%	One or more items in the matrix are dynamically updated based on which letters are most likely to be selected next.
Word completion/ prediction	100%	One or more items in the matrix are dynamically updated based on what word the user is most likely entering or is likely to enter next.

Source: Mankowski, R.E., *Predicting Communication Rates: Efficacy of a Scanning Model,* University of Pittsburgh, Pittsburgh, PA, 2009 [17].

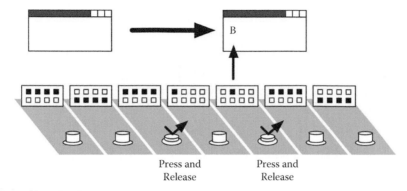

FIGURE 3.9   Automatic scanning.

different scanning modes before making a decision. For example, investigators have found that some individuals are much more accurate with inverse scanning [20].

3.6.1.1   Automatic Scanning

In *automatic scanning* (Figure 3.9), the system sequentially offers choices to the user. If the choice does not contain the desired item, the user waits for another choice to be offered. If the offered choice includes the desired item, the user activates a switch to make a selection. If the user selects a group of items, then the items within that group are scanned. Otherwise, the system generates the appropriate response to the selected item [2, 4, 12, 20]. Automatic scanning requires the least input from the user, but it does require him or her to wait until the appropriate moment to activate the switch [4]. The most efficient way to scan is to locate the desired item and wait until it is highlighted, rather than following the highlight [4].

3.6.1.2   Inverse Scanning

Inverse scanning (Figure 3.10) operates in an opposite manner from automatic scanning. The client activates the switch and the cursor highlights items in the array sequentially until he or she releases the switch to select the highlighted item or group of items [2, 4, 12, 20]. Inverse scanning is better for some clients who are able to relax a movement with more control than they are able to generate a movement at a precise time [4].

3.6.1.3   Step Scanning

In *step scanning* (Figure 3.11), the user controls the movement of input focus and the selection of items using one or two switches [2, 12]. In *one-switch step scanning*, the user presses the switch successively to move input focus between items. When the cursor is over the desired item, the user can select the item either by a longer switch press or by releasing the switch (i.e., dwell) [2, 4, 20]. In *two-switch step scanning*, one switch moves input focus and the second selects items [2].

3.6.2   Scan Patterns

The scan pattern (Figure 3.12) refers to the order in which items or groups of items are highlighted.

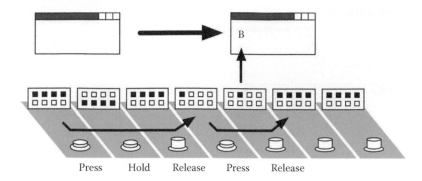

FIGURE 3.10   Inverse scanning.

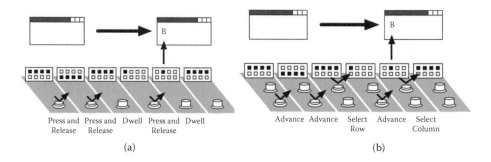

FIGURE 3.11   Step scanning: (a) one-switch step scanning and (b) two-switch step scanning.

3.6.2.1   Linear Scanning

In *linear scanning*, items are presented in a single group and the highlight moves through the group from left to right, presenting items one at a time [2, 12, 20, 21]. The advantage of linear scanning is its simplicity, but it is also the slowest scan pattern.

3.6.2.2   Hierarchical Scanning

As opposed to linear scan interfaces that use a single group, *hierarchical scanning* interfaces divide the selection set into hierarchical groups (or levels) of items that are individually selected. The user selects groups and then subgroups until a single item can be selected [2, 12, 21]. After the user selects the group containing the desired symbol, the symbol itself is chosen through linear scanning through the group [21]. If groups of items are spread across multiple pages, moving between pages normally happens by selecting "link" items that activate a new page [2]. Hierarchical scanning is faster than linear scanning but requires at least twice as many switch activations [21].

Row/column scanning is the most frequently used form of hierarchical scanning [2]. In row/column scanning, items are scanned in groups stacked in rows. A

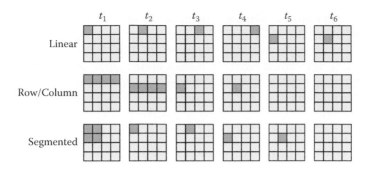

FIGURE 3.12 Scanning patterns.

common implementation of row/column scanning with one switch requires three switch hits to make one selection from a two-dimensional matrix of letters, numbers, symbols, words, or phrases. The first switch hit initiates a scan through the rows of the matrix. Each row of the matrix, beginning with the first, is highlighted in turn until the second switch hit is made to select a row. Each column of the row is then highlighted in turn until the target is highlighted, when the third switch hit is made to select the target [20].

3.6.2.3   Segmented Scanning

Segmented scanning is a form of group scanning in which the selection set is split into equal subgroups (quarters, halves, etc.) until a single item is chosen [2]. A segmenting scan is useful when there isn't a way to order items by frequency, or if items can be ordered by groups (e.g., letters, numbers, punctuation). Segmented scanning is also one way to do mouse operations by scanning.

3.6.2.4   In the Clinic: Choosing a Scanning Pattern

The factors to consider when choosing a scanning pattern are

- The client's cognitive skills. Linear scanning is less demanding cognitively than grouped scanning.
- The number of items in the scanning matrix. As the number of items increases, the number of scanning groups should increase. For example, 5 items can be scanned linearly in an efficient manner, 30 items probably require row/column scanning, and 128 items probably require at least one more level of scanning (e.g., group/row/column or segmented scanning).
- The client's physical skills. The number of scanning levels determines the number of switch presses required to select an item. For example, row/column scanning requires at least two switch presses and group/row/column scanning requires at least three switch presses. More importantly, multiple scanning levels introduce the need to generate multiple switch presses in succession. Scanning users who are unable to activate a switch three times in rapid succession may need to use row/column scanning.

- The organization of items within the scanning matrix. The order in which items are highlighted dictates how quickly each item can be selected. When items can be arranged by frequency of use (e.g., letters in a keyboard), a linear or hierarchical scanning pattern makes sense. When items can't be arranged by frequency, or when the position of items can change (e.g., icons on the computer desktop), then a segmented scanning pattern may be more appropriate.

3.6.3 SCANNING MATRIX

The items in the selection set and how those items are arranged play a significant role in text entry rate [21]. Items in a scanning matrix can be either *static* or *dynamic*. Static items always produce the same output. Examples of static keyboard items are

- Text entry (e.g., letters, numbers, punctuation)
- Editing (e.g., Backspace, Delete, arrow keys)
- Modifier keys (e.g., Shift, Control, Alt)
- Error correction (e.g., stop scanning, continue scanning)
- Navigation (e.g., a key that opens up a new keyboard layout, reverse scan direction)

Dynamic items, on the other hand, change based on the current context. Examples of dynamic selection set items are character prediction and word prediction.

Items are often arranged (1) alphabetically, (2) according to the arrangement of keys on a QWERTY keyboard, or (3) based on the frequency with which letters are used in the English language. An alphabetic or QWERTY layout will facilitate visual search of the matrix, but a letter-frequency arrangement will be significantly faster [21]. However, it can be difficult to determine which is the best frequency-based arrangement to use. Most frequency-based arrangements are derived from analyses of a corpus of written text, which often does not include punctuation and may or may not correspond well to everyday computer use. The ideal frequency-based matrix would be based on an individual client's actual computer activity, but it can be difficult to obtain this kind of data.

Koester's Frequency-Based Matrix

Sp	E	A	R	D	F
T	O	N	L	G	K
I	S	U	Y	B	X
H	C	P	Q	J	
M	W	V	Z		

Damper's Frequency-Based Matrix

Sp	E	A	R	D	U	V
T	O	I	L	G	K	
N	S	F	Y	X		
H	C	P	J			
M	W	Q				
B	Z					

Venkatagiri's Frequency-Based Matrix

Sp	T	I	H	F	B
E	O	R	C	P	Z
A	S	U	G	Q	
N	D	Y	J		
L	W	X			
M	K				
V					

Many clinicians choose an alphabetic or QWERTY arrangement, because that is more familiar to the client and reduces search time. If the client has the necessary cognitive skills and motivation to learn a frequency-based arrangement, then he or she will ultimately achieve a much greater text entry rate (TER).

3.6.4 SCAN RATE

Scan rate determines the time an item is highlighted and available for selection [2]. The scan rate is critical to text entry rate. If a person is capable of using a scan rate of 1.0 seconds, say, but their system is set to 2.0 seconds, their TER will be only half of what it could be. A case study by Koester in 1990 [22] demonstrated how modifications to both item layout and scan rate yielded a TER enhancement of 321% for one individual. For experienced users of single-switch scanning who have been proactive in adjusting their system configurations, gains may be more modest. For example, the five individuals in Bhattacharya's study [24] showed differences of 20% to 25% when using different configurations.

Working independently, two groups [23, 24] found that the ratio between a user's reaction time and an appropriate scan rate for that user is approximately 0.65 (which has been referred to as the 0.65 rule [18]), although neither group empirically demonstrated that the resulting scan rate was, in fact, literally optimal.

$$\text{Scan Rate} = \frac{\text{Average Switch Press Time}}{.65}$$

From a practical standpoint, the 0.65 rule makes sense. Given a person's average switch press time, the 0.65 rule provides a cushion that ensures that almost all presses occur within the desired scan period. The last 35% of the scan period serves as extra time, to accommodate presses that are slower than average. That seems like a reasonable cushion, but given that text entry rate is limited by scan rate, a smaller cushion would obviously be desirable.

The reason there needs to be any time cushion at all is that the scan rate is invariant, while switch press times are not. Part of this is due to natural variation inherent in human performance, and part of it is due to the fact that the scanning task may be somewhat different depending on the target (e.g., a first-column target may be chosen with a double-click, or a target not spotted until the last milliseconds). Switch press time generally follows a bell-shaped curve, with the highest-frequency press times occurring around the mean time, and a symmetrical decrease in frequency along both sides of the mean.

3.6.5   RECOVERY DELAY

The recovery delay is an extra delay after a selection is made before scanning resumes [2]. The point of the recovery delay is to allow recovery time between switch presses. A recovery delay is needed if the time required to recover from a switch press and then generate a second switch press is greater than the scan rate.

In general, a modest recovery delay imposes an extremely small drag on text entry rate. So, if there is uncertainty about whether or not to implement a recovery delay on a client's system, the clinician should lean toward using a recovery delay.

3.6.6   INITIATING SCANNING

For single-switch scanning, there are two options for initiating the scan [2]. In autostart, scanning restarts immediately after selection is made. In a manual start, the user must press a switch to initiate scanning. Autoscanning is convenient for individuals who have a hard time with two consecutive switch activations. A manual start is nice because it allows the user to control when scanning is active.

If a frequency-arranged matrix is used (and it should be), then the most frequently used items will be at the top of the matrix. A manual start will allow the user to begin the scanning process at the top of the matrix each time. Clinicians should therefore use a manual start unless the client has difficulty performing three consecutive switch activations (the first to initiate scanning, the second to select the first row, the third to select the first column).

3.6.7   WHERE SCANNING STARTS

In most systems, once the user makes a selection, scanning resumes at the topmost group (i.e., the first row for row/column scanning). Some systems provide alternatives, however, such as resuming scanning at the group where the selection took place (i.e., at the row where the selection occurred) or at the item that was selected (i.e., at the column that was previously selected).

If a frequency-arranged matrix is used (and it should be), then the most frequently used items will be at the top of the matrix. Scanning should thus begin on the first row.

3.6.8 REPEATING SELECTIONS

A small number of scanning systems allow the user to repeat selections [2]. Options include

- The user activates the switch as many times as the item is desired.
- The user holds the switch down until repeating initiates.
- The user presses the switch and the item starts repeating until the user presses the switch again.

Repeating selections comes up in a variety of situations:

- Moving the mouse cursor
- Using arrow keys to move the text cursor
- Scanning through menus
- Tabbing through links on a web page

3.6.9 ERROR CORRECTION

Errors in scanning differ from errors made when typing on a keyboard in that scanning errors do not necessarily generate text [4]. Scanning errors can be errors of *omission* (i.e., failing to activate the switch when the target is highlighted) or *commission* (i.e., activating the switch when the target is not highlighted). Developers have created several approaches to respond to each type of error.

When a user selects the wrong group, there must be a mechanism for correcting the error. The options available on commercial products are

- A fixed *loop count* that defines the number of times the items within a group are scanned before scanning recommences
- A *stop scanning* item (usually at the beginning of the row)
- Activating the switch for an extended time
- Selecting an (incorrect) item within the row

When the user selects the correct group, but fails to make a selection within that group, there must be some way to cause the system to scan through the group again. The options available on commercial products are

- A fixed *loop count* that defines the number of times the columns within each row are scanned before row scanning recommences
- A *continue scanning* item at the end of the row that can be selected to reinitiate scanning through the row

The only time an incorrect keystroke is generated is when the user selects the wrong item. Depending on the results of the keystroke within the application being used, it may or may not be possible to correct the error. The options available on commercial products include

- An undo option that may activate the Undo command within the underlying application
- A Backspace or Delete key
- Holding the switch once it is activated until a threshold is passed that restarts scanning without making a selection

To date, there is no empirical evidence that any of these error correction methods actually increase TER compared to a plain scanning matrix.

3.6.10   POINTING AND SCANNING

Using a switch interface to replace the computer mouse is remarkably inefficient. A client is usually much better off learning to operate the computer using keyboard commands. Another option is to integrate frequently used commands (e.g., save, print, quit) directly into the scanning selection set. Some on-screen keyboards include commands for automatically scanning through the items within an application's menu bar or the links on a web page (Figure 3.13).

3.6.10.1   Cartesian Scanning
Cartesian scanning uses linear movements to identify the target location for the cursor. When Cartesian scanning is activated, a line will move down the screen until the user activates the switch. The cursor then follows the line across the screen until the desired location is reached, at which point the switch is activated for a second time.

3.6.10.2   Polar Scanning
In polar scanning, the cursor rotates until a direction of travel is chosen. Rotation can be either continuous (which allows the cursor to move at any angle) or limited to four or eight compass directions [25]. Once a direction of travel is chosen, the cursor's

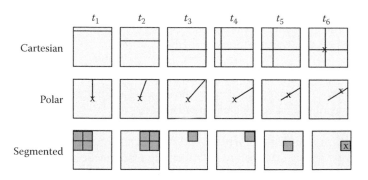

FIGURE 3.13   Pointing and scanning.

movement can be either a continuous motion or discrete steps (sometimes you're given a choice between small and large).

3.6.10.3 Segmented Scanning

In segmenting scanning the screen area is iteratively segmented into equal-sized subareas. The user has to select a subarea that contains the intended target [25].

3.7 MORSE CODE

Morse code (Figures 3.14 and 3.15) was invented in 1838 by Samuel F.B. Morse and Alfred Vail [26]. With one or two switches, Morse code is transmitted as a tone-silent time series. A tone element can be a *dot* (a short beep) or a *dash* (a long beep); a silent element can be a *dot-space* (a short pause between dots and dashes of a character) or a *character space* (a longer pause between characters) [27]. Dots are often referred to in writing as "dits" or an actual dot (.) and dashes are often referred to as "dahs" or hyphens (-). The ending *t* or *h* of dit and dah may not be included in the written representation of those sounds, unless it is the last dit or dah in that letter, number, or punctuation. For instance, the code for the letter *A* is didah and *I* is didit [28].

Morse code is designed for efficient communication at low bandwidth [29]. Morse code supports much faster text entry than scanning and does not require visual feedback [26]. Morse code also supports automaticity. Once a client becomes expert in Morse code, the codes for each letter can be produced automatically [4, 26].

Morse code derives its efficiency from the fact that the most frequently used letters have the shortest codes [30]. The average number of switch closures per letter in Morse code is 3.22, but is only 2.8 when frequency is taken into account [4, 27]. Morse figured out the frequencies of letters by weighing the bags of stamps at a printing press. He assumed the most frequently used letters would have the heaviest bags, because the printer would need more of those letters. Unfortunately, he didn't account for the fact that some letters (like the letter *i*) are physically smaller than other letters (like *y*), and thus weigh less. More importantly, there was no stamp for a space (or if there was, he didn't weigh it). Morse didn't care about spaces because there was a person receiving the codes who could identify the breaks between words based on timing or vocabulary.

Morse code takes time to learn and is no longer a common skill [26, 29]. Morse code also relies on timing to distinguish between dots and dashes, and emphasizes consistent switch activation [26], which can be difficult for some clients [31]. Morse code also lacks a natural means of mouse control.

One-switch Morse code uses the duration of switch activation to distinguish between dots and dashes. The standard for Morse code is [4]

- A dash is three times as long as a dot.
- A pause between characters is five times as long as a dot.

Two-switch Morse code uses one switch for dot and one switch for dash. A pause is used to indicate the end of a code. A feature of some two-switch Morse code

Character	Code	Character	Code
A	• ‒	N	‒ •
B	‒ • • •	O	‒ ‒ ‒
C	‒ • ‒ •	P	• ‒ ‒ •
D	‒ • •	Q	‒ ‒ • ‒
E	•	R	• ‒ •
F	• • ‒ •	S	• • •
G	‒ ‒ •	T	‒
H	• • • •	U	• • ‒
I	• •	V	• • • ‒
J	• ‒ ‒ ‒	W	• ‒ ‒
K	‒ • ‒	X	‒ • • ‒
L	• ‒ • •	Y	‒ • ‒ ‒
M	‒ ‒	Z	‒ ‒ • •
1	• ‒ ‒ ‒ ‒	6	‒ • • • •
2	• • ‒ ‒ ‒	7	‒ ‒ • • •
3	• • • ‒ ‒	8	‒ ‒ ‒ • •
4	• • • • ‒	9	‒ ‒ ‒ ‒ •
5	• • • • •	0	‒ ‒ ‒ ‒ ‒
Space	• • ‒ ‒	Period	• ‒ • ‒ • ‒

FIGURE 3.14   International Morse code.

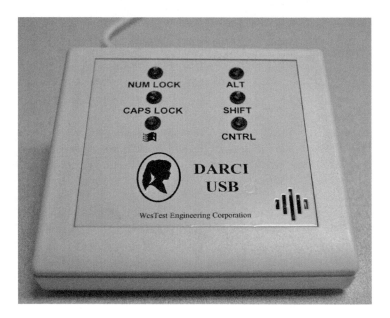

FIGURE 3.15   DARCI Morse code interface.

systems is *autokey*. The user can generate multiple dots or dashes by holding the switch down [4].

Three-switch Morse code uses a third switch to indicate the end of a character. Clients with increased muscle tone, spasticity, or tremor may have trouble with timing in Morse code. Adding a third switch to Morse code removes the timing element [4].

For evaluation, Anson recommends letting the client play games with a subset of Morse code for 1 hour [4]. For training, experts recommend against transcribing text with a code chart for reference because this will instill a three-step recall pattern (recall visual pattern, translate to auditory pattern, produce movements corresponding to auditory pattern). Instead, auditory training should be used [4, 28]. Teach the client to recognize Morse patterns, then teach the client to reproduce those patterns. Anson estimates a minimum of 10 to 20 hours of practice to reach proficiency [4].

3.8   MODELING SWITCH INPUT METHODS

3.8.1   ONE-SWITCH LINEAR SCANNING

Consider the simple scanning matrix with one row shown in Figure 3.16. Assume the client is using a linear scan pattern with scan delay t_d and it takes the client time t_s (on average) to press the switch. How much time does it take to select the letter D?

First, how many scan periods must elapse before the target letter is highlighted? As shown in Figure 3.17, three full scan steps must occur before the letter D is highlighted. If the scan delay is t_d, then the time elapsed before the letter D is highlighted is $3t_d$.

Once the target letter is highlighted, then the user must press the switch, which takes (on average) time t_s. So the average total time to select the letter D is

$$(3 \times t_d) + t_s$$

More generally, the average time to select a letter L_i is

$$T_i = (S_i \times t_d) + t_s$$

where S_i is the number of scan steps to letter L_i.

A	B	C	D	E

FIGURE 3.16   One-row scanning matrix.

0	1	2	3	4

FIGURE 3.17   Number of scan steps to reach each item within matrix.

Sp	E	A	R	D	U	V
T	O	I	L	G	K	
N	S	F	Y	X		
H	C	P	J			
M	W	Q				
B	Z					

FIGURE 3.18   Row/column scan matrix.

0	1	2	3	4	5	6
1	2	3	4	5	6	
2	3	4	5	6		
3	4	5	6			
4	5	6				
5	6					

FIGURE 3.19   Scan steps to reach each item in matrix.

3.8.2   ONE- AND TWO-SWITCH ROW/COLUMN SCANNING

Consider the row/column scanning matrix shown in Figure 3.18. Let:

- Scan delay $= t_d$
- Average switch press time $= t_s$

How much time does it take to select the letter *F*?

As shown in Figure 3.19, it will take four scan steps to reach the target letter. If the scan rate is t_d, then this will take time $4t_d$.

A total of two switch presses must also occur, once to select the row and once to select the letter. If switch press time is t_s, then this will take time $2t_s$. The total time, then, is

$$(4 \times t_d) + (2 \times t_s)$$

More generally, for any letter L_i,

$$T_i = (S_i \times t_d) + (2 \times t_s)$$

where S_i is the number of scan steps to L_i.

This model can also be modified to accommodate two-switch scanning by replacing t_d with t_s:

$$T_i = (S_i \times t_s) + (2 \times t_s) = (S_i + 2) \times t_s$$

3.8.3 ONE- AND TWO-SWITCH MORSE CODE

Consider the task of entering a single letter L using Morse code. Let:

- L_i = target letter
- X_i = number of dots in the Morse code for L_i
- Y_i = number of dashes in the Morse code for L_i
- t_{dot} = maximum time allowed for a dot
- t_{dash} = minimum time required for a dash
- t_{pause} = minimum time required between letters
- M = time required to remember the code

By convention:

$$t_{dash} = 3 \times t_{dot}$$

$$t_{pause} = 5 \times t_{dot}$$

The time T_i to enter the Morse code for letter L_i is

$$T_i = M + (X_i \times t_{dot}) + (Y_i \times t_{dash}) + t_{pause}$$

$$= M + (X_i \times t_{dot}) + (Y_i \times 3t_{dot}) + 5t_{dot}$$

$$= M + t_{dot}(X_i + 3Y_i + 5)$$

In a study of a similar model of Morse code [32], the value of M was found to vary greatly between subjects (from 17 to 332 msec), but the values for t_{dot} and t_{dash} were relatively consistent. The following model provides some insight into how one can increase text entry rate with Morse code:

- Reduce the time required to recall the code.
- Decrease the time required to generate a dot, dash, or pause.
- Decrease the 3:1 ratio of t_{dot} to t_{dash} and the 5:1 ratio of t_{dot} to t_{pause}.
- Use codes with more dots than dashes.

Similarly, two-switch Morse code can be modeled as follows:

L_i = target letter
X_i = number of dots in the Morse code for L_i
Y_i = number of dashes in the Morse code for L_i
t_{dot} = minimum time required for a dot or dash
t_{pause} = minimum time required between letters
M = time required to remember the code

By convention:

$$t_{pause} = 3 \times t_{dot}$$

The time T_i to enter the Morse code for letter L_i is

$$T_i = M + (X_i \times t_{dot}) + (Y_i \times t_{dash}) + t_{pause}$$

$$= M + t_{dot} \times (X_i + Y_i) + t_{pause}$$

$$= M + t_{dot} \times (X_i + Y_i + 3)$$

3.9   CHOOSING THE SCAN RATE

To accommodate the vast majority of switch presses with a fixed scan rate, a scan rate should be chosen that guarantees a high probability that any given press time for a user will be faster than the fixed scan rate. Any press times that are slower than the scan rate will result in an error, which is costly. If press times are assumed to follow a normal distribution, then the solution is fairly straightforward. For any normally distributed population, with mean m and standard deviation sd, there is a 95% chance that a randomly chosen member of the population is within two standard deviations of the mean, and there is a 97.5% chance that the value of a randomly chosen member is less than $(m + 2sd)$. Therefore, to ensure that at least 97.5% of press times are faster than the fixed scan rate, the scan rate (sr) should be set to $(m + 2sd)$, using the mean and standard deviation of the user's press times:

$$sr = (m + 2sd) \tag{3.1}$$

Furthermore, it is also known that it generally works well to use the 0.65 rule to set the scan rate as

$$sr = m/0.65 \tag{3.2}$$

If Equations (3.1) and (3.2) are combined, then, one can gain insight into why the 0.65 rule is effective for most people (or, at least, most people with approximately normally distributed switch press times). So:

$$m/0.65 = (m + 2sd) \tag{3.3}$$

which leads to

$$0.35m = (2)(0.65)sd \tag{3.4}$$

and

$$sd/m = 0.35/1.3 = 0.27 \tag{3.5}$$

Another name for (*sd/m*) is the coefficient of variation (CV). Based on the above analyses, whenever the CV of press times is at or below 27%, the 0.65 rule will establish a scan rate that is longer than 97.5% of the row press times. For individuals with higher variation in their switch press times, a scan rate set using the 0.65 rule would be expected to result in more than 2.5% errors, since it would be a faster scan rate than the (*m* + 2*sd*) method.

The statistical model described above assumes a scan rate ratio (r = *m/sr*) of 0.65 and an error rate of 97.5%. Recall that the error rate of 97.5% comes from a scan rate set at the mean press time plus two standard deviations. The number of standard deviations from the mean is called a *z*-score. So an error rate of 97.5% corresponds to a *z*-score of 2. If *z* is allowed to vary (as opposed to being fixed at 2), then the equation for *r* becomes

$$r = \frac{m}{sr} = \frac{m}{m + z(sd)} \tag{3.6}$$

Solving this equation for *sd* then yields

$$r = \frac{m}{m + z(sd)}$$

$$rm + rz(sd) = m \tag{3.7}$$

$$sd = \frac{m(1-r)}{rz}$$

Substituting this formulation of *sd* into the definition of CV, one can then derive the following relationship:

$$CV = \frac{sd}{m}$$

$$= \frac{m(1-r)}{rz} \cdot \frac{1}{m} \tag{3.8}$$

$$= \frac{1-r}{rz}$$

This more general relationship provides a model of how expected errors (due to the variation in switch press time) will increase with higher CV, under different scan rate ratios. If Equation (3.8) is solved for *z*:

$$z = \frac{1-r}{r(CV)} \tag{3.9}$$

Equation (3.9) can then be used to predict error rates as *r* and CV vary. Figure 3.20 illustrates this for three different scan rate ratios: 0.50, 0.65, and 0.80. The figure

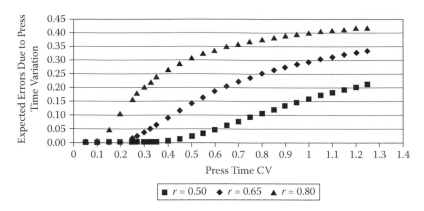

FIGURE 3.20 Predicted relationship between CV and errors.

provides some insight into why a ratio of 0.50 is a bit too conservative, and 0.80 is probably too aggressive. For example, at a ratio of 0.5, the press time CV must exceed 0.6 before errors due to press time variation exceed a modest 5%. Since actual user CVs are generally lower than that, the 0.50 ratio is unnecessarily conservative for most users. Conversely, boosting the ratio up to 0.80 in an attempt to increase productivity may backfire. In that case, variation-related errors will exceed 5% for CVs above 0.15.

REFERENCES

1. King, T.W. 1999. *Assistive technology: Essential human factors*. Boston: Allyn and Bacon, p. 303.
2. Colven, D., and S. Judge. 2006. *Switch access to technology: A comprehensive guide*. Oxford, UK: ACE Centre Advisory Trust.
3. Angelo, J. 2000. Factors affecting the use of a single switch with assistive technology devices. *Journal of Rehabiliation Research and Development* 37(5): 591–598.
4. Anson, D.K. 1997. *Alternative computer access: A guide to selection*. 1st ed. Philadelphia: F.A. Davis Company, p. 280.
5. Norman, D.A. 2002. *The design of everyday things*. New York: Basic Books.
6. Lancioni, G.E. et al. 2005. Microswitch programs for persons with multiple disabilities: An overview of the responses adopted for microswitch activation. *Cognitive Processing* 6(3): 177–188.
7. Romich, B., K. Hill, and B.W. Liffick. 2005. Free software for measuring single switch user performance. In *Technology and Persons with Disabilities Conference (CSUN)*. Los Angeles: California State University, Northridge.
8. Switch assessment and planning framework for individuals with physical disabilities. 2006. Oldham, UK: Ace Centre North.
9. Trewin, S., and H. Pain. 1999. Keyboard and mouse errors due to motor disabilities. *International Journal of Human-Computer Studies* 50(2): 109–144.
10. Trewin, S., and H. Pain. 1999. A model of keyboard configuration requirements. *Behaviour and Information Technology* 18(1): 27–35.
11. Trewin, S. 2002. Extending keyboard adaptability: An investigation. *Universal Access in the Information Society* 2(1): 44–55.
12. McCarthy, J. et al. 2006. Re-designing scanning to reduce learning demands: The performance of typically developing 2-year-olds. *Augmentative and Alternative Communication* 22(4): 269–283.

13. Koester, H., and S.P. Levine. 1994. Modeling the speed of text entry with a word prediction interface. *IEEE Transactions on Rehabilitation Engineering* 2(3): 177–187.
14. Lesher, G.W. et al. 2002. Acquisition of scanning skills: The use of an adpative scanning delay algorithm across four scanning displays. In *RESNA 2002 Annual Conference*. Minneapolis: RESNA Press, pp. 75–77.
15. Lesher, G.W., and G.J. Rinkus. 2002. Leveraging word prediction to improve character prediction in a scanning configuration. In *RESNA 2002 Annual Conference*. Minneapolis: RESNA Press.
16. Simpson, R.C., and H.H. Koester. 1999. Adaptive one-switch row-column scanning. *IEEE Transactions on Rehabilitation Engineering* 7: 464–473.
17. Mankowski, R.E. 2009. *Predicting communication rates: Efficacy of a scanning model*. Pittsburgh, PA: Department of Rehabilitation Science and Technology, University of Pittsburgh.
18. Simpson, R.C., H. Koester, and E.F. LoPresti. 2007. Selecting an appropriate scan rate: The ".65 rule." *Assistive Technology* 19(2): 51–60.
19. Simpson, R.C., H.H. Koester, and E.F. LoPresti. 2007. Evaluation of an adaptive row/column scanning system. *Technology and Disability* 18(3): 127–138.
20. Angelo, J. 1992. Comparison of three computer scanning modes as an interface method for persons with cerebral palsy. *American Journal of Occupational Therapy* 46(3): 217–222.
21. Venkatagiri, H.S. 1999. Efficient keyboard layouts for sequential access in augmentative and alternative communication. *Augmentative and Alternative Communication* 15(2): 126–134.
22. Horstmann, H.M. 1990. Quantitative modeling in augmentative communication—A case study. In *RESNA '90 Annual Conference*. Washington, DC: RESNA Press.
23. Cronk, S., and W. Wang. 2002. Investigating relationships between user performance and scan delays in aids that scan. In *Annual Conference on Rehabilitation Technology (RESNA)*. Minneapolis: RESNA Press.
24. Lesher, G.W., J. Higginbotham, and B.J. Moulton. 2000. Techniques for automatically updating scanning delays. In *Annual Conference on Rehabilitation Technology (RESNA)*. Orlando, FL: RESNA Press.
25. Biswas, P., S. Bhattacharya, and D. Samanta. 2005. User model to design adaptable interfaces for motor-impaired users. In *Tencon '05—IEEE Region 10 Conference*. Melbourne, Australia: IEEE, pp. 1801–1806.
26. King, T.W. 2000. *Modern Morse code in rehabilitation and education*. Boston: Allyn and Bacon.
27. Hsieh, M.-C., and C.-H. Luo. 1999. Morse code text typing training of a teenager with cerebral palsy using a six-switch Morse keyboard. *Technology and Disability* 10(3): 169–173.
28. Nellans, B. 1998. Learning and using Morse code. Available from http://www.morsex.com/cpy_code.htm (accessed 2006).
29. Johansen, A.S., and J.P. Hansen. 2006. Augmentative and alternative communication: The future of text on the move. *Universal Access in the Information Society* 5(2): 125–149.
30. Wickens, C.D., and J.G. Hollands. 2000. *Engineering psychology and human performance*. 3rd ed. Upper Saddle River, NJ: Prentice Hall, p. 573.
31. Hsieh, M.-C., and C.-H. Luo. 1999. Morse code typing training of an adolescent with cerebral palsy using microcomputer technology: Case study. *Augmentative and Alternative Communication* 15(4): 216–221.
32. Clerkin, P., S. Cronk, and P. Nimmagadda. 2005. GOMS modeling of Morse code. In *RESNA 28th Annual Conference*, S.G. Fitzgerald, ed. Atlanta, GA: RESNA.

4 Pointing

4.1 INTRODUCTION

Pointing in human–computer interaction consists of moving a cursor onto text or a graphical object with an input device and clicking a button [1]. Pointing is a fundamental operation in modern graphical user interfaces. Selecting a pointing device can have important implications for some computer users with disabilities. Clients with limited upper arm motion (particularly high-level spinal cord injury [SCI], multiple sclerosis [MS], or amyotrophic lateral sclerosis [ALS]) may not use a keyboard at all and may rely entirely on their pointing device (or a combination of their pointing device and speech recognition) for computer access. For these clients, choosing the wrong pointing device, or failing to properly configure the pointing device, can create unnecessary barriers to success. For all computer users with disabilities, providing access to the most appropriate pointing device can significantly increase efficiency while reducing frustration and fatigue.

There is a significant amount of scientific literature devoted to pointing and pointing devices. However, it's hard to draw conclusions about general classes of devices (e.g., mice, trackballs, joysticks) from a comparison of specific instances of each class [2]. Even if researchers want to address the fundamental differences between various classes of device, studies have to be done with specific products with fixed resolutions, sampling frequencies, form factors, sensor technologies, and transfer functions, and it can be hard to separate these engineering details from the underlying differences between two types of pointing devices [2]. This challenge is compounded when we understand that no two individuals are alike, even if they have been diagnosed with the same disability. In addition, results in the literature can grow outdated quickly. Do results obtained with a mouse that used a roller ball apply to an optical mouse? Do results obtained under Windows 95 apply to Windows 7?

Some clients may be better off using something other than a pointing device for certain operations. There are keyboard shortcuts for menus, voice recognition is an option, and there are keyboards and software that support gesture input. Another option is to make use of the command shell (discussed in Chapter 2), which is available in Windows, OS X, and Unix, even though the typical user may not know that it is there. The command shell may be the most efficient way to perform file manipulation tasks.

4.2 TYPES OF POINTING DEVICES

4.2.1 CONTROL DYNAMICS

Pointing devices can, for the most part, be divided into zero-order (position) control systems and first-order (velocity) control systems. The order of the system refers to the relationship between the force applied to the pointing device and the resulting

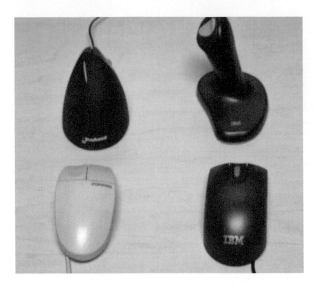

FIGURE 4.1   Examples of computer mice.

movement of the cursor on the screen [3, 4]. In a zero-order system, constant input produces a constant *position* [3, 4]. Examples of zero-order systems include mice and touch screens. In a first-order system, constant input produces a constant *velocity*. An example of a first-order system is a joystick [3, 4].

For zero-order systems, the user can adjust the *gain*, which is applied to the input. A gain larger than 1.0 means that movement of the device produces a proportionally larger movement of the cursor (e.g., a gain of 2 means that moving the device 1 inch moves the cursor 2 inches). A gain smaller than 1.0 produces a proportionally smaller movement of the cursor (e.g., a gain of 0.5 means that moving the device 1 inch moves the cursor 0.5 inch). For first-order systems, the user can adjust the *speed* and *acceleration* of the cursor.

Zero-order systems generally require greater movement (and greater range of motion) from the user than first-order systems. For example, reaching all points on the screen with a mouse typically requires moving the hand a much greater distance than using a joystick.

4.2.2 MOUSE

The mouse is by far the most popular type of pointing device. The mouse is a zero-order input device that converts linear displacement of the mouse into a corresponding linear displacement of the on-screen cursor (Figure 4.1).

4.2.3 TRACKBALL

Trackballs are zero-order systems that convert rotational displacement of a ball into a linear displacement of the on-screen cursor. Trackballs require less range of motion

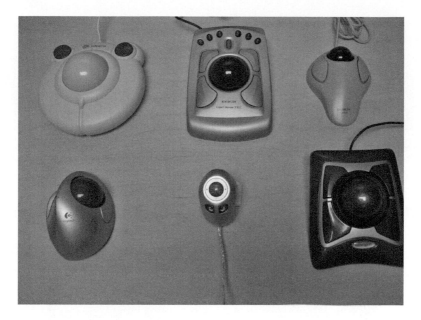

FIGURE 4.2   Examples of trackballs.

and require less desk space than traditional mice. Trackballs are nice because they don't require the user to grip and stabilize the device while generating a mouse click, which makes it easier to press or click the buttons without moving the mouse cursor. Consider using a trackball if your client has trouble keeping the mouse cursor over a target when clicking.

Trackballs are often considered to be more ergonomic than traditional mice. However, there are significant differences between models. Some are designed specifically for right- or left-handed users. Others require intense use of the thumb, and may pose their own ergonomic risks [5]. Many trackballs come with software that lets you program the various buttons to perform different functions, such as a drag lock or double-clicking. Trackballs can also be used with body parts other than the thumb or fingers (e.g., back of the hand, chin, foot) (Figure 4.2).

4.2.4 Trackpad/Touchpad

Trackpads are zero-order systems that convert linear displacement of the finger into a linear displacement of the on-screen cursor. Trackpads are most often associated with laptop computers, but trackpads for desktop computers are also available. Desktop trackpads can be useful because they allow orientations other than horizontal.

Trackpads are often able to distinguish single and double taps and tap-and-drag, while some provide a tapping area for a right-click as well, eliminating the need for mouse buttons. More recent trackpads are able to sense input from multiple simultaneous finger presses or motions (often called gestures), which has allowed for additional commands to be triggered from the trackpad (Figure 4.3).

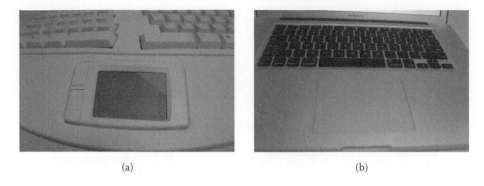

(a)   (b)

FIGURE 4.3   Examples of a trackpad (a) for desktop computers and (b) built into a laptop.

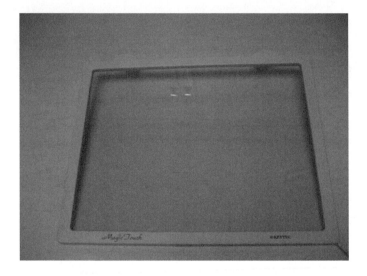

FIGURE 4.4   Touch screen.

4.2.5   TOUCH SCREEN

A touch screen is a zero-order system that converts finger position directly into cursor position. The touch screen can either be built in to the monitor or added on separately. Touch screens are good for young children and individuals with cognitive impairments who cannot understand the relationship between movement of a pointing device and movement of the on-screen cursor. Touch screens, particularly externally mounted touch screens, can require frequent calibration and their precision is lower than that of most other pointing devices. Touch screens are becoming increasingly common in "smart" cell phones, tablet computers, and all-in-one desktop computers (Figure 4.4).

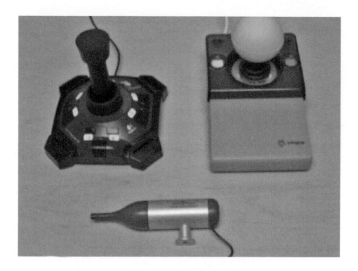

FIGURE 4.5 Joysticks: (a) Jouse and (b) Roller II Joystick.

4.2.6 Joystick

Joysticks are first-order systems. Joysticks can be either *displacement* or *isometric*. Displacement means that the cursor's speed and direction of travel are determined by the joystick's displacement from its center position, with greater displacement corresponding to greater speed. Most joysticks, including joysticks for wheelchairs and computer gaming, are displacement joysticks. An isometric joystick sets the cursor's speed and direction of travel based on force, with greater force corresponding to greater speed. The trackpoints on laptop computers are usually isometric joysticks.

Joysticks can be operated by the hand, but also by the tongue, chin, or any other body part. Wheelchair joysticks can be used to control the mouse, but it requires specific hardware on the wheelchair. Some joysticks can control the mouse cursor without any additional software. Software also exists that allows regular gaming joysticks to be used to control the mouse cursor (Figure 4.5).

4.2.7 Mouse Keys

Mouse keys allows the user to control the mouse cursor using the number pad on the keyboard. Mouse keys is a first-order input method that converts key presses to cursor velocity. The directions of movement are controlled using the number pad keys as shown in Figure 4.6 [6].

While mouse keys is almost always slower than using an actual mouse [7], it can be a good option for those without sufficient hand dexterity or steadiness to use other hand-controlled devices. It can also be used as a supplement to a standard mouse by using its mouse button keys.

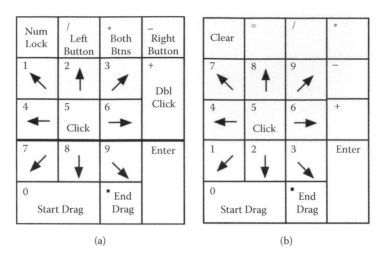

(a)   (b)

FIGURE 4.6   Mouse keys for (a) Windows and (b) OS X.

4.2.8   HEAD-CONTROLLED MOUSE EMULATOR

Head-controlled mouse emulators use the position of the head to control the position of the mouse cursor. Head-controlled mouse emulators are usually zero-order systems that map the orientation of the head (neck rotation and neck flexion/extension) to a cursor position on the screen. The biggest challenge with using a head-controlled mouse emulator is keeping the on-screen cursor still. With most pointing devices, the user can remove his or her hand from the device, preventing further movement. With a head-controlled mouse emulator, however, that isn't possible.

A second challenge with a head-controlled device is performing mouse button operations. The alternatives are external switches and dwell-clicking software. External switches typically require a cord that "tethers" the user to the computer, although wireless switches are available. A client may also require assistance mounting an external switch each time he or she wants to use the computer. Dwell-clicking (described in more detail in Section 4.4.6) requires the user to steady the cursor on the target for a preset amount of time. While it eliminates the cord and the need for mounting assistance, it is easy to generate unwanted mouse clicks, which can lead to inefficiency and frustration. Therefore, dwell-clicking is typically only used by those who cannot operate an external switch.

Another concern with using a head mouse is the need to make large head movements both side to side and up and down to move the cursor across the whole screen and then hold it steady. A user may find that it initially increases the strain on his or her neck. Consequently, more extended trial periods are advisable (Figure 4.7).

4.2.9   FOOT MOUSE

It is possible to perform pointing tasks with one's feet. There are foot mouse devices designed specifically for operation by feet. It is also possible to use a trackball with

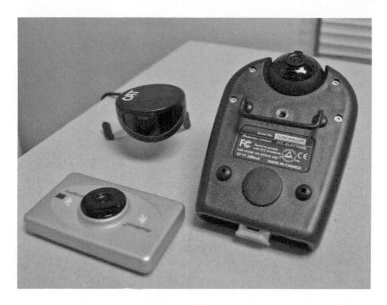

FIGURE 4.7 Head-controlled mouse emulators.

one's foot. While the idea of using a different part of the body to control a mouse is appealing to many, it is important to keep in mind that good balance while sitting favors having both feet placed firmly on the ground. Additionally, the leg muscles are longer and designed for more gross motor function than the arms and hands, while wrists are generally more flexible than ankles.

4.3 MODELING PERFORMANCE ON POINTING TASKS

4.3.1 Fitts's Law

Fitts's law is based on the fundamental truth that the time to acquire a target is a function of the size of the target and the distance to the target [8–10]. Fitts's intention was to model this relationship as a transmission of information. A movement to a target (of a specific size at a specific distance) is assigned an index of difficulty (in units of bits). If the number of bits is divided by the time to move, then a rate of transmission in bits per second can be ascertained [8–10]. This is analogous to information capacity (C; in bits/second) in Shannon's theorem [8–10]:

$$C = B \times \log_2 \frac{S + N}{N}$$

where B is the channel's bandwidth, S is the signal power, and N is the noise power [8–10].

Fitts's law relates movement time (MT) to target size (width; W) and distance (movement amplitude; A) [8–10]. There are many formulations of Fitts's law. One often used formulation was derived by MacKenzie [8]:

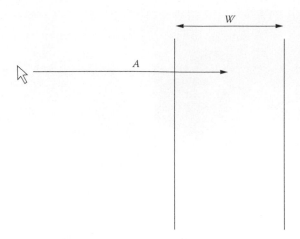

FIGURE 4.8   Fitts's law.

$$MT = a + b \log_2\left(\frac{A}{W} + 1\right)$$

The index of difficulty (ID) is defined as [8–10]

$$ID = \log_2\left(\frac{A}{W} + 1\right)$$

A concept that is central to Fitts's law is *index of performance* (Figure 4.8), which is analogous to channel capacity in information theory:

$$IP = ID/MT$$

4.3.1.1   Effective Width, Distance, and Throughput

In a Fitts's law task, in which a person is asked to move from a starting point to a target, there are actually two different widths [8, 11–13]:

- The actual width of the target, W, which represents what subjects were *asked* to do
- The effective width of the target, W_e, which represents what subjects actually *did*

The effective target width represents the level of precision achieved in selecting a target. The more precise the movement is, the smaller the effective target width will be [8, 11–13] (Figure 4.9).

The calculation of W_e relies on the fact that the spread of hits in a targeting task is normally distributed about the target center [8, 11]. If the standard deviation of the endpoint coordinates (σ) is known, the formula is [8, 9, 11]

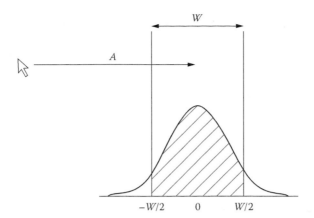

FIGURE 4.9 Effective width.

$$W_e - 4.133 \times \sigma$$

One potential drawback to this method is that it assumes that the person is aiming for the center of the target, rather than for any point within the target, which may not be true for larger targets.

The second method is based on the error rate rather than selection points. The nice thing about this method is that it focuses on errors (which is what counts), rather than distance from the center of the target. The problem is this method breaks down when there are no errors.

To calculate W_e based on the error rate [8, 9, 11],

$$W_e = \begin{cases} W \times \dfrac{2.066}{z(1 - Err/2)} & \text{if } Err > 0.0049\% \\ W \times 0.5089 & \text{otherwise} \end{cases}$$

where Err is the observed error rate, and $z(x)$ represents the inverse of the standard normal cumulative distribution, or the z-score that corresponds to the point where the area under the normal curve is $x\%$.

The effective distance, A_e, is calculated as the mean movement distance from the start-of-movement position to the endpoints [9].

ID_e is the *effective index of difficulty*, based on the effective width of the target and the effective distance to the target [9, 12]:

$$ID_e = \log_2\left(\frac{A_e}{W_e} + 1\right)$$

Fitts's law was derived empirically, and is not based on an underlying understanding of motion. This is important because the ID values used for predicting movement times with a Fitts's law equation should lie strictly within the range of ID_e values that were used when constructing the model [14]. Fitts's law does not help us predict the performance of new devices because it is a *post hoc* descriptive measure of performance [15].

4.3.1.2 Limitations of Fitts's Law

Fitts's law describes a very specific situation. There is an assumption that the movement from the starting position is rapid and aimed, which means it's always in a straight line and confident (starts with high initial velocity as if there were no other targets and you know exactly where you need to go) [10]. Fitts's model, in its original form, is also one-dimensional, with the target width W the only movement constraint, colinear with the direction of movement [10, 16]. Selecting an object with the mouse is a two-dimensional (bivariate) pointing task, constrained by both the target's width and height, and the location of the target relative to the cursor position is a two-dimensional vector [16] (Figure 4.10).

Investigators often lose sight of the fact that Fitts's law is more *explanatory* than *predictive*. Fitts's law summarizes the relationship between movement time, target size, and target distance based on observations of a person performing a specific task with a specific device. Movement time refers to the time subjects spend moving the pointing device, and does not include homing time, dwell time, or reaction time [8, 9]. Attempts to generalize to other people, other tasks, or other devices should be viewed skeptically [9, 15].

Numerous investigators (e.g., [3, 17–24]) have used Fitts's law to document the performance of individuals with disabilities when performing point-and-click tasks on a computer. Movement by both able-bodied and disabled subjects who have cerebral palsy (CP) with both position and isometric joysticks conformed to Fitts's law [3]. Discrete target acquisition for both the mouse and the head-controlled pointer was aptly described for able-bodied and disabled subjects using Fitts's law [24]. Children with CP adhered to Fitts's law in a discrete tapping task on a touch tablet [25]. Across investigators, however, there have been large differences in task implementation and performance measures. These differences make it difficult to compare results between studies [9], reducing their clinical utility.

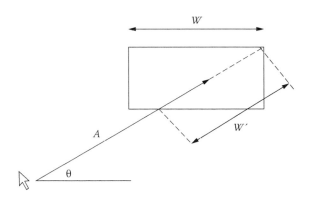

FIGURE 4.10   Two-dimensional Fitts's law task.

Prior research differs in the extent to which it claims that movements by people with motor impairments can be modeled by Fitts's law, since such people's ability to make closed-loop corrections during movement may be compromised [17]. Several investigators have found that, for some individuals with disabilities, Fitts's law does not fit observed data as accurately as other models [23, 26]. Sears et al. [27] found that (for large enough targets) selection time was proportional to distance but not target size when the cursor is controlled by voice commands. Cook et al. [21] found that selection time was proportional to target size but not distance for subjects with CP.

4.3.1.3 Psychomotor Movement Models

Many psychomotor theories have been put forward to explain Fitts's law, but none have been totally satisfactory [28]. Pointer movement can be separated into two components [3, 8, 10, 15, 29, 30]:

- A ballistic movement with the greatest velocity that covers most of the movement distance
- A "homing" phase in which more movement control is required and cursor velocity is slower

Within the ballistic and homing phases there can still be submovements defined by changes in velocity [30]. Efficient cursor movements have ballistic and homing phases of equal duration, only one submovement, and only one cycle of acceleration and deceleration [30]. Individuals with mobility impairments tend to cover less distance with their primary submovement compared with able-bodied computer users and make many more submovements [19]. Even for able-bodied computer users, however, cursor trajectories produced by a mouse are characterized by prolonged homing phases with large numbers of cycles of acceleration and deceleration [30].

4.3.2 STEERING LAW

Fitts's law is not an adequate model for trajectory-based tasks [31]. Steering through a very narrow tunnel without going out of the boundaries at any point of the trial is much more difficult than tapping on small targets [31] (Figure 4.11).

The steering law applies to situations in which the path followed by the cursor matters as much as the final destination. Tasks such as drawing, writing, navigating through nested menus, moving in three-dimensional virtual worlds, and avoiding "mouse-over" areas on web pages are similar in that they are all based on movement trajectories, not targets [2, 32].

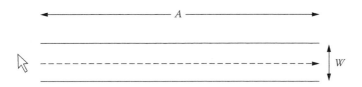

FIGURE 4.11 Steering law.

The steering law is an extension of Fitts's law in which there are an infinite number of goals between the start and finish points [31]. For a one-dimensional movement within a tunnel of constant width [2, 31]:

$$MT = a + b\left(\frac{A}{W}\right)$$

where A is the length of the tunnel and W is the width.

It should be pointed out that the steering law predicts the time it takes to *successfully* steer through a tunnel with a given difficulty quantified by ID. In Accot and Zhai's original study, if the mouse cursor went over the boundaries of the tunnel before completion, the trial was aborted [2]. In that study [2], the number of trials in which the cursor left the tunnel were 9, 18.8, 18.7, 17.5, and 18.9%, respectively, for the mouse, tablet, trackball, touchpad, and trackpoint in the linear steering task.

4.4   INTERVENTIONS

4.4.1   MAKE THINGS CLOSER

One obvious approach to making a pointing task more efficient is to decrease the distance the cursor must move [33]. Unfortunately, we can't keep all the targets close to the mouse cursor all of the time. One way to limit the maximum possible movement distance, however, is to decrease the screen resolution. Decreasing the screen resolution makes targets appear larger by increasing the size of each pixel (thus decreasing the number of pixels on the screen), but does not change the relationship between the movement of the mouse and the corresponding number of pixels moved by the on-screen cursor, so the difficulty of the movement task does not change. One thing changing the screen resolution does do, however, is reduce the number of pixels available on the display, which eliminates the possibility of movements with greater amplitude.

4.4.2   MAKE THINGS BIGGER

Another approach to making a pointing task more efficient is to increase the size of the target [10, 29, 32–37]. However, we want to make the targets bigger without changing the distance to the target. Sometimes, such as with the items in a menu, changing the size of each item also changes the distance to the item. In other words, as each item in a menu gets bigger, the distance between the pointer and the last item in the menu gets bigger, too. This means that increasing the size of menu items will only improve performance if the effect of target size on movement time is greater than the effect of distance. Investigators have found that size has a greater effect on movement time [8, 11, 36, 37], so this seems reasonable.

It is possible to change the size of several on-screen objects (e.g., icons, text, buttons) independently, but we also have limited space to work with on a computer display, so there are limits to how big we can make things. There is a trade-off between aesthetics, intelligibility, and target size. We also need to keep some open space in which new icons can be created. In short, we want some space between items, but not too much space. As a general rule, the size of an object on the screen should be proportional to its expected frequency of use [10].

4.4.3 CONTROL-DISPLAY GAIN

Control-display gain (CDG) is a unit-free coefficient that translates movement of a pointing device to movement of the mouse cursor [38]. CDG is typically referred to as *gain* or *sensitivity*, and determines how far the cursor moves on the screen in response to a movement of the pointing device [29]. If CDG is 1, the mouse cursor moves exactly the same distance and speed as the pointing device; if CDG is greater than 1, the mouse cursor moves proportionally farther and faster than the pointing device; and if CDG is less than 1, the mouse cursor moves more slowly and a shorter distance than the pointing device [38] (Figure 4.12).

CDG is computed from the ratio of the mouse cursor velocity to device velocity [38]:

$$CDG = \frac{V_{pointer}}{V_{device}}$$

The simplest form of CDG is a linear relationship. In modern operating systems, however, the CDG options consist of a family of curves with varying speed and acceleration properties [39]. Pointer acceleration (also referred to as enhanced pointer precision) dynamically manipulates CDG based on the speed at which the user moves the pointing device: when the pointing device is moved quickly, CDG is high; when the pointing device is moved slowly, CDG is low. The underlying assumption is that fast device movement implies the target is far from the mouse cursor, so cursor movement can be amplified to cover the distance more quickly. Conversely, slow device movement implies that the target is near the mouse cursor, so cursor movement should be slow to support accurate adjustments [38]. Investigators have found that pointer acceleration can improve performance for both able-bodied computer users [39] and computer users with disabilities [40].

Arnaut and Greenstein [29] systematically explored the relationship between CDG and target width on performance with a pointing device. They found that changing gain simultaneously changes target width and movement distance, which means performance is unlikely to change much. Even large changes in CDG are unlikely to produce big changes in task time. This is because people adapt their behavior to compensate for changes in CDG.

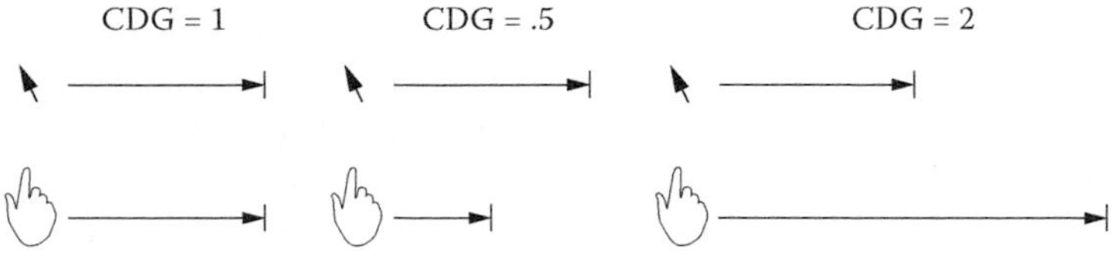

FIGURE 4.12   Control-display gain.

There are three CDG regions [20, 21, 36, 38]:

- Too low: Task time increases because the user has to make multiple ballistic movements to cover the same distance.
- Good enough: User can get to target in a single ballistic movement and can still make adequate fine movements to hit target.
- Too high: Task time increases because of difficulty with fine motor movements.

The question, then, is what's best in the good enough region? One possible answer is that the best is what minimizes the user's effort. A simple approach to choosing CDG is to pick the smallest gain that still allows the user to move the cursor across the entire screen in one movement.

4.4.4   ClickLock

The ClickLock (aka drag lock) feature is intended for computer users who have trouble holding down the left mouse button and moving the mouse at the same time (i.e., clicking and dragging). ClickLock allows the user to hold the mouse button for longer than a threshold time, move the mouse to the new location, and then click the mouse button again. The effect is the same as a drag and drop, but without having to keep the mouse button depressed for the entire duration of the move.

4.4.5   External Switches

There are pointing devices that have jacks for one or more external switches. By adding the external switch it can be possible to control one or more click functions with the help of another body part, or for special needs learners, the help of another person. In addition, there are separate interfaces that connect a switch to the computer through the USB port (Figure 4.13).

4.4.6   Dwell-Clicking

Dwell-clicking software allows the user to perform a mouse operation by positioning the on-screen cursor within the bounds of a target (or icon) for a period of time, instead of clicking to indicate target selection [9]. A tool palette enables the user to switch between left, right, and ClickLock mouse button actions.

Dwell-clicking software is most often used by consumers who are using head-mounted mouse emulators. Dwell-clicking requires the user to steady the cursor on the target for a preset amount of time. While it eliminates the cord and the need for mounting assistance, it is easy to generate unwanted mouse clicks, which can lead to inefficiency and frustration. Therefore, it is typically only used by those who cannot operate an external switch.

The greatest advantage of dwell-clicking software is that it allows the user to pull up to the computer and start working, without having to position an external switch for mouse button operations. The greatest challenge with dwell-clicking is setting

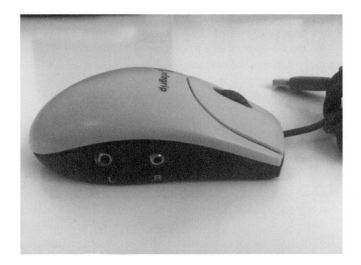

FIGURE 4.13   Switch-adapted mouse. (From http://www.infogrip.com.)

an appropriate dwell time that is long enough to minimize unintended clicks but not so long that clicking intentionally is too difficult. One approach to dealing with problems with dwell-select with a head-mounted mouse emulator is a joystick mode, in which there is a relatively large dead zone of head movement before cursor movement is activated [21].

4.4.7   Position Targets on Edges

Locating targets along edges decreases target selection time [1, 34]. The screen edge is, for all practical purposes, infinitely deep. It doesn't matter how fast that mouse is going when it hits the screen edge, that pointer absolutely will not overshoot [10, 32, 33]. All four corners can be used as well [32].

Although placing the menus at the top of the display does leverage Fitts's law nicely, it also presents its own set of problems [33]. Detaching applications from their menu bar seems to violate the idea that related things should be together. On a multimonitor system, the distance between the application and its menu could be quite large unless the application window is maximized. Additionally, the edges of the screen are typically harder for the head mouse or eye gaze users to reach.

4.4.8   Snap to

Snap to refers to software, either built in to an operating system or installed as a separate program, that automatically moves the mouse cursor to the default button in a window or dialog box. This typically means the cursor automatically moves to the OK or Cancel button of a dialog box as soon as it is displayed. For dialog boxes that are displaying information, this can be quite a time saver.

4.4.9 TRAINING

Knowledge and strategy deficits (e.g., learning that it is the very tip of the arrow cursor where mouse button operations occur) can be overcome by training. However, significant training time may be necessary to learn to use a device successfully [21] or improve performance. In addition, experience or practice cannot necessarily compensate for physical difficulties in operating input devices [20].

4.5 IN THE CLINIC

It can take hours to optimize the settings for a pointing device, even for able-bodied subjects, and there can also be complex interactions among the multiple dimensions of an input method [2]. Before choosing a pointing device, the clinician needs to determine what is important to the client. The client's priorities may include

- Being able to drive up to the computer and start work independently
- Speed
- Precision
- Overall effort required
- Pain management
- Portability
- Reliability
- Cost

It is also important to understand what sorts of activities the client will engage in. Some activities, like video games, place a premium on speed. Other activities, like drawing or computer-aided design (CAD), emphasize accuracy.

Also keep in mind that many individuals will prefer the mouse to alternative pointing devices, despite difficulties in operating it. Many people only have access to, or are required to use, standard computers with ordinary keyboards and mice [17, 20]. They may share a computer with others who use a mouse, or have used a mouse before acquiring a disability. They may find alternatives too expensive, or simply find that the mouse is easier to understand than other devices [41].

4.5.1 PROBLEMS GRASPING AND MANIPULATING A MOUSE

Physical disabilities can result in difficulty in grasping and manipulating the mouse [20]. Users with disabilities can also have difficulty lifting and repositioning a mouse [20]. One obvious approach to these types of problems is to choose a device other than a mouse. A first-order control device, which requires less hand movement, may be particularly useful in this situation. A device like a trackball, which is a zero-order device that also requires limited hand movement, may also be an option.

4.5.2 PROBLEMS MAKING LONG OR STRAIGHT MOVEMENTS

For some individuals, large mouse movements can be difficult or tiring [20]. In particular, moving the mouse over a long distance while maintaining a straight path can be difficult [35]. There are several alternatives for compensating for these types of difficulties:

- Reduce the maximum possible distance between the mouse cursor and the target
- Increase the CDG
- Use a first-order control pointing device
- Provide additional training

4.5.3   PROBLEMS POSITIONING THE CURSOR INSIDE TARGETS

Pointing is the most fundamental mouse operation, and yet also one of the most difficult [20]. Users may experience difficulty in moving the mouse cursor to within a target [20, 35, 42], particularly if the target is small [1]. Possible interventions include

- Make the targets bigger
- Decrease the CDG
- Position targets along the screen edge
- Provide additional training

4.5.4   PROBLEMS WITH SINGLE- AND DOUBLE-CLICKING

Single- or double-clicking can be difficult for a variety of reasons. Users may slip outside a target when pressing the mouse button [1, 20, 35, 42]. In one study involving computer users with disabilities, the position where the mouse button was released was not the same as the position where it was pressed in 28.1% of mouse clicks [20]. Interventions for problems with single-clicking inside a target include

- Using a pointing device (e.g., trackball, joystick) that separates the mouse buttons from the part of the device that causes cursor movement
- Reducing the CDG
- Using an external switch
- Using dwell-clicking software
- Providing additional training

Additional interventions for problems with double-clicking inside a target include

- Using a pointing device (e.g., trackball, joystick) that has a programmable button that can be assigned to double-click
- Increasing time allowed between clicks

Another difficulty that some computer users with disabilities experience is activating a mouse button unintentionally during movement. Unintentional mouse clicks can have unwanted side effects, with time-consuming recovery [20]. Interventions include

- Using a pointing device (e.g., trackball, joystick) that separates the mouse buttons from the part of the device that causes cursor movement
- Using an external switch
- Using dwell-clicking software
- Providing additional training

4.5.5   PROBLEMS WITH CLICKING AND DRAGGING

Dragging (holding down the mouse button while moving the mouse) can be very difficult [21]. While the able-bodied subjects performed 94.9% of drag operations correctly in Trewin's study, only 45% of drags by disabled subjects were successful [21]. Once a drag has been started, a common difficulty is raising the mouse button in the correct position at the end of the drag. The mouse may be positioned correctly, but then slip as the user releases the button. Another common problem is difficulty in holding down the mouse button while moving the mouse [20]. A third difficulty is that some users can get stuck and have to abandon a drag. This may be because they run out of space to move the mouse and cannot lift it up while holding down the mouse button, or they may reach a position where they are physically unable to make the required movement in order to complete the drag [20].

Interventions for problems with clicking and dragging include

- Activating the ClickLock feature
- Using an external switch (possibly with a switch latch)
- Using dwell-clicking software
- Providing additional training

4.6   MEASURING PERFORMANCE ON POINTING TASKS

4.6.1   TIME, ACCURACY, AND THROUGHPUT

The traditional approach to measuring performance with pointing devices is to record the time required to select a target on the screen and the accuracy with which this is accomplished. When reading the literature or discussing a client, however, it is important to be clear on what was actually recorded. Be careful when applying results from the scientific literature to a specific client. What was measured and how it was measured need to correspond to the factors of interest for that client. Also be careful when comparing results between studies. Studies may use the same terms (movement time, accuracy) to refer to different things.

Selecting a target on the computer screen with a pointing device can be divided into the following component actions:

- Reaction: The time from the onset of the stimulus to the beginning of cursor movement [9]
- Homing: Moving one's hand from the keyboard to the pointing device and grasping it [9]

Measure	Gripping Mouse, Manipulating Mouse, Repositioning Mouse	Long Mouse Movements (Fatigue, ROM)	Straight Mouse Movements	Positioning Cursor inside Target	Moving Mouse during Clicking	Double-Clicks	Unintentional Clicks	Dragging
Target reentry				X	X	X		
Task axis crossing			X					
Movement direction change			X					
Orthogonal direction change			X					
Movement variability			X					
Movement error			X					
Movement offset			X					
Distance traveled relative to cursor displacement			X					
Cursor distance traveled away from the target			X					
Verification time				X				
Number of submovements		X	X					
Number of submovements following final target entry				X	X	X		
Number of slip-offs				X	X	X		
Coincident error		X	X					
Perpendicular error		X	X					
Overshoot error			X	X				
Mean counterproductive submovements		X	X					
Ratio of path length to task axis length		X	X					

TABLE 4.1
Pointing Problems and Potential Interventions

	Bigger	Closer	CDG	First-Order Control	ClickLock	External Switches	Dwell-Clicking	Edges	Training
Gripping mouse, manipulating mouse, repositioning mouse				X					
Long mouse movements (fatigue, ROM)		X	X	X					
Straight mouse movements				X					X
Positioning cursor inside target	X		X					X	X
Moving mouse during clicking						X	X		X
Double-clicking						X	X		X
Unintentional clicks						X	X		X
Dragging					X	X	X		X

- Moving: Moving the mouse cursor from its starting position into/over the target [9, 43]
- Verification: Verifying that the mouse cursor is in/over the target before target selection [19, 34, 44]
- Selection: Identifying the target with an explicit action (e.g., pressing the mouse button) [9]

The scientific literature is inconsistent regarding which of these components is included in the total time measured. For example, homing is often not included in empirical research, which typically consists of a series of consecutive pointing tasks without any text entry, but homing can be a significant problem for some consumers. Similarly, many studies combine movement, verification, and selection time, although each of these tasks presents its own unique challenges to users.

Accuracy is typically measured as the percent of selections (e.g., mouse clicks) that occur when the pointer is inside the target [43]. An alternative measure of accuracy that is sometimes used is the percentage of trials that end with a successful selection, regardless of how many clicks occurred outside the target during each trial. Once again, the scientific literature is inconsistent in its use of these measures.

The human factors community moved to reduce variability between studies by incorporating a specific evaluation protocol for pointing devices into the ISO9241-9 standard [45]. The standard specifies the use of *throughput* (measured in bits/second) as the dependent measure compared between devices. Throughput (also referred to as the *index of performance*) is given by the formula [2, 8, 9, 12, 43, 46]

$$TP = \frac{ID}{MT}$$

where *MT* is movement time and *ID* is the *index of difficulty*, calculated as [2, 8, 9, 12, 43, 46]

$$ID = \log_2\left(\frac{A}{W} + 1\right)$$

where *A* is the distance to the target (the *amplitude* of movement) and *W* is the target size (the *width*).

Investigators have found that throughput is independent of the speed–accuracy trade-off [47]. In other words, the same person performing the same pointing task with the same pointing device will obtain the same throughput when performing the task quickly (with less accuracy) or slowly (with greater accuracy). In addition, since throughput is independent of the specific task parameters (target size and distance), it is *theoretically* possible to compare results across studies that do not use identical settings [2, 46]

Keep in mind, however, that the guidelines within the ISO9241-9 standard were developed for human factors research, which is almost the exact opposite of clinical practice. In human factors research, investigators are evaluating devices over a large group of homogeneous able-bodied participants and want a single number that is based on a consistent measure that can be applied to all participants and is amenable to group statistical analyses.

In the clinic, on the other hand, the focus is on a single client (generally someone who is atypical in some way that affects function), and reducing performance to a single number is less important than fully characterizing the client's unique needs. There is also little need to employ the exact same measure of performance across all clients and devices. Clinicians should feel free to pursue whatever measure or measures best document a client's specific needs.

4.6.2 TRAJECTORY ANALYSIS

Tasks such as drawing, writing, navigating through nested menus, gesturing, and moving in three-dimensional virtual worlds are increasingly common. A common feature of these tasks is that they are all based on movement *trajectories*, not targets [2]. A drawback to relying exclusively on throughput as a basis for comparing devices is that throughput bases accuracy entirely on the endpoint of the cursor's motion and ignores the cursor's path of travel during each trial [2, 43]. A device that is slightly slower but produces a much straighter path of travel may be preferable to a slightly faster device with a less optimal path of travel for tasks where the cursor's actual path of travel is just as important as the final destination. As shown in Figure 4.14, accessing the submenu of a drop-down menu requires first selecting the menu item, then moving the cursor across that item to the submenu while keeping the mouse cursor within the bounds of the menu item. If the cursor leaves the menu item, then the submenu will disappear.

Several investigators have recognized the limitations of using throughput as the only performance measure, and have proposed additional, complementary measures (see Table 4.2) [9, 12, 18, 43, 44, 48, 49]. These measures can provide the client and clinician with a great deal of additional information, but it is likely that a distinct subset of measures will be of greatest interest for each client, device, and task. For example, a client with tremor but otherwise relatively good aim is likely to have high movement variability. A client with spasticity, on the other hand, may move in

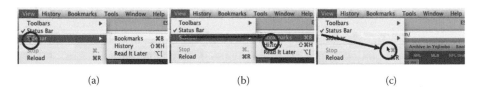

(a)   (b)   (c)

FIGURE 4.14 An illustration of when the path of the mouse cursor matters. (a) The cursor has selected the Sidebar item, which has a submenu of three items. (b) The cursor has successfully moved into the submenu without leaving the blue "tunnel" of the Sidebar item. (c) The cursor fails to stay within the tunnel and the submenu disappears.

TABLE 4.2
Performance Measures Reported in the Literature

Measure	Definition
Target reentry	If the pointer enters the target region, leaves, then reenters the target region, then target reentry occurs [43].
Task axis crossing	The pointer crosses the task axis on the way to the target [43].
Movement direction change	The pointer's path relative to the task axis changes direction [43].
Orthogonal direction change	Direction changes along the axis orthogonal to the task axis [43].
Movement variability	Represents the extent to which the sample points lie in a straight line along an axis parallel to the task axis [43].
Movement error	The average deviation of the sample points from the task axis, irrespective of whether the points are above or below the axis [43].
Movement offset	Represents the tendency of the pointer to veer left or right of the task axis during a movement [43].
Distance traveled relative to cursor displacement	Captures how closely the cursor path follows a straight line [12].
Cursor distance traveled away from the target	The total distance traveled by the cursor in a direction that takes it farther away from the target [12].
Verification time	The time from the end of the last submovement (i.e., the cursor has stopped moving) to the end of the trial (i.e., the user has successfully clicked inside the target) [44].
Number of submovements	Captures the fluidity of motion by indicating how often the cursor has to stop and start on the way to the target [44].
Number of submovements following final target entry	Even after the cursor has landed inside the target, additional submovements may still occur inside the target [44].
Number of slip-offs	A slip-off is a submovement that begins inside the target, but ends outside [44].
Coincident error	The difference of the submovement's component along the instantaneous task axis (ITA) minus the submovement's starting distance from the target's center [44].
Perpendicular error	The distance between the submovement's endpoint and the ITA, measured in a direction normal to the ITA [44].
Overshoot error	If the cursor moves farther along the desired direction of motion than was required, an overshoot occurs [44].
Mean counterproductive submovements	If the submovement moves the cursor in a direction directly away from the target, then a counterproductive submovement occurs [44].
Ratio of path length to task axis length	The path length is the sum total distance moved by the cursor from the point of origin to the target, and the task axis length is the shortest distance between the start point and the target [44].

relatively straight lines (and thus have low movement variability) but have poor aim, and thus have high movement error and movement offset. A client with difficulty operating the mouse button, but no difficulty placing the mouse cursor in the target, would have low movement variability, movement error, and movement offset, but a high number of slip-offs, target reentries, and submovements following final target entry (Figure 4.15).

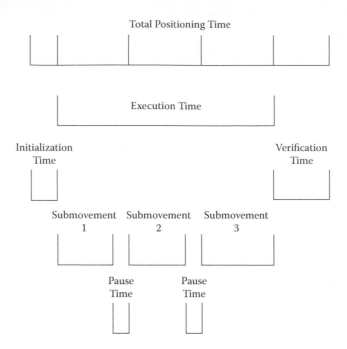

FIGURE 4.15 Dividing a movement into submovements. (Based on Walker, N., D.E. Meyer, and J.B. Smelcer, *Human Factors,* 35(3), 431–458, 1993 [34]; Hwang, F. et al., *6th International ACM SIGACCESS Conference on Computers and Accessibility,* ACM Press, Atlanta, GA, 2004 [44].)

4.6.3   SUBMOVEMENT ANALYSIS

Unless the distance between starting point and target is very short, the movement of the cursor from starting point to the target is typically broken into a series of discrete submovements. The analysis of submovements has several potential clinical applications. For example, submovement analysis can be used to quantify the effects of tremors and spasticity on performance *and* the effects of device and device configuration on tremors and spasticity. For an individual client, a particular position or movement may be particularly likely to induce tremors or spasticity. Documentation of this fact is important to justify the additional cost of mounting equipment.

In practice, determining how to divide a movement into submovements is tricky, and multiple definitions of a submovement have been reported in the scientific literature [12, 17, 44, 48, 49]. Submovements are generally defined based on cursor speed or acceleration. Some devices, like head-mounted mouse emulators, are never truly at rest, which makes it particularly difficult to identify submovements.

4.6.3.1   Number of Submovements

The number of submovements within a trial reflects the fluidity of motion by indicating how often the cursor stops and starts on the way to the target [12, 49]. Individuals with motor impairments compensate for greater noise in their motor system by using more submovements [3, 17, 19, 35]. Even after the cursor has landed within the target, additional submovements may still occur [44]. As with long verification times, high numbers of these may reflect perception or selection difficulties [44].

4.6.3.2 Pauses

A pause is a period in which no mouse movement is reported [19, 34]. Note that pauses do not correspond precisely to submovements, since submovements may be combined without pausing the motion of the cursor, but wherever a pause occurs, a submovement break occurs [19]. A large number of pauses can indicate difficulty in physically manipulating the pointing device. A long pause duration can indicate problems with movement planning or with finding the target.

4.6.3.3 Verification Time

Verification time represents the amount of time that a subject takes to check the location of the cursor after movement has ended but before a selection is made [19, 34, 44]. The duration of the verification phase of a mouse movement is dependent on target width and height (but not distance) [34]. Long verification times may reflect difficulties with perceiving that the cursor is inside the target, or difficulties performing the selection portion of the task [44].

4.6.4 Measures of Overall Movement Relative to the Target

The measures in this section summarize the entire trajectory of the cursor from the starting position to the target.

4.6.4.1 Spatial Distribution

The range of possible distances from the target's center at which the cursor may be located can be divided into bands, represented graphically as concentric rings centered on the target. As the cursor moves toward the target, it travels a certain distance in each band [18]. For a straight path, the distribution will be uniform across all radii up to the cursor's initial distance from the target. This characteristic is intended to capture the "spatial spread" of the cursor movement about the target and may indicate where along the trajectory difficulties in cursor control most often occur. For example, the characteristic would distinguish between difficulties in selecting a target compared with difficulties in navigating to the target [12].

4.6.4.2 Distribution of Distance Traveled for a Range of Cursor Speeds

This is a distribution that indicates how far the cursor traveled while moving at a particular speed. This measure may be effective at capturing the occurrence of spasms, which often result in high-speed movements [12, 49].

4.6.4.3 Cursor Distance Traveled Away from the Target

This is the total distance traveled by the cursor in a direction that takes it farther away from the target. It is intended to capture how well the user is able to move the cursor directly toward the target [49].

4.6.4.4 Distribution of Distance Traveled for a Range of Curvatures

This is a distribution indicating how far the cursor traveled at a particular radius of curvature, and capturing how highly curved a path is. For example, the distribution for a straight path will have 100% of the distance traveled at a radius of curvature of infinity [12].

4.6.4.5 Erroneous Selections

An erroneous selection is a selection (e.g., mouse button click) registered outside of the target [12, 49]. Erroneous selections can occur for several reasons [20]:

- The cursor slips out of the target during selection.
- The user incorrectly believes the cursor is in the target when selecting.
- The user unintentionally makes a selection during cursor movement.

4.6.5 COMPARING THE CURSOR'S TRAJECTORY TO A FIXED TASK AXIS

The task axis is defined as the straight line from the start point to the target center. The task axis is the shortest distance between the start point and the target (Figure 4.16). The measures in this section evaluate performance relative to the optimal path the cursor could follow from the starting position to the target. This optimal path is typically a straight line between the starting position and target, but some tasks (e.g., menu navigation, shape tracing) may have a very different type of optimal path.

4.6.5.1 Ratio of Path Length to Task Axis Length

This is defined as $D1/D2$, where $D1$ is the distance traveled by the cursor and $D2$ is the length of the task axis. This measure is intended to capture how closely the cursor path follows the optimal path. A value of 1 indicates motion directly toward the target, and larger values indicate greater deviations [12, 19].

4.6.5.2 Task Axis Crossing (TAC)

This is an instance where the pointer's actual path crosses the ideal path. The pointer crosses the task axis on the way to the target. TAC may be valuable if, for example, the task is to trace along a predefined path as closely as possible [12, 43] (Figure 4.17).

Movement Variability	Low	Low	High	High
Movement Error	Low	Very High	High	Very High
Movement Offset	Low	High	Low	High

FIGURE 4.16 Movement variability, movement error, and movement offset.

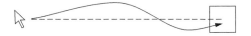

FIGURE 4.17 Task axis crossing.

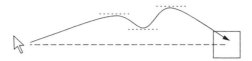

FIGURE 4.18 Movement direction change.

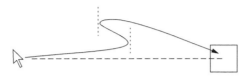

FIGURE 4.19 Orthogonal direction change.

4.6.5.3 Movement Direction Change

This is an instance where the pointer's actual path changes direction either toward or away from the ideal path (i.e., the slope of the actual path is 0) [43]. A movement direction change occurs when the tangent to the cursor path becomes parallel to the task axis [12] (Figure 4.18).

4.6.5.4 Orthogonal Direction Change

This is an instance where the pointer's actual path changes direction either toward or away from the axis orthogonal to the ideal path (i.e., the slope of the actual path is infinite) [43]. An orthogonal direction change occurs when the tangent to the cursor path becomes perpendicular to the task axis [12] (Figure 4.19).

4.6.5.5 Movement Variability

This is a continuous measure computed from the x-y coordinates of the pointer during a movement task. It represents the extent to which the sample points lie in a straight line along an axis parallel to the task axis. It is computed as the standard deviation in the distances of the sample points from the optimal path [12, 43]. In the case of a traditional Fitts's law task, where the cursor moves in one direction (say, along the x axis), movement variability is given by

$$MV = \sqrt{\frac{\sum (y_i - \bar{y})^2}{n-1}}$$

Given an optimal path that starts at point (x_s, y_s) and ends at point (x_e, y_e), movement variability is given by

$$MV = \sqrt{\frac{\sum d_i^2}{n-1}}$$

where

$$a = \frac{y_e - y_s}{x_e - x_s}$$

$$c = y_s - ax_s$$

and, for each point (x_i, y_i):

$$d_i = \frac{ax_i - y_i + c}{\sqrt{a^2 + b^2}}$$

4.6.5.6   Movement Error

This is the average deviation of the sample points from the task axis, irrespective of whether the points are above or below the optimal path [12, 43]. In the case of a traditional Fitts's law task, where the cursor moves in one direction (say, along the x axis), movement error is given by

$$ME = \frac{\sum |y_i - y_i'|}{n}$$

Given an optimal path that starts at point (x_s, y_s) and ends at point (x_e, y_e), movement error is given by

$$ME = \sqrt{\frac{\sum |d_i|}{n}}$$

4.6.5.7   Movement Offset

This is the average distance (directional) between the actual path and the ideal path. Movement offset represents the tendency of the pointer to veer left or right of the task axis during a movement [43]. Unlike movement error, this measure is related to whether the points are above or below the axis [12]. In the case of a traditional Fitts's law task, where the cursor moves in one direction (say, along the x axis), movement offset is given by

$$MO = \frac{\sum (y_i - y_i')}{n}$$

Given an optimal path that starts at point (x_s, y_s) and ends at point (x_e, y_e), movement offset is given by

$$MO = \sqrt{\frac{\sum d_i}{n}}$$

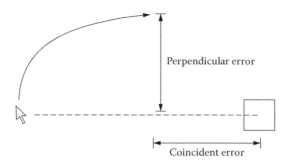

FIGURE 4.20   Instantaneous task axis. (Based on Hwang, F. et al., *6th International ACM SIGACCESS Conference on Computers and Accessibility*, ACM Press, Atlanta, GA, 2004 [44].)

4.6.5.8   Maximum Orthogonal Displacement

Maximum orthogonal displacement is the greatest distance by which the cursor becomes displaced from the tuck axis [34].

4.6.6   COMPARING THE CURSOR'S TRAJECTORY TO AN INSTANTANEOUS TASK AXIS

The instantaneous task axis (ITA) (Figure 4.20) is defined as the line connecting a submovement's starting point to the target's center [44]. The ITA varies with cursor position, reflecting the fact that the desired direction of travel at a point in time is dependent on the cursor position at that time, and not on the cursor position at the start of the task [44, 49]. After each submovement, two error values can be calculated [44]:

- Coincident error: The difference of the submovement's component along the ITA minus the submovement's starting distance from the target's center [44].
- Perpendicular error: The distance between the submovement's endpoint and the ITA, measured in a direction normal to the ITA [44].

4.6.6.1   Counterproductive Submovements

If the submovement moves the cursor in a direction directly away from the target, then a counterproductive submovement occurs. In these cases, the coincident error will be negative and have a magnitude larger than the submovement's starting distance from the target [44].

4.6.6.2   Slip-offs

A slip-off is a submovement that begins inside the target, but ends outside. This measure counts the number of slip-offs in one trial [44]. Slip-offs may be indicative of difficulties with cursor stabilization [12, 19, 43, 44, 48] (Figure 4.21).

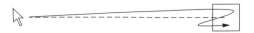

FIGURE 4.21   Slip-offs.

4.6.6.3   Overshoots

Overshoots occur when the user moves past the target. It's easy to define overshoot for one-dimensional tasks, but it can be tougher for two-dimensional tasks because the cursor can overshoot the target without passing through the target. Overshoots differ from undershoots in that an overshoot can occur without a selection (mouse click) occurring, but it's hard to identify undershoots in the absence of selections [44].

4.7   SPEED–ACCURACY OPERATING CHARACTERISTIC (SAOC)

In 1899, Woodworth demonstrated the fundamental truth that (in pointing, at least) it is impossible to be fast and accurate at the same time [50]. This *speed–accuracy trade-off* forces computer users to accept either an increase in the time spent during movement or a lesser degree of terminal accuracy [46]. Clients can change their performance under the same experimental conditions (i.e., using the same device to perform tasks of equal difficulty) by adjusting their emphasis between speed and accuracy between trials [51].

There are two problems with using this in the clinic, however. First, by compressing the results into a single number, throughput effectively hides the effect of the speed/accuracy trade-off. However, clients and clinicians may be interested in performance under high- and low-speed conditions because some real-world pointing tasks require greater precision than others, and this should be considered during clinical assessments. For example, working with computer-aided design (CAD) programs or drawing programs that require precise targeting places a much greater than normal emphasis on accuracy.

Second, the nature of the speed/accuracy trade-off dictates that, at low error rates, small changes in error rates can be accompanied by extremely large variations in movement time [51]. In other words, the difference in movement time between two devices may be much greater when one device is operated at 2% error and the other is operated at 3% error than when one device is operated at 20% error and the other is operated at 21% error. Since many clients attempt to minimize errors when trying devices in the clinic, this effect has relevance for clinical practice.

The solution is to have clients use each device under a range of speed/accuracy settings [4, 11, 52], and to present data from these trials separately for each device, rather than as a single statistic (Figure 4.22).

The SAOC is a graphical representation of the trade-off between speed and accuracy [4]. Pew [53] originally used the SAOC to describe accuracy in choice reaction tasks, but it has since been used (though not widely) in a range of timed reaction tasks. Rival [54] is one of the few investigators who has used the SAOC to show performance in a pointing task under different speed–accuracy settings.

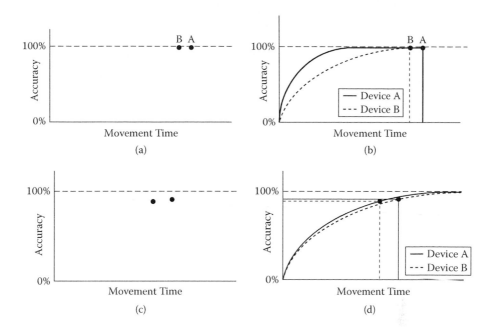

FIGURE 4.22 Collecting a single speed/accuracy data point for each device can produce data that are difficult to interpret. (a, b) A situation where the faster device can actually appear slower at 100% accuracy. (c, d) A situation where a small difference in accuracy leads to a relatively large difference in movement time, even though the underlying speed–accuracy curves are nearly identical.

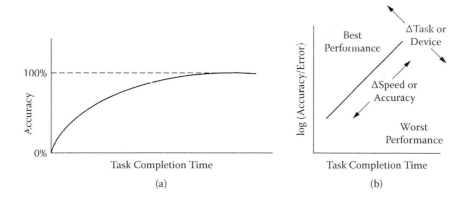

FIGURE 4.23 Speed–accuracy operating characteristic. (a) Task completion time plotted against accuracy. (b) Task completion time against the log of the ratio of accuracy to error.

As shown in Figure 4.23, there are two ways to plot the SAOC. The curved relationship between speed and accuracy (shown in the left panel of Figure 4.23) is more intuitive, but is less conducive to comparisons between devices. The linear relationship between speed and the log of the ratio of accuracy to error (shown in the right panel of Figure 4.23) lends itself more easily to device comparisons.

When inspecting the SAOC, curves lying toward the lower right represent the least desirable performance (i.e., long task completion time and low accuracy), while curves closer to the upper left corner represent the most desirable performance (i.e., short task completion time and high accuracy) [4, 55]. Performance is varied *along* a single curve by changing the emphasis on speed and accuracy [4]. Performance is varied *between* two curves by changes to the task (e.g., changing the pointing device, the pointing device's operating parameters, or the difficulty of the targets) [4]. The goal of a computer access assessment then is to identify the solution (pointing device, device configuration, task requirements) that produces the curve closest to the upper left while conforming to additional nonperformance criteria established between client and clinician (e.g., reducing pain, avoiding fatigue, maximizing portability, simplifying setup, minimizing local support requirements).

REFERENCES

1. Accot, J., and S. Zhai. 2002. More than dotting the i's— Foundations for crossing-based interfaces. In *Conference on Human Factors in Computing Systems*, D. Wixon, ed. Minneapolis: ACM, pp. 73–80.
2. Accot, J., and S. Zhai. 1999. Performance evaluation of input devices in trajectory-based tasks: An application of the steering law. In *Proceedings of the SIGCHI Conference on Human Factors in Computing Systems: The CHI Is the Limit*. Pittsburgh, PA: ACM Press.
3. Rao, R.S., and R. Seliktar. 2000. Evaluation of an isometric and a position joystick in a target acquisition task for individuals with cerebral palsy. *IEEE Transactions on Rehabilitation Engineering* 8(1): 118–125.
4. Wickens, C.D., and J.G. Hollands. 2000. *Engineering psychology and human performance*. 3rd ed. Upper Saddle River, NJ: Prentice Hall, p. 573.
5. *Musculoskeletal disorders in the U.S. office workforce*. 2001. Zeeland, MI: Herman Miller.
6. Colven, D. 2006. *Accessing Windows with a keyboard*. Oxford, UK: ACE Centre Advisory Trust.
7. Cantor, A. 2006. Windows keyboard access FAQ v1.4. Available from http://www.cantoraccess.com/keyaccess/keyaccessfaq.htm (accessed 2006).
8. MacKenzie, I.S. 1992. Fitts's law as a research and design tool in human-computer interaction. *Human-Computer Interaction* 7(1): 91–139.
9. Soukoreff, R.W., and I.S. MacKenzie. 2004. Towards a standard for pointing device evaluation, perspectives on 27 years of Fitts's law research in HCI. *International Journal of Human-Computer Studies* 61(6): 751–789.
10. Hale, K. 2007. Visualizing Fitts's law. Available from http://particletree.com/features/visualizing-fittss-law/ (accessed April 8, 2008).
11. Wobbrock, J.O. et al. 2008. An error model for pointing based on Fitts's law. In *Twenty-Sixth Annual SIGCHI Conference on Human Factors in Computing Systems*, M. Czerwinski, A. Lund, and D.S. Tan, eds. Florence, Italy: ACM Press, pp. 1613–1622.
12. Keates, S. et al. 2002. Cursor measures for motion-impaired computer users. In *Proceedings of the Fifth International ACM Conference on Assistive Technologies*, V.L. Hanson and J. Jacko, eds. Edinburgh, Scotland: ACM Press, pp. 135–142.
13. Murata, A., and H. Iwase. 1999. Proposal of two-dimensional effective target width in Fitts's law. In *IEEE International Conference on Systems, Man, and Cybernetics*. Tokyo: IEEE Press.

14. Soukoreff, R.W., and I.S. MacKenzie. 2004. Towards a standard for pointing device evaluation, perspectives on 27 years of Fitts's law research in HCI. *International Journal of Human-Computer Studies* 61: 751–789.

15. Mithal, A.K. 1995. Using psychomotor models of movement in the analysis and design of computer pointing devices. In *Conference on Human Factors in Computing Systems*. Denver, CO: ACM Press.

16. Grossman, T., and R. Balakrishnan. 2005. A probabilistic approach to modeling two-dimensional pointing. *ACM Transactions on Computer-Human Interaction* 12(3): 435–459.

17. Wobbrock, J.O., and K.Z. Gajos. 2008. Goal crossing with mice and trackballs for people with motor impairments: Performance, submovements and design directions. *ACM Transactions on Access Computing* 1(1): 1–37.

18. Hwang, F. 2002. A study of cursor trajectories of motion-impaired users. In *CHI '02 Extended Abstracts on Human Factors in Computing Systems*, L. Terveen and D. Wixon, eds. Minneapolis: ACM Press, pp. 842–843.

19. Keates, S., and S. Trewin. 2005. Effect of age and Parkinson's disease on cursor positioning using a mouse. In *7th International ACM SIGACCESS Conference on Computers and Accessibility*, A. Sears and E. Pontelli, eds. Baltimore: ACM Press, pp. 68–75.

20. Trewin, S., and H. Pain. 1999. Keyboard and mouse errors due to motor disabilities. *International Journal of Human-Computer Studies* 50(2): 109–144.

21. Cook, A.M. et al. 2005. Measuring target acquisition utilizing Madentec's tracker system in individuals with cerebral palsy. *Technology and Disability* 17(3): 155–163.

22. Gajos, K.Z., J.O. Wobbrock, and D.S. Weld. 2007. Automatically generating user interfaces adapted to users' motor and vision capabilities. In *ACM Symposium on User Interface Software and Technology*, C. Shen and R. Jacob, eds. Newport, RI: ACM Press, pp. 231–240.

23. Bravo, P.E. et al. 1993. A study of the application of Fitts's law to selected cerebral palsied adults. *Perceptual and Motor Skills* 77(3 Pt 2): 1107–1117.

24. Radwin, R.G., G.C. Vanderheiden, and M.-L. Lin. 1990. A method for evaluating head-controlled computer input devices using Fitts's law. *Human Factors* 32(4): 423–438.

25. Smits-Engelsman, B.C.M., and E.A.A. Rameckers. 2007. Children with congenital spastic hemiplegia obey Fitts's law in a visually guided tapping task. *Experimental Brain Research* 177: 431–439.

26. Gajos, K.Z., J.O. Wobbrock, and D.S. Weld. 2008. Improving the performance of motor-impaired users with automatically-generated, ability-based interfaces. In *Twenty-Sixth Annual SIGCHI Conference on Human Factors in Computing Systems*, M. Czerwinski, A. Lund, and D.S. Tan, eds. Florence, Italy: ACM, pp. 1257–1266.

27. Sears, A., M. Lin, and A.S. Karimullah. 2002. Speech-based cursor control: Understanding the effects of target size, cursor speed, and command selection. *Universal Access in the Information Society* 2(1): 30–43.

28. Plamondon, R., and A.M. Alimi. 1997. Speed/accuracy trade-offs in target-directed movements. *Behavioral and Brain Sciences* 20(2): 279–349.

29. Arnaut, L.Y., and J.S. Greenstein. 1990. Is display/control gain a useful metric for optimizing an interface? *Human Factors* 32(6): 651–663.

30. Phillips, J.G., and T.J. Triggs. 2001. Characteristics of cursor trajectories controlled by the computer mouse. *Ergonomics* 44(5): 527–536.

31. Accot, J., and S. Zhai. 1997. Beyond Fitts's law: Models for trajectory-based HCI tasks. In *SIGCHI Conference on Human Factors in Computing Systems*, S. Pemberton, ed. Atlanta, GA: ACM Press, pp. 295–302.

32. Tognazzini, B. 1999, February. A quiz designed to give you Fitts. Available from http://www.asktog.com/columns/022DesignedToGiveFitts.html (accessed April 8, 2008).

33. Atwood, J. 2006, August 9. Fitts's law and infinite width. Available from http://www.codinghorror.com/blog/archives/000642.html (accessed April 7, 2008).

34. Walker, N., D.E. Meyer, and J.B. Smelcer. 1993. Spatial and temporal characteristics of rapid cursor-positioning movements with electromechanical mice in human-computer interaction. *Human Factors* 35(3): 431–458.

35. Smith, M.W., J. Sharit, and S.J. Czaja. 1999. Aging, motor control, and the performance of computer mouse tasks. *Human Factors* 41(3): 389–396.

36. Sandfeld, J., and B. Jensen. 2005. Effect of computer mouse gain and visual demand on mouse clicking performance and muscle activation in a young and elderly group of experienced computer users. *Applied Ergonomics* 36(5): 547–555.

37. Stafford, T. 2005, January 20. Size and selection times: Fitts's law. Available from http://www.mindhacks.com/blog/2005/01/size_and_selection_t.html (accessed April 8, 2008).

38. Casiez, G. et al. 2008. The impact of control-display gain on user performance in pointing tasks. *Human-Computer Interaction* 23: 215–250.

39. Pointer Ballistics for Windows XP. 2002, October 31. Available from http://www.microsoft.com/whdc/archive/pointer-bal.mspx (accessed July 14, 2008).

40. LoPresti, E.F., H.H. Koester, and R.C. Simpson. 2008. Toward automatic adjustment of pointing device configuration to accommodate physical impairment. *Disability and Rehabilitation: Assistive Technology* 3(4): 221–235.

41. Trewin, S., S. Keates, and K. Moffatt. 2006. Developing steady clicks: A method of cursor assistance for people with motor impairments. In *8th International ACM SIGACCESS Conference on Computers and Accessibility*, S. Keates, ed. Portland, OR: ACM, pp. 26–33.

42. Choe, E.K. et al. 2009. Exploring the design of accessible goal crossing desktop widgets. In *Conference on Human Factors in Computing Systems*, D.R. Olsen and R.B. Arthur, eds. Boston: ACM Press, pp. 3733–3738.

43. MacKenzie, I.S., T. Kauppinen, and M. Silfverberg. 2001. Accuracy measures for evaluating computer pointing devices. In *SIGCHI Conference on Human Factors in Computing Systems*. Seattle, WA: ACM Press.

44. Hwang, F. et al. 2004. Mouse movements of motion-impaired users: A submovement analysis. In *6th International ACM SIGACCESS Conference on Computers and Accessibility*. Atlanta, GA: ACM Press.

45. International Standards Organization, ed. 2002. Ergonomic requirements for office work with visual display terminals (VDTs). Part 9. Requirements for non-keyboard input devices. In 9241-9:2000(E). Geneva: International Standards Organization, p. 54.

46. Bootsma, R.J., L. Fernandez, and D. Mottet. 2004. Behind Fitts's law: Kinematic patterns in goal-directed movements. *International Journal of Human-Computer Studies* 61(6): 811–821.

47. MacKenzie, I.S., and P. Isokoski. 2008. Fitts's throughput and the speed–accuracy trade-off. In *CHI 2008*. Florence, Italy: ACM Press, pp. 1633–1636.

48. Hwang, F. 2003. Partitioning cursor movements in "point and click" tasks. In *CHI '03 extended abstracts on human factors in computing systems*, G. Cockton and P. Korhonen, eds. Ft. Lauderdale, FL: ACM Press, pp. 682–683.

49. Keates, S. et al. 2002. The use of cursor measures for motion-impaired computer users. *Universal Access in the Information Society* 2(1): 18–29.

50. Woodworth, R. 1899. The accuracy of voluntary movement. *Psychological Review* 3: 1–106.

51. Wickelgren, W.A. 1976. Speed–accuracy tradeoff and information processing dynamics. *Acta Psychologica* 41(1): 67–85.

52. Simpson, R.C. 2009. Using the speed–accuracy operating characteristic to visualize performance with pointing devices. *Open Rehabilitation Journal* 2: 58–63.

53. Pew, R.W. 1969. The speed–accuracy operating characteristic. *Acta Psychologica* 30(1): 16–26.
54. Rival, C., I. Olivier, and H. Ceyte. 2003. Effects of temporal and/or spatial instructions on the speed–accuracy trade-off of pointing movements in children. *Neuroscience Letters* 336(1): 65–69.
55. Pew, R.A., and A.S. Mavor, eds. 1998. *Modeling human and organizational behavior: Application to military simulations*. Washington, DC: National Academy Press, p. 432.

5 Text Entry

5.1 INTRODUCTION

This chapter covers hardware and software for entering text into a computer. Text entry devices come in many shapes and sizes, including some that bear little or no resemblance to a traditional keyboard. Text entry devices can be physical objects (e.g., a keyboard) or virtual objects displayed on the computer screen.

Input methods exist on a continuum. At the slowest end of the spectrum are *scanning input methods*, which are covered in Chapter 3. At the other end of the spectrum are *direct selection input methods*, which are covered in this chapter. Direct selection means that the desired input (e.g., a letter, number, punctuation mark) is chosen by the user without the need to reject any other potential items. Direct selection is the fastest and simplest form of input, but requires more motor control than scanning.

5.2 DESCRIBING KEYS

Most (but not all) text entry devices have keys, buttons, or switches that the user must activate (either singly or in combination) to produce text. In this section we discuss the terminology used for describing and comparing the keys on text entry devices.

5.2.1 SIZE

Keys come in different sizes, and there are typically different-sized keys on the same text entry device. Some devices, however, are designed with keys that are especially large or especially small. Large keys are advantageous because they allow for larger labels and graphics, and can be activated by larger body parts (e.g., knuckles, toes) [1]. On the other hand, large keys mean that the device itself must be larger or use fewer keys [1] (Figure 5.1).

5.2.2 RESOLUTION

A key's *resolution* is the amount of surface area that responds to user input (e.g., pressing or touching) [2]. Resolution *is not relative* to the size of the key [2]. Adding space between keys on the keyboard does not change resolution, but a keyguard (see Section 5.2) does if it covers part of each key (Figure 5.2).

5.2.3 SENSITIVITY

Sensitivity refers to the amount of force or time required to activate a key [3]. Keys that are very sensitive respond to very little force or activate immediately after being

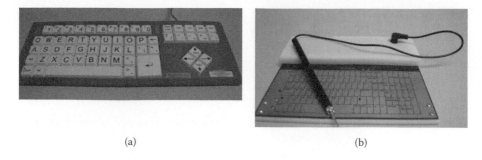

(a)   (b)

FIGURE 5.1   Key size: Keyboard with (a) large keys and (b) small keys.

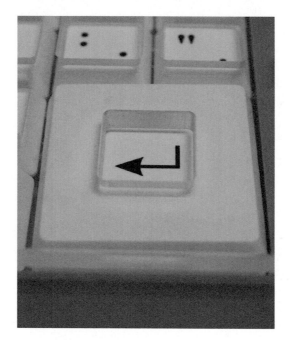

FIGURE 5.2   A keyguard changes a key's resolution.

touched. Keys with reduced sensitivity, on the other hand, require greater force or time to activate.

Setting the sensitivity for the keys of a keyboard requires balancing between *false positive* keystroke errors (a key activates when it should not) and *false negative* keystroke errors (a key fails to activate when it should). Decreasing sensitivity will reduce false positive keystroke errors, but may introduce additional false negative keystroke errors. Increasing sensitivity will decrease false negative keystroke errors but possibly increase false positive keystroke errors. For example, if a client has tremors that cause him to press the desired key several times, instead of just once, then decreasing key sensitivity can eliminate unwanted keystrokes. At the same time, however, decreasing key sensitivity may also increase the number of instances

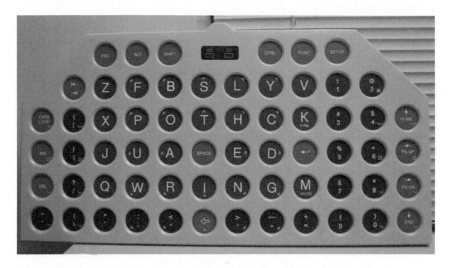

FIGURE 5.3 Contrast can be visual, tactile, or proprioceptive.

where the client presses the key but fails to press hard or long enough, and no key-stroke is produced (a false negative keystroke error). Similarly, a client with limited strength may need a keyboard with very sensitive keys, at the expense of additional unintended keystrokes (false positive keyboard errors).

5.2.4 CONTRAST

Contrast refers to the distinctiveness of the key in comparison to the background and surrounding keys [3]. Contrast can be (Figure 5.3)

- Visual: Keys can use different colors, labels, or graphics.
- Tactile: Keys can have different surface materials or textures.
- Proprioceptive: Special keys can be distinguished by locating them in partic-ular locations (e.g., the Escape key in the upper left corner of the keyboard).

The reason to increase the contrast of a key is to make a key faster and easier to find or to incorporate more sensory cues to support accurate keystrokes.

5.2.5 FEEDBACK

Feedback describes a key's response to activation [3]. Feedback can be

- Visual: A key can change color or light up when activated.
- Kinesthetic: A key can move when activated.
- Auditory: A key can generate a click or other sound when activated.

Feedback is important to let users know when they have activated a key, and to help users figure out whether or not they have activated the desired key. This is typically more important for clients adjusting to a new text entry device. The need for feedback often dissipates with learning because experienced users usually trust that the keystroke was accepted.

5.2.6 Functional Transparency

Functional transparency refers to the extent to which a user can determine what a key actually does when activated [3]. Functional transparency is most directly determined by a key's label, but can also be influenced by a key's location, arrangement with other keys, and convention. For example, an unlabeled key that is much longer than other keys and located at the bottom center of the keyboard is assumed to produce a space.

Functional transparency is a continuum with items that are *transparent* (the purpose of a key is obvious) on one end and *opaque* (the purpose cannot be deduced and must be taught) on the other, with the items in between being *translucent* (the purpose isn't obvious but can be deduced). Note that the functional transparency of a key can vary between people. Something that is transparent to one person may be opaque to another [3].

Transparency is good, because it allows clients to use a keyboard without training. However, making a text entry device completely transparent usually means getting rid of functions that aren't immediately intuitive. Sometimes, a little effort learning an opaque interface can produce much better results. For example, the function keys on many laptops are labeled ambiguously, but that makes it easier to assign multiple functions to them arbitrarily (Figure 5.4).

5.2.7 Affordance

The affordances of an item are the *perceptions* it creates about how it can be used [3, 4]. This is different than how an item can *actually* be used in that an item may imply that it can be used in ways that it can't or may hide functionality it actually has. In the case of a keyboard key, its affordance is the way in which it is activated. Most keyboard keys are activated by being pushed and then released; i.e., they *afford* pushing. Some keys, however, are activated by touch and do not actually depress.

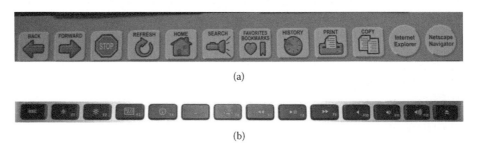

(a)

(b)

FIGURE 5.4 Functional transparency describes how easy or hard it is to figure out what a key actually *does*. The function of some keys is (a) transparent, while for others it can be (b) opaque.

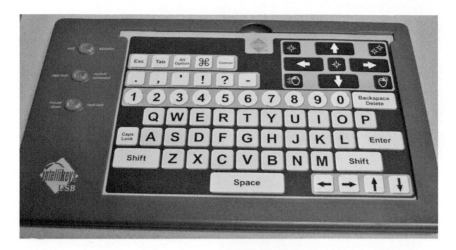

FIGURE 5.5 Not all keyboard keys are activated by being depressed. Keys on a membrane keyboard are activated by touch.

These keys do not afford pushing and, in fact, can break if pushed too hard. Other keys are activated by light, and will not respond to touch or pressure (Figure 5.5).

5.3 DESCRIBING KEYBOARDS

Just as there is a vocabulary for describing individual keys, there is a vocabulary for describing and comparing keyboards.

5.3.1 TRANSFERABILITY

Transferability refers to the extent that (1) a keyboard allows existing knowledge to be applied (or transferred) to its operation and (2) the knowledge of a keyboard can be applied to future interactions with other devices [5]. A keyboard that closely resembles a standard keyboard with a QWERTY layout has greater transferability than a text entry device that is dramatically different. From a design perspective, high transferability makes a keyboard easier to use initially and reduces training time but also reduces design flexibility (Figure 5.6).

5.3.2 AFFORDANCE

Keyboards that do more than just enter text need to provide affordances that indicate their additional functionality. For example, some keyboards include built-in mouse control, and other keyboards provide special function keys for launching programs. These keys need to be clearly labeled to make their function clear. On the other hand, these additional functions sometimes require additional software to be installed on the computer to actually work. If the additional software isn't installed, the affordances of these keys can create false promises of functions that aren't available.

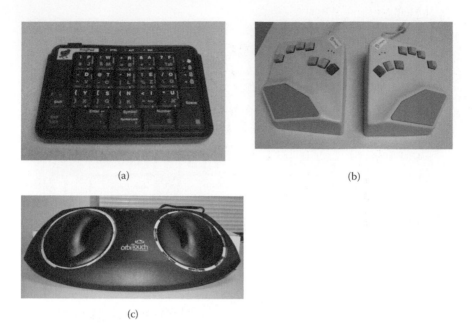

(a)   (b)

(c)

FIGURE 5.6   Some text entry devices have very low transferability: (a) FrogPad keyboard, (b) BAT keyboard, (c) orbiTouch keyboard.

5.3.3   OPERATING MODES

Keyboards use different operating modes to allow the same key to perform multiple functions [5]. Familiar examples of two operating modes are typing in lowercase and typing in capital letters. In lowercase mode, the letter keys produce lowercase letters and the number keys produce numbers. In uppercase mode (which is accessed by holding down the shift key), the same letter keys produce uppercase letters and the number keys produce punctuation marks. Laptop computers typically provide an "fn" key that allows the number keys to perform as function keys.

Some keyboards provide numerous task- or program-specific operating modes. An important factor to consider when using these keyboards is the mechanism provided for switching between modes. The IntelliKeys keyboard, for example, requires the user to manually switch among overlays to change operating modes. The Discover on-screen keyboard, on the other hand, automatically switches between modes each time a new program is activated.

The advantage of providing multiple operating modes is that the keyboard needs fewer keys, which allows the keyboard to be smaller or the keys to be bigger. Imagine how large a keyboard would be if it had separate keys for upper- and lowercase letters and separate keys for numbers and punctuation. On the other hand, having multiple operating modes can lead to errors when the user is unaware which operating mode is active (as anyone who has mistakenly pressed the caps lock key can attest) (Figure 5.7).

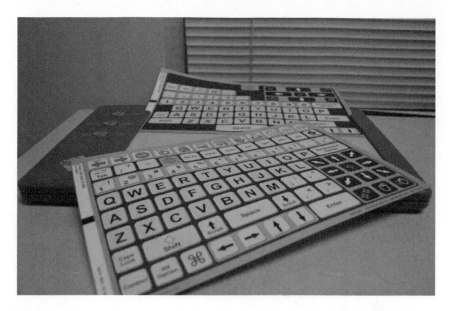

FIGURE 5.7 Most keyboards have multiple modes of operation, but some are especially flexible.

5.4 PHYSICAL TEXT ENTRY DEVICES

Text entry devices can be physical devices or virtual devices presented on a computer screen. In this section we present vocabulary for describing physical text entry devices.

5.4.1 SIZE

Small-footprint keyboards typically have keys that are the same size as a standard keyboard, but take up less physical space [6]. Small-footprint keyboards make it easier for a one-hand or one-finger typist to reach all the keys, particularly the command keys (e.g., home, insert, arrows). Small-footprint keyboards can also reduce the amount of reaching required to use a pointing device.

Small-footprint keyboards usually reduce their size by eliminating some keys (like the number pad) and rearranging others. Some small-footprint keyboards make use of smaller keys to further reduce the size of the keyboard, making them useful for individuals with limited range of motion or very small hands. On the other hand, by eliminating keys, these keyboards must either eliminate functions or add additional operating modes (the fn key on many laptop keyboards is an example of adding another operating mode).

At the opposite extreme, some keyboards provide extra-large keys to accommodate users with poor aim or impaired vision [1]. In order to include enough keys to operate a modern computer, these keyboards either add additional operating modes or are much larger than a standard keyboard. Larger keyboards take up more space on the desk and require greater range of motion. A larger keyboard will also require the pointing device to be moved farther away from the user (Figure 5.8).

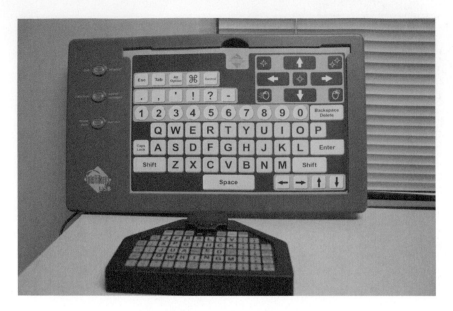

FIGURE 5.8   Keyboards of different sizes.

5.4.2 SURFACE

Text entry devices can either use individual keys or a flat membrane. Individual keys provide tactile feedback (from the key edges) and kinesthetic feedback (by moving up and down as they are pressed). Individual keys can also be designed to provide auditory feedback by clicking when pressed. One significant drawback to individual keys is that they provide space for food, liquids, and saliva to enter the keyboard [1]. Another drawback to individual keys is that they limit a keyboard's flexibility. Individual keys are a fixed size and in a fixed location, making it difficult to redesign the keyboard.

Membrane keyboards provide a single flat surface. The keys on a membrane keyboard do not provide kinesthetic or auditory feedback [1], but can provide tactile feedback by using different materials for each key (and auditory feedback can come from a speaker on the computer or keyboard). A membrane keyboard is more robust in the face of food and liquids [1]. Some membrane keyboards allow the user to create new keyboards with keys of any size or shape through interchangeable overlays or software the creates customized keyboards [1]. Membrane keyboards are especially appropriate when the client:

- Would benefit from task-specific keyboard overlays
- Uses the keyboard with only one computer or doesn't mind carrying the keyboard between computers
- Would benefit from a smaller, larger, or custom layout

Membrane keyboards that do not provide tactile feedback are often used because they do not require significant force to activate. However, a low-force membrane

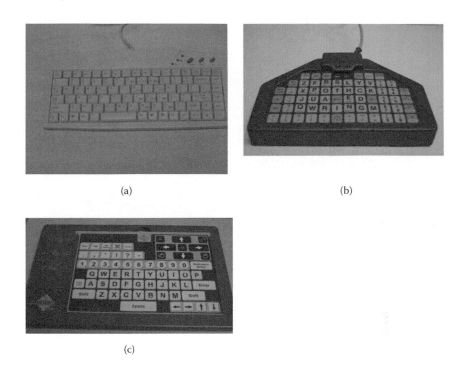

(a)   (b)

(c)

FIGURE 5.9   Keyboards can have (a) individual keys, (b) a membrane surface, or (c) a membrane surface with interchangeable overlays.

keyboard that imposes a long acceptance delay can actually lead to harder key presses. If the client is not aware of the time delay, he or she may begin by pressing lightly on a target key but increase the pressure until the key is activated. The client may then assume that it was the increased pressure, not the elapsed time, that led to the key being activated, leading to an increasing spiral of key press force (Figure 5.9).

5.4.3   Fixed or Interchangeable Layouts

A keyboard's layout (i.e., the arrangement of its keys) can be either fixed or interchangeable (Figure 5.10). Keyboards with individual keys typically have fixed layouts. Some membrane keyboards have fixed layouts, but others support multiple layouts through interchangeable overlays.

The advantages of static layouts are that they facilitate learning/automaticity (i.e., learning the motor pattern required for key activation as in touch typing) and do not require the user to swap overlays for different activities or programs. On the other hand, a static layout must have all the keys it will ever need on the keyboard all the time, which makes it difficult to simplify the keyboard by eliminating unnecessary keys. Static keyboards are also more likely to need multiple operating modes. The primary advantage of interchangeable layouts is that they allow task-specific keyboards. On the other hand, the overlays must be stored and manipulated by the user and task-specific keyboards have limited transferability.

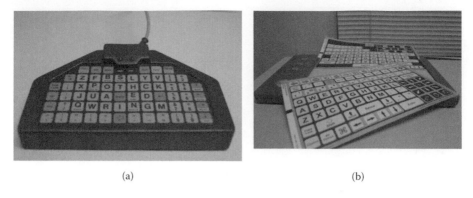

(a)   (b)

FIGURE 5.10   Some membrane keyboards (a) have fixed layouts, while others (b) allow the user to switch between different keyboards by swapping different overlays printed on sheets of vinyl.

5.4.4   CHORD KEYBOARDS

Chord keying (Figure 5.11) was first proposed in 1942 [7]. Chord keyboards use combinations of keys (with each combination of keys referred to as a chord, like a chord on a piano) to generate all of the letters, punctuation marks, and digits of a traditional keyboard with a fraction of the number of keys [8–10]. Chord keyboards thus require less overall hand and arm movement but increased coordination and fine motor control [1, 8].

Chord keyboards can be beneficial for people with the use of only one hand who retain independent movement in each of their fingers [6, 8], and for individuals with visual impairments (because chord keyboards eliminate the need to remember the location of numerous keys) [9]. On the other hand, chord keyboards have low transferability and functional transparency, which means they have a significant learning curve. Research also indicates they rarely allow users to type as fast as on a conventional keyboard because conventional keyboards allow the user to coordinate and overlap finger movements for multiple letters [1, 8, 9]. Chording keyboards also don't provide any visual cues about how to generate each letter [1].

5.5   KEYBOARD MODIFICATIONS

5.5.1   TYPING AIDS

A typing aid is a rod that is used to activate keys (Figure 5.12). A typing aid can be positioned on nearly any part of the body. The most common positions are

- On the hand (with a cuff or velcro strap)
- In the mouth (with a mouth guard)
- On the head (with a helmet or straps)

Typing aids have much to recommend them. They are simple, reliable, easy to understand, and portable [11]. One drawback to typing aids is that they can be difficult for a user to put on and take off independently (particularly the head-mounted

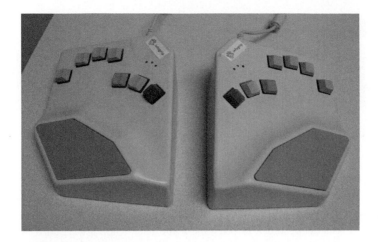

FIGURE 5.11 A chord keyboard.

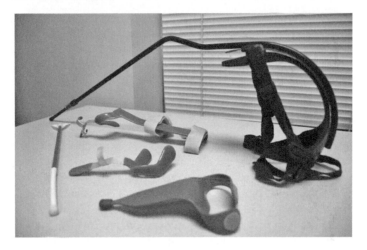

FIGURE 5.12 Typing aids.

versions). Another drawback is that typing aids do not work with input devices that require skin contact, like the screens on smart phones and the trackpads on most laptops. Mouthsticks can also lead to temporomandibular joint dysfunction or tooth migration in long-term users, so custom bite molds are often recommended.

Typing aids are particularly useful as emergency backup options for those occasions when a client's primary access methods crash, break, or are otherwise unavailable. For example, a mouthstick can be left in a cup or mouthstick dock next to the keyboard for emergencies.

5.5.2 KEYGUARDS

Keyguards are thick plastic sheets that are positioned on top of a keyboard, with holes in the sheet providing access to the keys beneath [1] (Figure 5.13). A keyguard

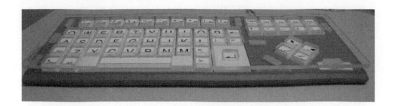

FIGURE 5.13   Keyguard.

allows a user to place his or her hands on the keyboard without activating any keys. It also isolates the keys to help people with tremors or without good hand control to hit individual keys without activating adjacent ones by mistake. As with typing aids, the greatest virtue of a keyguard is its simplicity. Keyguards are easy to understand, no software is needed, and it is obvious to the user when a keyguard is in use [1]. Keyguards are also an effective method of preventing access to certain keyboard keys.

However, many users who try keyguards do not like them [12]. Keyguards can slow typing and can make it difficult to see the labels on the keys [12]. A keyguard must be made for the keyboard on which it is used in order for the holes to align properly with the keys, so it can be difficult to transfer keyguards between computers [1, 12]. Keyguards can also be problematic for clients with large fingers [1].

5.5.3   KEYBOARD LAYOUT

On a computer, the operating system defines the connection between the keys on the keyboard and the characters that result from pressing those keys. This makes it fairly easy to redefine what each key does [1]. Alternative layouts have been designed for typists who use one finger, one hand, or both hands. It is estimated to take 90 to 100 hours to learn a new keyboard layout, but this hasn't been tested [1]. If you need to change layouts a lot (for example, in the clinic or a computer lab), consider getting "keyboard skins" and pasting the labels on those [1].

5.5.4   STICKY KEYS

Sticky Keys is an accessibility feature within computer operating systems that is designed to help people who find it difficult to hold down one key while pressing another [1, 13]. Sticky Keys causes modifier keys (e.g., Shift, Alt, Control, Windows key) to latch until the next alphanumeric key has been pressed [1, 14]. For example, with Sticky Keys, a user presses the Shift key and then the *a* key to produce a capital *A*.

Note that Sticky Keys does not work with the fn key on many laptops. That's because the operating system never sees the fn key. Instead, the laptop hardware uses the fn key to change the meaning of some of the keyboard keys. This is typically only a problem if a client wants to use Mouse Keys with a laptop, and the laptop requires the fn key to be held down in order to access the number pad.

Noteworthy settings within Sticky Keys for Windows 7 include (Figures 5.14 and 5.15)

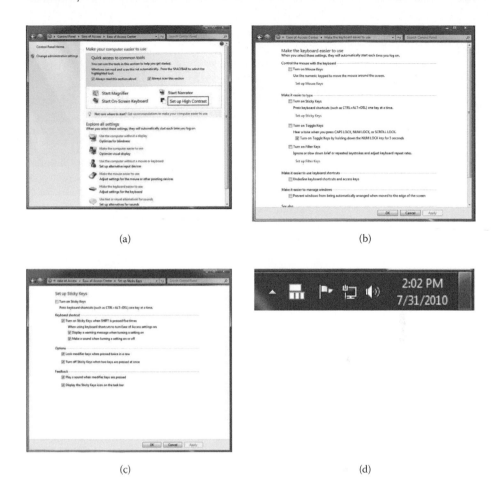

FIGURE 5.14 Sticky Keys in Windows 7.

- Turn Sticky Keys off if two keys are pressed at once. This is important when a client shares a computer with more than one person (when you may want to activate this feature). Other users of the computer can find the Sticky Keys feature annoying. If they use the keyboard in the standard way Sticky Keys will automatically turn off. This can, however, be a problem for the user who does need Sticky Keys when a helper uses the keyboard and this setting turns Sticky Keys off [15]. On the other hand, if a client occasionally uses more than one digit to type, then it might be important to turn this feature off.
- Press modifier key twice to lock. Pressing a modifier key twice will lock down that modifier key until it is pressed for a third time. This can make typing things like "BBC" a bit easier [15]. Note, however, that this feature can sometimes be problematic, as it can generate accidental situations where a modifier key is latched down unintentionally.
- This setting activates audible and visible indications of sticky keys status [15].

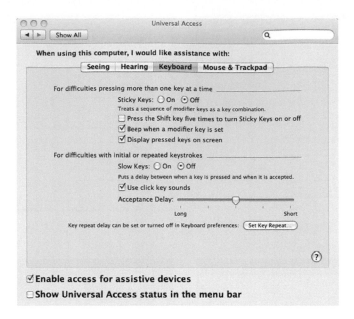

FIGURE 5.15   Sticky keys in Mac OS X.

5.5.5 FILTER KEYS

The Filter Keys feature combines what used to be three separate operating system features (Figures 5.16 and 5.17):

- Bounce Keys: Designed for users who unintentionally press the same key repeatedly.
- Repeat Keys: Designed for users who unintentionally hold down keys for an extended period of time.
- Slow Keys: Designed for users who frequently press the wrong key unintentionally.

5.5.5.1   Bounce Keys

Bounce Keys is often used for clients with intention or essential tremors. When a keystroke is accepted, the key that was pressed is "deactivated" for a specified time. Additional keystrokes on the same key during this time are ignored, but keystrokes on different keys are accepted [1, 14, 16]. This means that two different keys can be pressed in sequence without any delay, but a delay is required between *two presses of the same key* (Figure 5.18).

5.5.5.2   Repeat Keys

Repeat Keys allows users to adjust the time a key must be held down before it will start to repeat. This allows those who find it difficult to release a key quickly after pressing it to avoid errors caused by unwanted repeats [13]. Key repeating can be

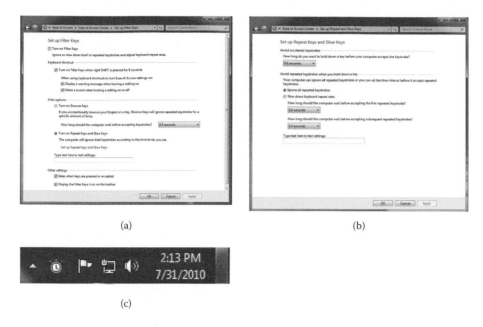

FIGURE 5.16   Filter Keys in Windows 7.

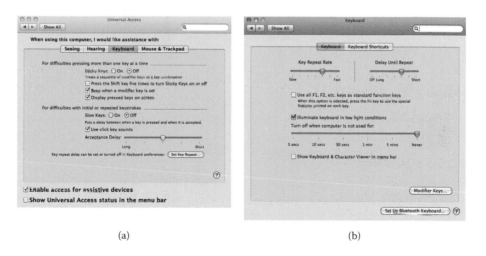

FIGURE 5.17   Filter Keys in Mac OS X.

turned off entirely, or the timing can be slowed. There are two repeat key settings [16] (Figure 5.19):

- Repeat delay. The time for which a key must be pressed before the repeat starts.
- Repeat rate. The time between successive key repeats once repeating has started.

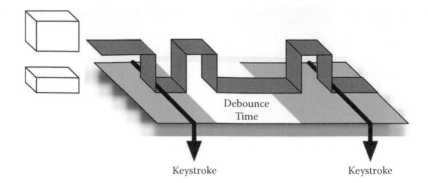

FIGURE 5.18   Bounce Keys.

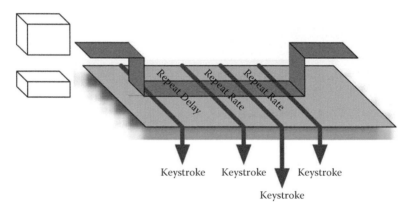

FIGURE 5.19   Repeat Keys.

Keep in mind that changing the repeat settings will also affect the arrow keys and delete keys.

5.5.5.3   Slow Keys

Slow Keys increases the time a key must be held down before the system recognizes a key press [14]. Slow Keys is typically used to ignore brief key presses from poor targeting or dragging the fingers or hand across the keyboard [12, 16]. Slow Keys determines the time for the first keystroke to be recognized. Repeat Keys determines the time for all subsequent keystrokes to be recognized if the key is held down.

When using Slow Keys, the setting for "Beep when keys pressed or accepted" becomes very important. When Slow Keys is active, the feedback from the keyboard can be misleading. The click from the keys and the kinesthetic feedback from movement no longer correspond to a keystroke being accepted. Unfortunately, the beep isn't very loud and there's no way to get feedback just for acceptance, rather than both key press and acceptance (Figure 5.20).

Unlike Bounce Keys and Repeat Keys, Slow Keys sets an upper bound on text entry rate. The user cannot enter text any faster than allowed by Slow Keys. For example, if the Slow Keys threshold is set to 0.5 second, the maximum possible text entry rate is

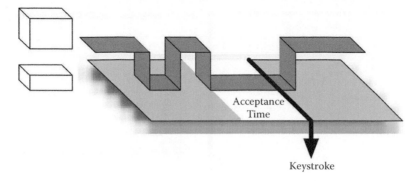

FIGURE 5.20   Slow Keys.

$$\frac{1 \text{ char}}{.5 \text{ sec}} \times \frac{60 \text{ sec}}{1 \text{ min}} \times \frac{1 \text{ word}}{5 \text{ char}} = 24 \text{ wpm}$$

5.5.6   USING THE WINDOWS REGISTRY

The Filter Keys settings place an upper bound on how fast someone can enter text, so it is important to set the value as accurately as possible. Sometimes, the values that Windows 7 makes available in the control panel don't match up well with a client's needs. It is possible to specify a custom value in the registry using the "regedit" program.

Windows stores all of its configuration information in the registry. The control panels are just applications that modify the registry. Keep in mind that if you do modify the registry directly using regedit you will need to reboot before your changes take effect. Also keep in mind that editing the registry can be dangerous if you do not know what you are doing (Figure 5.21).

5.6   ON-SCREEN KEYBOARDS

On-screen (or virtual) keyboards are software-based keyboards presented directly on the computer screen (Figure 5.22). On-screen keyboards are familiar to anyone who has entered text into a cell phone not equipped with a physical keypad. On-screen keyboards on computers can be operated by a pointing device or switch and allow the client to use a single device for computer control. A nice feature of on-screen keyboards is their ability to be highly context sensitive, including changing their display to reflect changing modes (e.g., when Shift or Caps Lock is pressed).

On-screen keyboards can take up a lot of space on the screen, blocking access to other programs [1]. One solution is to use two monitors, one for the on-screen keyboard and the other for all other software. On-screen keyboards can also be confusing for clients, because they don't follow normal user interface conventions [1]. Normally, the window that is frontmost on the screen is the window that has input focus and will receive the user's input. On-screen keyboards are always frontmost, however, but redirect their input to another window. On-screen keyboards also use their own internal settings, and don't follow the settings in the Accessibility control panel.

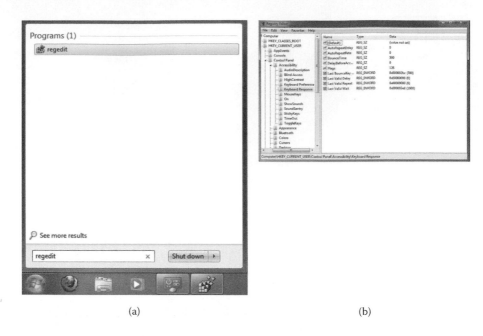

(a)   (b)

FIGURE 5.21   Using the Registry Editor program in Windows 7 to set Filter Keys values.

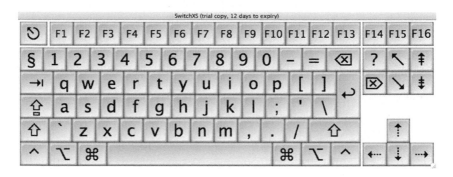

FIGURE 5.22   On-screen keyboard.

5.6.1 Static or Dynamic Layout

Because on-screen keyboards are software based, they can be remarkably flexible. Most on-screen keyboards allow the user to choose between multiple keyboard layouts. Often, a key on one layout will branch to a different layout. For example, a layout with letters and punctuation will branch to a layout with numbers and function keys. Some products will automatically switch between different keyboard layouts depending on which application is active. If a client can benefit from multiple task-specific keyboards, it's important to consider how easy it is to switch between keyboards. Another important thing to consider is whether your client has the cognitive skills needed to manage multiple keyboards. Some clients may benefit from a single, static keyboard.

5.6.2 DESIGN TOOLS

Many on-screen keyboards allow the user to edit existing keyboard layouts or even create their own keyboards. However, few on-screen keyboards provide user-friendly tools for editing. If editing keyboards is important, choose an on-screen keyboard that includes a user-friendly editor. Most programs offer a free trial period that allows you to explore their features before purchasing.

5.6.3 DWELL SELECTION

An alternative to selecting keys by clicking on them is to select keys by positioning the cursor over a key (i.e., dwelling) for a specified period of time. Dwell selection is needed when the user can't generate mouse clicks or when clicking the mouse button causes the mouse cursor to move. Dwell clicking is slower and less reliable than clicking, and places an upper limit on text entry rate. If speed is important, and the client can perform any kind of click within a few hundred milliseconds, click interaction is likely to be more efficient than dwell activation [17].

On screen keyboards typically provide two configuration options for dwell selection:

- Dwell period: How long the cursor needs to hover over a key before the key is selected.
- Dwell tolerance: How much the cursor can move (measured in pixels) before it is no longer considered to be dwelling.

Configuring dwell selection requires a balance between high sensitivity (setting the dwell period too short or the dwell tolerance too large, which will make it easier to generate intended clicks but increase the likelihood of unintended clicks) and low sensitivity (setting the dwell period too long or dwell tolerance too low, which will reduce unintentional clicks but make it difficult to keep the cursor still enough for long enough to generate intended clicks).

5.6.4 AMBIGUOUS KEYBOARDS

One approach to reducing the number of keys on a keyboard, and the keyboard's resulting size, is to assign multiple characters to each key (Figure 5.23). These are referred to as *ambiguous keyboards*, because the actual character that is produced each time a key is pressed is determined as the user is typing. Since each key press can correspond to several letters, software must be used to map keystrokes to words (i.e., *disambiguate* the user's input) [18].

Ambiguous keyboards are most familiar in the context of telephones, where there are fewer keys than letters of the alphabet [18]. By exploiting the statistics of English, software can correctly disambiguate characters on a nine-key telephone keypad approximately 88% of the time [19]. Disambiguation can happen either *by letter* or *by word*. In by-letter disambiguation, the user must check each letter that is entered to determine if the correct letter was chosen [17, 18]. In by-word disambiguation, the system presents the user with all possible words that could be constructed based on the sequence of keystrokes that was entered, and the user selects the desired word [17, 18].

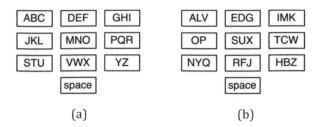

(a)   (b)

FIGURE 5.23   Ambiguous keyboard layouts: (a) alphabetic arrangement and (b) frequency-of-use arrangement. (Based on Lesher, G.W., B.J. Moulton, and D.J. Higginbotham, *IEEE Transactions on Rehabilitation Engineering*, 6(4), 415–423, 1998 [18].)

5.7   ONE-DIGIT TEXT ENTRY

5.7.1   INTRODUCTION

One-digit text entry refers to any text entry method in which

- Keys on a keyboard are directly selected (as opposed to selected through scanning)
- Only one key can be selected at a time (as opposed to simultaneously holding down a modifier key like Ctrl or Shift and pressing a letter key)
- Only one "thing" is used to select keys (as opposed to hunt-and-peck typing with multiple fingers)

Examples of one-digit text entry methods include

- One-finger typing
- Operating an on-screen keyboard with a pointing device
- Eye gaze

The most important characteristic of one-digit text entry is *the inability to press multiple keys at the same time.*

5.7.2   ONE-DIGIT KEYBOARDS

One-digit keyboard layouts are an active area of research, because of the increased use of smart phones for instant messaging and email. Keyboards for one-digit typing take a much different approach than keyboards designed for two-handed (or even one-handed) typing. Two-handed keyboards split frequently used pairs of letters on opposite sides of the keyboard, to take advantage of multiple fingers moving in parallel. A one-digit keyboard, on the other hand, positions commonly used letters close together to minimize travel between keys [20]. Similarly, the standard QWERTY keyboard is rectangular, to accommodate both hands. One-digit keyboards are often square or even somewhat circular, to limit the maximum possible distance between keys [20] (Figure 5.24).

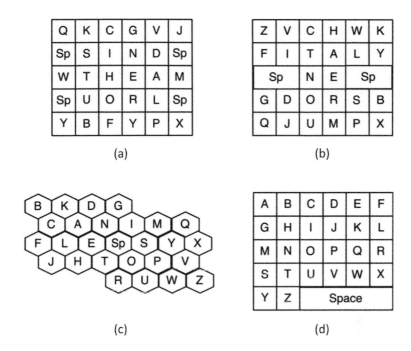

FIGURE 5.24   One-digit keyboard layouts: (a) OPTI II, (b) FITALY, (c) ATOMIK, and (d) alphabetic. (Based on Zhai, S., M. Hunter, and B.A. Smith, *Human–Computer Interaction,* 17(2/3), 229–269, 2002 [20].)

[	]	3	2	1	V	U	P	6	7	8	9
;	4	Q	M	I	T	S	C	K	Z	Back	
5	J	G	N	R	E	H	B	Y	X	0	↵
/	'	F	O	A	D	L	W	,	.	↑	
Shift	Ctrl	Alt	Space			Shift		←	↓	→	

FIGURE 5.25   Chubon keyboard layout. (Based on Anson, D.K. et al., *Assistive Technology,* 31(1), 40–45, 2001 [21].)

Numbers and punctuation present another design decision for one-digit keyboards. Many one-digit keyboards separate out numbers and punctuation to another mode or page. This approach simplifies the layout of the keyboard for novices but can have performance implications because some punctuation keys (e.g., the period) are actually used more often than some letter keys [20]. Integrating punctuation or number keys may increase efficiency, but will increase the complexity of the keyboard [20].

The Chubon layout (Figure 5.25) was designed specifically for one-digit typing. The Chubon layout positions the most frequently used letters in the center of the keyboard. The Chubon keyboard is nice in that it's designed for standard keyboards. On the other hand, sticking with the standard keyboard hardware limits the layout's flexibility in terms of the shape, size, and arrangement of the keys [1].

The Chubon layout reduces total digit travel for average text [1, 21] but does not necessarily improve performance over the standard QWERTY keyboard layout. In 2001, Anson and colleagues compared the Chubon keyboard with the standard QWERTY keyboard [21] in a study involving nine able-bodied subjects. The Chubon layout did not increase subjects' text entry rate or decrease errors [21].

5.7.3 Modeling User Performance during One-Digit Text Entry

One-digit typing has two parts: finding the key and activating the key. Finding the key is a visual search task. Activating the key is a targeting task that is modeled by Fitts' law.

5.7.3.1 Modeling Visual Search

Models of visual search within structured but unfamiliar environments assume people search left to right and top to bottom [5]. In these models, visual search time is directly proportional to target position:

$$T_s = a \times n$$

where a is the amount of time to review a single item and n is the position of the item.

The obvious shortcoming of this model is that it does not accommodate learning [17, 22]. As a person becomes familiar with the keyboard, visual search time will decrease. At the extreme, touch typists don't engage in any visual search. This is unlikely to be the case for most one-digit typists, however, because they use visual, rather than tactile or proprioceptive, cues to locate their target.

Sears et al. [23] studied visual search time for six keyboards that can be operated with a single digit. Two keyboards used familiar layouts (QWERTY and alphabetic) and two keyboards were ambiguous (i.e., assigned more than one symbol to each key). Not surprisingly, the familiar layouts resulted in lower visual search times than unfamiliar layouts and ambiguous keyboards had longer visual search times than keyboards that assigned one symbol to each key [23].

There are practical implications for clinicians in these results. For a given keyboard, it is possible to increase familiarity through practice, but the design choice of one symbol per key or multiple symbols per key is fixed. In addition, choosing an efficient, but unfamiliar, keyboard layout may result in slower performance initially, but performance is likely to improve as familiarity increases.

5.7.3.2 Modeling Key Activation

Moving a mouse cursor or finger from one key to another is typically modeled as a pointing task using Fitts' law (see Section 4.3.1 and Figure 5.26) [20]. The general approach is

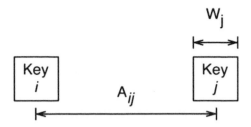

FIGURE 5.26 Fitts' law applied to the movement between two keys [20].

1. Use Fitts' law to calculate the average movement time between each pair of keys.
2. Multiply the average movement time between each pair of keys by the frequency that the corresponding pair of letters is used in the English language.
3. Add it all up to get the average time to enter a letter.

$$MT = a + b \log_2 \left(\frac{A_{ij}}{W_j} + 1 \right)$$

For example, consider the standard telephone keypad:

1	2	3
4	5	6
7	8	9
*	0	#

Assume you know the frequency with which each pair of keys is pressed:

		\...then, this key is pressed.										
		1	2	3	4	5	6	7	8	9	*	0	#
First, this key is pressed...	1	0.06%	0.11%	0.09%	0.07%	0.08%	0.09%	0.07%	0.08%	0.09%	0.01%	0.05%	0.01%
	2	0.08%	0.10%	0.09%	0.07%	0.09%	0.06%	0.11%	0.08%	0.10%	0.01%	0.05%	0.01%
	3	0.09%	0.07%	0.08%	0.09%	0.07%	0.09%	0.06%	0.11%	0.09%	0.01%	0.05%	0.01%
	4	0.09%	0.07%	0.09%	0.07%	0.08%	0.09%	0.07%	0.08%	0.09%	0.01%	0.05%	0.01%
	5	0.06%	0.11%	0.07%	0.09%	0.08%	0.10%	0.09%	0.06%	0.11%	0.01%	0.05%	0.01%
	6	0.07%	0.09%	0.09%	0.09%	0.06%	0.11%	0.07%	0.08%	0.09%	0.01%	0.05%	0.01%
	7	0.09%	0.07%	0.08%	0.07%	0.09%	0.08%	0.10%	0.07%	0.09%	0.01%	0.05%	0.01%
	8	0.07%	0.09%	0.09%	0.06%	0.11%	0.08%	0.10%	0.07%	0.08%	0.01%	0.05%	0.01%
	9	0.09%	0.06%	0.11%	0.09%	0.07%	0.08%	0.09%	0.07%	0.09%	0.01%	0.05%	0.01%
	*	0.001%	0.001%	0.001%	0.001%	0.001%	0.001%	0.001%	0.001%	0.001%	0.001%	0.001%	0.001%
	0	0.07%	0.08%	0.06%	0.11%	0.08%	0.10%	0.07%	0.09%	0.09%	0.01%	0.05%	0.01%
	#	0.001%	0.001%	0.001%	0.001%	0.001%	0.001%	0.001%	0.001%	0.001%	0.001%	0.001%	0.001%

The average time to move between the 3 key and the 7 key ($MT_{3,7}$) is predicted using Fitts' law. The frequency ($f_{3,7}$) with which this movement occurs (i.e., the frequency with which a 7 follows a 3 in a phone number) is 0.06% (shown in bold in the table above). The weighted average movement time is then:

$$0.0006 * MT_{3,7}$$

The overall average key press time can be calculated as

$$\overline{MT} = \sum_i \sum_j f_{i,j} \times MT_{i,j}$$

5.7.3.3   Predicting Text Entry Rate

The resulting model for text entry consists of two steps, repeated for each character of the text to be entered:

1. Find the key corresponding to the next character to be entered (a visual search).
2. Press the next key (a movement).

This leads to the following mathematical model:

$$TER = \frac{60}{T_s + \overline{MT}}$$

5.8   ONE-HANDED TEXT ENTRY

It is possible to touch-type with a single hand. Touch typing is defined by the automaticity of the user's movements:

- Eliminating visual search
- Minimizing hand movement
- Overlapping finger movements

If you're not doing this, then you're really just single-digit typing with more than one digit. Wiklund, Dumas, and Hoffman [24] found an average speed for one-handed hunt-and-peck typing on a standard keyboard of approximately 23 words per minute (wpm) [25].

Situations in which one-handed patterns might be considered include [1]

- A client with severely limited function in one hand but normal strength and movement in the other
- A client who needs to use one hand for something other than typing

Nobody has studied whether using a one-handed keyboard increases the risk of musculoskeletal disorder (MSD).

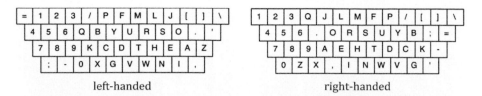

left-handed   right-handed

FIGURE 5.27 One-handed Dvorak keyboard layouts.

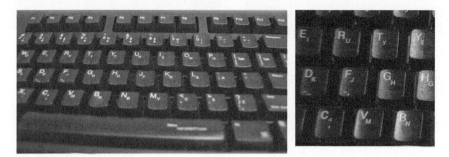

FIGURE 5.28 Half-QWERTY keyboard.

5.8.1 Using a Standard Keyboard

It is possible to touch-type with one hand on a regular keyboard with no overlays or assistive devices. However, typing with one hand on a standard keyboard can be slow, and it is hard to stretch to reach all of the keys without losing the "home" position [10]. Single-handed users may benefit from using smaller keyboards that present keys in a more compact area, and therefore require less movement and stretching [6, 10].

The one-handed Dvorak layouts (Figure 5.27) place the alphabetic keys to one side of the keyboard, with the numbers positioned to the side rather than being a single line above the letters. The highest-frequency letters are positioned under the index finger and lower-frequency letters are placed away from the home row and are typed with fingers that have less strength and mobility. Right- and left-handed versions are available [1, 26].

5.8.2 One-Handed Keyboards

Several alternative designs for one-handed keyboards are available. The half-QWERTY (Figure 5.28) uses the same kinds of keys that are found on a regular keyboard, but each key can generate either of two characters depending on whether or not a mode key is depressed [25]. In one study, able-bodied subjects achieved an average speed of 34.7 wpm after 10 training sessions [25]. Maltron sells single-handed keyboards for both the right and left hand (Figure 5.29).

One-handed chord keyboards are also available [9]. Gopher and Raij [27] tested subjects' rates of skill acquisition on both one-handed and two-handed chord keyboards, as well as standard QWERTY. None of their subjects had any previous experience in typing. After 10 hours, their one-handed group was typing at approximately 21 wpm [25, 27].

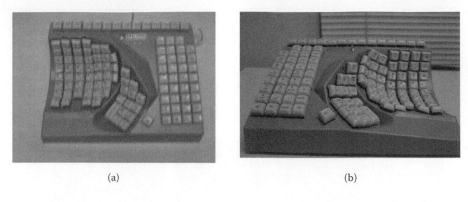

     (a)   (b)

FIGURE 5.29 One-handed keyboard (a) for left hand and (b) for right hand.

5.9 TWO-HANDED TEXT ENTRY

Numerous designers have attempted to improve upon the QWERTY keyboard layout. The design criteria for an optimal keyboard layout for two-handed use include

- Most frequently used letters on the home row
- Frequency of use of both hands balanced
- Most frequently used letters accessed by stronger/more dexterous fingers
- Alternate use of both hands maximized
- Consecutive use of a single finger minimized
- Movement of fingers from home row minimized
- Frequently used letter combinations arranged to maximize alternate use of hands

The most popular alternative to the QWERTY layout is the Dvorak layout (Figure 5.30). Dvorak patented his "typewriter keyboard" in 1936 (U.S. patent 2040248). The Dvorak simplified keyboard positions the most frequently used letters on the home row, with the most frequently used letters under the strongest fingers and low-frequency letters farther from the resting position of the hands [1]. To increase alternation between the hands, the five vowels are on the left side of the home row, and the five most common consonants are on the right [28].

The Dvorak keyboard can type about 400 of the most common English words using only the keys on the home (middle) row of letter keys [28]. For the QWERTY keyboard the comparable number is about 100 [28]. However, there is no definitive proof that the Dvorak keyboard increases typing speed or reduces the risk of MSD [1].

5.10 ASSESSMENT ISSUES

5.10.1 Choosing between Keyboards

When deciding on a keyboard for a client, there are several potential goals:

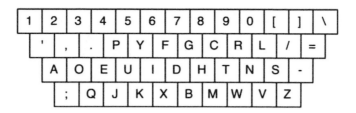

FIGURE 5.30 Dvorak keyboard layout.

- Maximizing text entry rate
- Minimizing errors
- Avoiding pain
- Prolonging activity

The specific goals and their relative priority depend on the client.

Keep in mind that the niftiest technology may not be the best solution. Often, the best way to increase text entry rates in realistic scenarios is to strive for simplicity and clarity in the user interface, rather than opting for including every possible time-saving feature in the system [17]. A standard keyboard may still be the most efficient input mechanism for your client, when the time and effort required to switch to a new input device are taken into account [12].

In addition, many clients have good reasons to *want* to use a standard keyboard [12, 21]. Most clients will already be familiar with a standard keyboard, and using a standard keyboard means they don't need to transfer equipment between computers. Some clients (especially adolescents) want to avoid the stigma associated with being different or using technology for people with disabilities. Further, some clients may not accept their need to use an alternative input method.

Finally, some clients may simply lack the motivation or ability to learn how to use a new input device. Most clients, when presented with a novel input device, are going to enter text slowly and less accurately [21]. It can be difficult to convince clients to invest time now for uncertain future gains in productivity. Clinicians must also keep in mind the fact that, especially after a neurological injury, some clients will display limitations in new learning. In these cases, the advantages of relying on old learning (the standard keyboard) may outweigh the potential benefits of a new input method [21].

Factor	On the One Hand	On the Other Hand
Size	Increasing the size lets you add more buttons or make the existing buttons bigger. Bigger buttons are easier to hit and can be operated with larger activation sites.	Increasing the size of the keyboard increases the range of motion needed to strike all the keys.
Membrane or individual keys	Membrane keyboards can be waterproof. Membrane keyboards are also easier to switch visual displays for key definitions in and out.	Using a membrane keyboard means you don't get kinesthetic or auditory feedback *from the keyboard* (although auditory feedback could be provided by the PC).

Factor	On the One Hand	On the Other Hand
Transferability	A keyboard with high transferability makes it easier for the user to switch between different computers and activities without getting confused.	High transferability constrains the options available to the keyboard designer.
Multiple operating modes	Assigning multiple meanings to keys lets you have fewer keys, so the keys can be bigger or the keyboard can be smaller.	It can be difficult to know which mode the keyboard is in, which can lead to errors and frustration.
Functional transparency	The more transparent the system is, the easier it is to just pick up and use. The more it looks like a keyboard, the easier it is to pick up and use.	Increasing functional transparency usually means getting rid of features that aren't immediately intuitive. Sometimes a little effort in learning an opaque interface can produce much better results.

TABLE 5.1

Types of Errors That Result in Substitutions, Omissions, and Insertions

	Error	Target Text	Resulting Text
Substitution	Additional key press error	And	Abd
	Dropping error	And	and
	Transposition error	And	Adn
Omission	Missing key error	And	Ad
Insertion	Overlap error	And	Abnd
	Long key press error	And	Annnd
	Bounce errors	And	Annnd
	Remote errors	And	Afnd

5.10.2 Configuring a Keyboard

Most keyboard configuration options are designed to reduce errors. The specific configuration change for each client depends on the types of errors the client is most likely to make. Errors can be divided into three categories (Table 5.1):

- Substitutions: Aiming for one key but activating another.
- Omissions: Failing to activate the desired key.
- Insertions: Activating keys in addition to the desired key.

A substitution can result from several distinct causes. An *additional key press error* results when a key near the target key is pressed by mistake [12, 13]. Potential interventions for clients who make large numbers of additional key press errors are

- Make the key easier to hit by increasing key size
- Make the key easier to distinguish from surrounding keys by increasing key contrast
- Make the wrong key harder to activate by decreasing key sensitivity using Slow Keys.
- Increase the dead space in between keys by decreasing key resolution using a keyguard or by increasing the space between keys.

A *dropping error* is caused by the failure to press down more than one key at once [12, 13], either when a user fails to maintain pressure on a modifier key (e.g., Shift, Alt, Ctrl) or when the modifier key is never pressed in the first place. In one study, individuals with motor disabilities reported that simultaneously pressing multiple keys was the most difficult keyboard operation [12, 13]. Fifty percent of participants with motor disabilities in the study avoided simultaneous key presses. The principal intervention for dropping errors is Sticky Keys.

A *transposition error* results when two or more characters are typed in the wrong order [13]. This is a cognitive error in which the correct characters are targeted in the wrong order. Interventions for clients prone to transposition errors are spell checkers (which catch errors after they occur) and word prediction utilities (which eliminate the need to completely spell out words).

Omissions result from *missing key errors*, in which a movement intended to press a key did not produce a character, either because the key was not pressed with sufficient force or because the user missed the key entirely [12, 13]. Potential interventions for missing key errors are

- Make keys easier to hit by making the keys larger or increasing key resolution
- Make keys easier to reach by using a smaller keyboard
- Make keys easier to activate by decreasing key sensitivity by using a keyboard that requires less key press force
- Provide increased feedback when a key has been activated, through either the computer or the keyboard itself

An insertion can result from several distinct causes. In an *overlap error*, two adjacent keys are pressed at once due to poor accuracy on the part of the user [12]. There are several possible underlying causes, including poor movement control, intention tremor, or disrupted proprioceptive or visual feedback mechanisms [12]. Interventions for overlap errors include

- Increase the dead space in between keys by decreasing key resolution using a keyguard or by increasing the space between keys
- Make the wrong key harder to activate by decreasing key sensitivity using Slow Keys
- Make the key easier to distinguish from surrounding keys by increasing key contrast

Long key press errors are caused when a key is activated for longer than the key repeat delay [12, 13]. Long key presses are potentially the most significant source of performance errors for keyboard users with motor disabilities [13]. The intervention for long key press errors is to reduce key sensitivity by using Repeat Keys to either increase the repeat delay or eliminate key repeat altogether [14].

Bounce errors result when the user unintentionally presses the intended key more than once [12, 13]. The intervention for bounce errors is to reduce key sensitivity by using Bounce Keys.

Remote errors occur when a key is pressed with a digit or body part other than the one that was intended to touch the keyboard [12, 13]. Clients who tend to drag their hands across the keyboard are especially prone to this type of error. Interventions for remote errors include

- Make the wrong key harder to activate by decreasing key sensitivity using Slow Keys
- Increase the dead space in between keys by decreasing key resolution using a keyguard or by increasing the space between keys

5.10.3 EVALUATING PERFORMANCE

There are several reasons to have a client complete a typing test:

- Identifying what problems the client has
- Comparing the efficacy of different potential interventions
- Documenting the need for an intervention
- Evaluating the effect of an intervention over time

In all cases, it's important to actually observe the client entering text. People are good at developing compensation mechanisms for their disability, so problems may not be apparent from a transcript of their typing. This is one reason why clinicians won't be replaced by automated tools any time soon.

5.11 UNCONSTRAINED TEXT ENTRY TASKS

Most typing tests focus on text entry speed and ignore accuracy. However, individuals with disabilities can devote a significant amount of time to error correction. In one study, participants with disabilities spent 7.3% of their time correcting keyboard errors as opposed to an average of 1.7% in the nondisabled group [13]. Identifying the sources of errors and the appropriate configuration choices to suppress errors could therefore provide significant increases in productivity for some users [13].

Measuring performance with text entry devices therefore needs to incorporate both speed and accuracy [29]. Measuring speed is straightforward, but measuring errors is not [29]. One approach is to count errors by hand [30, 31], which can make it difficult to compare results across studies that use different counting methods. Counting by hand can also be extremely time-consuming.

Another common approach is to reject incorrect keystrokes, forcing the transcribed text to match the presented text exactly [29, 32–35]. A frequent side effect of this approach is that users will often not notice their first incorrect keystroke and produce a string of subsequent incorrect keystrokes. Another issue with this approach is the difficulty it presents in dealing with techniques like word completion or abbreviation expansion where a single keystroke can produce multiple characters, only some of which may be incorrect. For example, if a user is expected to enter the word *fall*, a reasonable strategy might be to type the letter *f*, then select *falls* from the word completion list and then erase the trailing *s*. However, it's not clear in this case how to treat this input. The input could be treated as a single incorrect character (either the keystroke to select the wrong word from the word completion list or the *s* at the end of *falls*) or four incorrect characters (*alls*). It's also not clear how to distinguish this case from the case where a user selects the wrong word from the word completion list by mistake. Finally, rejecting incorrect keystrokes also eliminates the ability to examine:

- What strategies the user adopts to identify and correct errors
- The relative cost of error correction for different text entry methods
- Whether certain target characters are more likely to lead to errors than other characters

A different approach is to limit the text entry task to transcribing single characters, rather than whole words or sentences. This approach also fails to accommodate techniques like word prediction. Other approaches include measuring errors at the word level, discarding trials with errors, or ignoring errors altogether.

As an alternative, investigators within the field of human factors have recently begun employing unconstrained text entry protocols [29, 32–35] in which the user is allowed to make errors and decide whether or not to correct the errors that occur. The primary advantage of this approach is that it allows users to enter text under more natural, realistic conditions [29, 32–35]. This approach also allows investigators to analyze the entire input stream, including errors and error corrections [35], thus providing a more detailed picture of text entry.

5.11.1 EVALUATING ACCURACY

Each trial within an unconstrained text entry protocol involves the following strings [29, 32–34, 36]:

- The presented text (P) is the string of characters the participant was asked to reproduce.
- The input stream (IS) consists of all of the keys that were pressed by the participant in the order that the keystrokes occurred.
- The transcribed text (T) consists of the text that the participant entered and did not subsequently delete.

The difference between what the client was asked to enter (P) and what was actually entered (T) can be calculated using the Levenshtein string distance (LSD)—also called the minimum string distance (MSD)—which calculates the minimum distance between two strings defined in terms of three editing primitives: insertion, omission, and substitution [29] (Figure 5.31).

P = For	P = For	P = For
T = Fox	T = Forx	T = Fo
(a)	(b)	(c)

FIGURE 5.31   Editing primitives: (a) substitutions, (b) insertions, and (c) omissions.

For any two strings P and T, more than one minimum set of transformations (i.e., combinations of insertions, omissions, and substitutions) may exist for the computed MSD. Each transformation is called an alignment and represents a possible explanation of the transcription errors made [32]. The set of alignments with the fewest transformations is referred to as the set of optimal alignments. For example, given [32]:

- P: quickly
- T: qucehkly

there are four optimal alignments, each involving three transformations (MSD = 3):

P: quic— kly	P: quic-kly	P: qui-ckly	P: qu-ickly
T: qu-cehkly	T: qucehkly	T: qucehkly	T: qucehkly

In each alignment, a dash in the top string represents an insertion and a dash in the bottom string represents an omission. Where letters differ in the top and bottom, a substitution occurred [32].

5.11.2   Evaluating Performance at the Trial Level by Comparing P and T

5.11.2.1   Transcription Error Rate (E_{TR})

Using the MSD statistic, transcription error rate (E_{TR}), given a presented text string (P) and a transcribed text string (T), is [32]

$$E_{TR} = \frac{MSD(P,T)}{\overline{S}_A} \times 100\%$$

where $\overline{S}_A$ is the mean number of characters in the optimal alignments.

5.11.2.2   Keystrokes per Character (KSPC)

Keystrokes per character (KSPC) is a measure of the effort required to generate text with a given text entry method:

$$KSPC = \frac{|IS|}{|T|}$$

KSPC will be higher for less skilled users and for text entry methods that require more keystrokes to enter text or correct errors [29]. For example, Morse code will have a higher KSPC than a standard QWERTY keyboard for most users, because multiple switch presses are required for all but two of the letters of the alphabet.

There is a problem with KSPC, however. KSPC reflects the *combined* cost of committing errors and fixing them. A large KSPC value could mean that many errors were committed but correction was easy (took few keystrokes), or it could mean that few errors were committed but correcting them was arduous (requiring many keystrokes) [33].

5.11.2.3 Transcription Rate (R_T)

The transcription rate (R_T), measured in characters per second, is calculated from the appearance of the presented text, P, to the time the participant ends the trial [36]:

$$TER = \frac{|T|}{t}$$

where $|T|$ is the length of (i.e., number of characters in) the transcribed text and t is the transcription time. R_T focuses on the resulting text, T, ignoring text that was erased by the participant.

5.11.3 EVALUATING PERFORMANCE AT THE TRIAL LEVEL USING THE INPUT STREAM

5.11.3.1 Decomposing the Input Stream

IS can be decomposed into [29, 32–34]:

- Correct characters (C). The correct key pressed at the correct time.
- Incorrect and not fixed characters (INF). Any errors that are not rectified by the client—extra characters (insertions) in T, incorrect characters (substitutions) in T, and omitted characters (deletions) *not* in T.
- Fixed characters (F). Characters that are removed from T in the process of correcting errors. This includes both characters that were typed in error and *characters that were correct but removed anyway.*
- Edits (E). Keystrokes used to remove characters or reposition the cursor (e.g., backspace, delete, arrow keys) as well as modifier keys (Shift, Alt, and Control) when used in conjunction with these editing functions.

Identifying the keystrokes that are in E is trivial. It can be a lot harder to tease out which characters in T belong in C and which belong in INF. However, the number of characters in C and INF ($|C|$ and $|INF|$, respectively) can be calculated using the MSD function [33]:

$$|INF| = MSD(P, T)$$

$$|C| = max(|P|, |T|) - MSD(P, T).$$

F can be further decomposed into [34]:

- Fixed keystrokes that were correct (F_c) but removed in the process of fixing errors
- Fixed keystrokes that were in error (F_e) and were removed

5.11.3.2   Total Error Rate (E_{TO})

Examining the components of the input stream allows us to include fixed errors in the total error rate (E_{TO}) [33]:

$$E_{TO} = \frac{|INF| + |F|}{|C| + |INF| + |F|} \times 100\%$$

E_{TO} can be divided into the not corrected error rate (E_{NC}) [33]:

$$E_{NC} = \frac{|INF|}{|C| + |INF| + |F|}$$

and the corrected error rate (E_C) [33]:

$$E_C = \frac{|F|}{|C| + |INF| + |F|}$$

Looking at the components of F, the corrected but right error rate (E_{CBR}) [34] is

$$E_{CBR} = \frac{|F_c|}{|C| + |INF| + |F|} \times 100\%$$

and the corrected and wrong error rate (E_{CAW}) [34] is

$$E_{CAW} = \frac{|F_e|}{|C| + |INF| + |F|} \times 100\%$$

E_{TR} can also be written in terms of the components of IS as [33]

$$E_{TR} = \frac{|INF|}{|C| + |INF|} \times 100\%$$

E_{TO} is valuable for obvious reasons, but E_C and E_{NC} also have clinical utility. In particular, if E_{TO} is similar across conditions, then a large difference in E_C or E_{NC} across conditions is likely to be of interest to the clinician. The change may be due to different strategies employed by the client (i.e., increased/decreased vigilance toward identifying typos), or there may be a difference between conditions in the difficulty associated with correcting errors.

5.11.3.3   Keystrokes per Character (KSPC)

Keystrokes per Character (*KSPC*) can also be calculated based on the components of *IS* [33]:

$$KSPC = \frac{|C| + |INF| + |F| + |E|}{|C + INF|}$$

5.11.3.4   Bandwidth

If text entry is viewed as information transfer, then *C* represents the amount of useful information transferred, and *INF*, *IF*, and *F* represent wasted bandwidth [33].

Utilized bandwidth (B_U):

$$B_U = \frac{C}{C + INF + F + E}$$

Wasted bandwidth (B_W):

$$B_W = \frac{INF + F + E}{C + INF + F + E}$$

B_U and B_W provide measures of text entry efficiency that are independent of time. These measures are useful for research purposes when comparing performance between participants with and without disabilities. By eliminating speed, differences in movement time between participants are removed [36].

These measures are also useful clinically when evaluating devices with steep learning curves, where speed is initially slow but is likely to increase with practice. In addition, B_U and B_W, in combination with E_C and E_{TO}, can provide insight into how efficiently a client can correct errors. If E_C and E_{TO} are similar between two conditions, but B_W increases, this indicates an increased number of keystrokes devoted to fixing errors [36].

5.11.3.5   Keystroke Rate (R_K)

Keystroke rate (R_K), measured in keystrokes per second, is the total number of keystrokes entered divided by the total amount of time for transcription in seconds [36]:

$$R_K = \frac{|IS|}{t}$$

where |*IS*| is the length of the input stream. R_K is thus distinguished from R_T in that it reflects all keystrokes generated by the user. R_K is particularly useful when a client's goal is to reduce the *number* of keystrokes (perhaps due to issues of pain or fatigue) [36].

5.11.3.6 Examples

Consider the following situation, where < represents the backspace key (from [33]):

- Presented text: the quick brown
- Input stream: th quix<ck brpown
- Transcribed text: th quick brpown

There are three errors:

1. An *e* is omitted.
2. There is an extra *x* that is corrected with a backspace.
3. There is an extra *p* that remains uncorrected.

We can then categorize the keystrokes within the input stream as follows:

- *C*: t, h, space, q, u, i, c, k, space, b, r, o, w, n
- *INF*: missing e after th, p
- *F*: x
- *E*: Backspace

It follows that

- $|C| = 14$
- $|INF| = 2$
- $|F| = 1$
- $|E| = 1$
- $MSD = 2/(14 + 2) \times 100\% = 12.5\%$
- $KSPC = (14 + 2 + 1 + 1)/(14 + 2) = 1.125$
- $E_{TO} = 3/(14 + 2 + 1) = 17.6\%$
- $E_{NC} = 2/(14 + 2 + 1) = 11.8\%$
- $E_C = 1/(14 + 2 + 1) = 5.9\%$

Now consider this situation (from [34]):

- Presented text: the quick brown
- Input stream: thw quick<<<<<<<e quick brown
- Transcribed text: the quick brown

We can then categorize the keystrokes within the input stream as follows:

- *C*: t, h, e, space, q, u, i, c, k, space, b, r, o, w, n
- *INF*: None
- *F*: w, space, q, u, i, c, k
- *E*: Backspace (seven times)

It follows that

- $|C| = 15$
- $|INF| = 0$
- $|F| = 7$
- $|E| = 7$
- $|F_c| = 6$
- $|F_e| = 1$
- $KSPC = (15 + 0 + 7 + 7)/(15 + 0) = 1.125$
- $E_{TO} = (7 + 0)/(15 + 0 + 7) = 31.8\%$
- $E_{NC} = 0/(15 + 0 + 7) = 0\%$
- $E_C = 7/(15 + 0 + 7) = 31.8\%$
- $E_{CBR} = 6/(15 + 0 + 7) = 27.3\%$
- $E_{CAW} = 1/(15 + 0 + 7) = 4.5\%$

5.11.4 EVALUATING PERFORMANCE AT THE CHARACTER LEVEL

5.11.4.1 Types of Errors

When comparing P and T, there are only three types of errors: insertions, omissions, and substitutions. These are the *uncorrected errors* that comprise *INF*. When analyzing *IS*, several more types of *corrected errors* (F_e) are possible, along with characters that were correct but deleted (F_c) during error correction [35].

In a *corrected substitution*, the user meant to press one key but pressed another and (some time later) corrected the error. This is what we typically think of as a typo. In a *corrected insertion*, an extra character was entered unintentionally and then removed. In a *corrected omission*, a character in P is initially skipped, but then replaced [35].

This leaves us with the following categories for characters within *IS*:

1. Correct letters that were not erased (C)
2. Uncorrected substitutions (INF_s)
3. Uncorrected insertions (INF_i)
4. Uncorrected omissions (INF_o)
5. Corrected letters that were erased (F_c)
6. Corrected substitutions (F_s)
7. Corrected insertions (F_i)
8. Corrected omissions (F_o)
9. Editing keystrokes for navigation and correction (E)

5.11.4.2 Errors of Commission: Insertions and Substitutions

Errors of commission include both insertions and substitutions. There are three measures of interest: uncorrected errors of commission, corrected errors of commission, and total errors of commission [35]. The uncorrected errors of commission rate (EC_U) answers the question: Of the characters remaining in T, what percent were erroneous? EC_U is calculated as [35]

$$ECU = 1 - \frac{|C|}{|T|}$$

The corrected errors of commission rate (EC_C) answers: Of the erased characters, what percent were erroneous? EC_C is calculated as [35]

$$EC_C = 1 - \frac{|F_c|}{|IS| - |T|}$$

where $|F_c|$ is the number of characters that were entered correctly and subsequently erased.

The total errors of commission rate (EC_T) answers: Of all entered characters, what percent were erroneous? EC_T is calculated as [35]

$$EC_T = 1 - \frac{EC_U + EC_C}{|IS|}$$

Note that EC_T does not capture omission errors. It focuses on the question: Given that a character was entered, what are the chances that character was correct?

5.11.4.3   Targeting Accuracy: Substitution Error Rates

Looking at the number of substitutions allows us to answer the following question: What is the probability of getting character c when trying for c [35]? Another way of looking at this, particularly for keyboards, is targeting accuracy. In other words, given that the user was aiming for the key corresponding to c, what was the probability of activating that key?

Three substitution rates can be calculated [35]. The uncorrected substitution rate (ES_U) answers the question: When trying for c, what is the probability that we produce an uncorrected substitution for c? ES_U is calculated as [35]

$$ES_U = \frac{|INF_s|}{|P|}$$

The corrected substitution rate (ES_C) answers the question: When trying for c, what is the probability that we produce a substitution for c that is subsequently corrected? ES_C is calculated as [35]

$$ES_C = \frac{|F_s|}{|P|}$$

The total substitution rate (ES_T) answers the question: When trying for c, what is the probability that we get something other than c? ES_T is calculated as [35]

$$ES_T = \frac{|INF_s| + |F_s|}{|P|}$$

5.11.4.4 Omission Error Rates

The omission rate reflects how likely the user is to fail to enter a character c when it is the target character [35]. The equations for omission rates are [35]

$$EO_U = \frac{|INF_o|}{|P|}$$

$$EO_C = \frac{|F_o|}{|P|}$$

$$EO_I = \frac{|INF_o| + |F_o|}{|P|}$$

5.11.4.5 Insertion Error Rates

The insertion rate reflects how likely the user is to enter a character unintentionally [35]:

$$EI_U = \frac{|INF_i|}{|IS|}$$

$$EI_C = \frac{|F_i|}{|IS|}$$

$$EI_T = \frac{|INF_i| + |F_i|}{|IS|}$$

5.12 SIGNAL DETECTION THEORY

Signal detection theory (SDT) is used to model tasks where an observer must classify items as either *signal* (i.e., what the observer is looking for) or *noise* (i.e., not what the observer is looking for). SDT applies to problems as varied as screening luggage at the airport, diagnosing cancer, and inspecting products on an assembly line. SDT describes these classification problems in terms of a cutoff or criterion value (X_C) that the observer establishes to decide how to classify an item based on the available evidence. If the evidence falls below the cutoff value, then the item is classified as noise. If the evidence exceeds the cutoff value, then the item is classified as signal. Exactly how the observer quantifies the evidence and sets the cutoff value depends on the task at hand. In computer access, we are most often concerned about numerical observations like pixels and time, making it easy to display the SDT problem graphically (Figure 5.32).

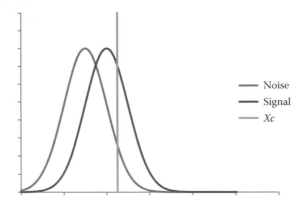

FIGURE 5.32   **(See color insert.)** Graphical depiction of signal detection theory problem.

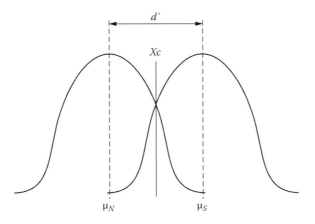

FIGURE 5.33   Sensitivity.

The distance between signal and noise is called *sensitivity* (d') and is measured in standard deviations from the mean values of signal and noise. As sensitivity increases, the difference in means grows and it becomes easier to distinguish between signal and noise. Conversely, as sensitivity decreases, signal and noise become more similar and the classification problem becomes harder (Figure 5.33).

Every time the observer classifies an item as signal or noise, there are four possible outcomes (Figure 5.34 and Table 5.2):

- Hit: The observer classifies the item as signal and it really is what the observer is looking for.
- Correct rejection: The observer classifies the item as noise and it really isn't what the observer is looking for.
- False alarm: The observer classifies the item as signal but it isn't really what the observer is looking for.
- Miss: The observer classifies the item as noise but it actually is what the observer is looking for.

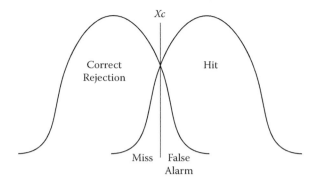

FIGURE 5.34 Possible outcomes of SDT classifications.

TABLE 5.2

Possible Outcomes of a Classification Decision

	Accept	Reject
Signal	Hit	Miss
Noise	False alarm	Correct reject

If the data for signal and noise are normally distributed (i.e., signal ~ N(μ_S,σ_S^2); Noise ~ N(μ_N,σ_N^2)) then we can calculate the probability of each outcome:

$$P(H) = P(x \geq X_C|S) = 1 - \Phi_S(X_C)$$

$$P(M) = P(x \leq X_C|S) = \Phi_S(X_C)$$

$$P(FA) = P(x \geq X_C|N) = 1 - \Phi_N(X_C)$$

$$P(CR) = P(x \leq X_C|N) = \Phi_N(X_C)$$

where Φ_S and Φ_N are the cumulative distribution functions for signal and noise, respectively. In Microsoft Excel, $\Phi_S(X_C)$ is calculated using the INVDIST function:

$$INVDIST(X_C,\mu_N,\sigma_N,TRUE)$$

When choosing X_C, the observer can be *conservative* and set the cutoff value very high (i.e., farther to the right). A conservative cutoff value would reject more noise items but would also lead to more misses (misclassifying signal items as noise). A *liberal* cutoff (i.e., farther to the left) would correctly classify more items as signal but would also produce more false alarms (Figure 5.35).

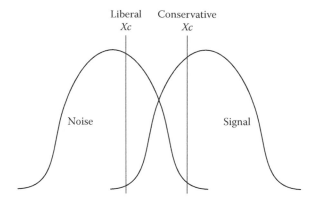

FIGURE 5.35   The cutoff value can be liberal or conservative.

We can depict the implications of different cutoff values on performance using the receiver operating characteristic (ROC) [5]. The ROC plots the likelihood of a hit (on the y axis) against the likelihood of a false alarm (on the x axis) for different values of X_C. The ROC thus provides a visual representation of the trade-off between a conservative cutoff value and a liberal cutoff value.

To construct the ROC, begin with X_C all the way to the left of the frequency distribution. As you move X_C to the right, calculate the probability of a hit (the area under the signal curve to the right of X_C) and a false alarm (the area under the noise curve to the right of X_C) and plot those values. The end result is the ROC.

To plot the ROC in Microsoft Excel, first recall that

$$P(H) = P(x \geq X_C | S) = 1 - \Phi_S(X_C) = 1 - INVDIST(X_C, \mu_S, \sigma_S, TRUE)$$

$$P(FA) = P(x \geq X_C | N) = 1 - \Phi_N(X_C) = 1 - INVDIST(X_C, \mu_N, \sigma_N, TRUE)$$

Create a table in Excel with three columns:

- The first column is potential values for X_C.
- The second column contains the equation for $P(H)$.
- The third column contains the equation for $P(FA)$.

Then create an XY scatter plot using the resulting columns (Figure 5.36).

Perfect performance on an SDT task would be 100% probability of a hit and 0% probability of a false alarm, which would position the ROC in the upper left corner of the graph. As signal and noise diverge, and the classification task becomes easier, the ROC moves toward the upper left corner. Classification performance is maximized when X_C is chosen at the point on the ROC that is closest to the upper left corner. The value of X_C that is actually adopted, however, may not be chosen to maximize classification performance.

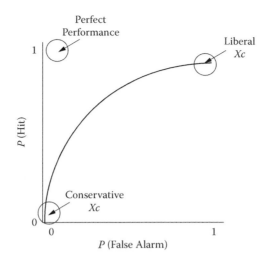

FIGURE 5.36   Receiver operating characteristic.

One consideration is the cost of making a mistake. If false alarms are a big deal, then X_C will be chosen to reduce false alarms. Similarly, if misses are a big deal, then X_C will be chosen to reduce misses. A second consideration is how often signal and noise occur. If noise is uncommon, then X_C may be slightly more liberal. If noise is very common, then X_C may be slightly more conservative (Figure 5.37).

SDT can be used to describe the problem of choosing several values for Filter Keys:

- Bounce Keys: Distinguishing between an intentional key press and an unintentional key press based on the time since the last press of the same key.
- Slow Keys: Distinguishing when a user has held down a key long enough to trigger a single keystroke.
- Repeat Keys: Distinguishing when a user has held down a key long enough after the initial keystroke to trigger repeated keystrokes.

In each case, intentional presses on the key are the signal, unintentional presses on the key are noise, and the task is to distinguish between the two. A time cutoff must be chosen that balances between *false alarms* (a key activates when it should not) and *misses* (a key fails to activate when it should). Decreasing the cutoff will reduce misses but may introduce additional false alarms. Increasing the cutoff will decrease misses but possibly increase false alarms.

For example, if a client has tremors that cause him to press the desired key several times, instead of just once, then increasing the Bounce Keys delay can eliminate unwanted keystrokes. At the same time, however, increasing the delay may also increase the number of instances where the client presses the key intentionally but fails to wait long enough, and no keystroke is produced (a miss). The trade-off is between speed (TER) and accuracy (errors), and the value you choose depends on the priority assigned to each.

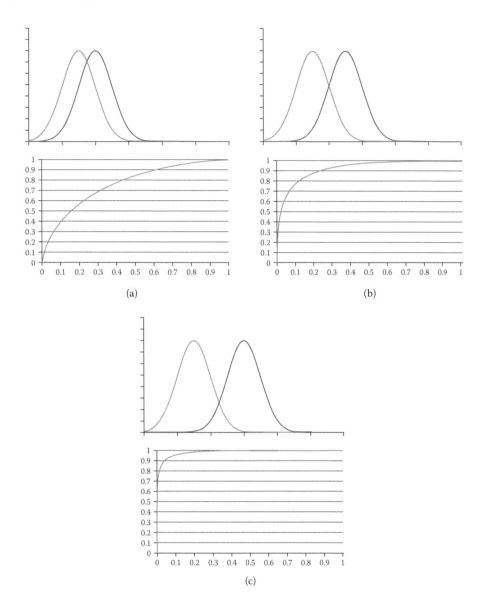

FIGURE 5.37   **(See color insert.)** When sensitivity is (a) low, performance on the SDT task is poor; performance on the SDT task improves as sensitivity (b) increases; when sensitivity is (c) high, performance improves.

There is also another thing to consider about the SDT problem for Filter Keys: by choosing X_C, we are also likely to influence the signal itself. Noise can't really be influenced because it represents unintentional keystrokes. Signal, on the other hand, is intentional. If we increase the time threshold, then the user is likely to change his or her behavior in response. This means we increase sensitivity (d') and the mean value of signal.

In order to actually apply SDT in the clinic, we start by measuring the following values:

- The probability of noise occurring ($P(N)$), the mean of the noise (μ_N), and the standard deviation of the noise (σ_N)
- The probability of signal occurring ($P(S)$), the mean of the signal (μ_S), and the standard deviation of the signal (σ_S)

Next, calculate β_{OPT}:

$$\beta_{OPT} = \frac{P(S)}{P(N)} \times \frac{I(S)}{I(N)}$$

where $I(S)/I(N)$ is the relative importance of correctly identifying signal and identifying noise. Often, these are of equal importance, so $I(S) = I(N)$.

Then, find the value X_C such that

$$\frac{P(X_C|N)}{P(X_C|S)} = \beta_{OPT}$$

Since both signal and noise are normally distributed:

- $P(X_C|N)$ can be interpreted as the probability that the observed keystroke duration was at least as large as X_C given that the keystroke was a typo—in other words, the probability that a typo will be misclassified as a correct keystroke (a false alarm).
- $P(X_C|S)$ can be interpreted as the probability that the observed keystroke duration was less than X_C given that it was a correct keystroke—in other words, the probability that a correct keystroke will be misclassified as a typo (a miss).

We can then rewrite the equation above as

$$\frac{P(X_C|N)}{P(X_C|S)} = \frac{1 - \varphi_N(X_C)}{\varphi_S(X_C)} = \beta_{OPT}$$

where $\varphi_N(X_C)$ is the cumulative distribution function for the noise signal and $\varphi_S(X_C)$ is the cumulative distribution function for the signal function. In Microsoft Excel, this means finding a value of X_C such that

$$\frac{1 - INVDIST(X_C, \mu_N, \sigma_N, TRUE)}{INVDIST(X_C, \mu_S, \sigma_S, TRUE)} = \beta_{OPT}$$

We can also examine how different values for X_C will affect text entry rate. Doing so, however, requires making a few assumptions:

1. We assume that the value for X_C does not change the visual search time required to find a key on the keyboard or the time required to move between keys on the keyboard. In other words, a slower X_C won't make a person take longer to find the next key or move to the next key.
2. We assume the user will correct each incorrectly accepted keystroke by immediately deleting it. This is common behavior for augmentative communication device users who are trying to create well-formed utterances and who may be using word completion, but may not be true for computer users, who might rely on spell checkers to fix errors after the fact.
3. We assume the user will immediately notice any correct keystrokes that are erroneously rejected because they failed to exceed the X_C threshold.

Let T_M be the average time (in seconds) to move between keys (which includes recalling what the next key is, finding the next key, and moving to the next key). T_M can be measured as the time between releasing one key and activating the next key.

We can use the probability of a correct keystroke, $P(S)$, to calculate the average number of correct keystrokes per minute (K_{cor}):

$$K_{cor} = P(S) \times \frac{60}{T_M + \mu_S}$$

Similarly, we can use the probability of a typo ($P(N)$) to calculate the average number of typos per minute (K_{typo}):

$$K_{typo} = P(N) \times \frac{60}{T_M + \mu_N}$$

The average total number of keystrokes per minute (K_{avg}) is then

$$K_{avg} = K_{cor} + K_{typo}$$

The number of correct keystrokes that will be erroneously filtered out (misses) for a given value of X_C will then be

$$K_{miss} = K_{cor} \times P(M) = K_{cor} \times \varphi_S(X_C)$$

and the number of correct keystrokes that will be correctly accepted (hits) for a given value of X_C will be

$$K_{hit} = K_{cor} \times P(H) = K_{cor} \times (1 - \varphi_S(X_C))$$

Similarly, the number of typos that will be erroneously accepted (false alarms) will be

$$K_{FA} = K_{typo} \times P(FA) = K_{typo} \times \left(1 - \varphi_N\left(X_C\right)\right)$$

and the number of typos that will be correctly filtered out (correct rejections) will be

$$K_{CR} = K_{typo} \times P(CR) = K_{typo} \times \varphi_N\left(X_C\right)$$

The average number of characters per minute that will be accepted (K_{acc}) is the sum of hits and false alarms:

$$K_{acc} = K_{hit} + K_{FA}$$

K_{acc} represents the average number of keystrokes that will be accepted in a minute. Recall from assumption 2 that any incorrectly accepted keystroke will be immediately deleted. This means that an incorrectly accepted keystroke takes up two total keystrokes without resulting in any net text entered. Similarly, an incorrectly rejected keystroke will need to be repeated, meaning an incorrectly rejected keystroke takes up two total keystrokes to generate one net character. Average net text entered per minute is thus

$$K_{net} = K_{acc} - 2 \times K_{FA} - K_{miss}$$

Thus, we want to choose a value for X_C that maximizes K_{net}.

5.12.1 EXAMPLES

EXAMPLE 5.1

You have a client complete a typing test and observe numerous incorrect keystrokes in which the client pressed the key next to the desired key. These typos could have been prevented if slow keys was used. What should be the acceptance delay for slow keys?

Here are the data from the client's typing test for the duration (i.e., how long the key was *held down*, not the time *between* keystrokes) of correct and incorrect keystrokes:

	Mean Keystroke Duration (ms)	Standard Deviation	Frequency
Typos	40.00	23.80	0.40
Correct keystrokes	131.56	49.60	0.60

Step 1. Based on these data, we can calculate the frequency distributions for the duration of typos and the duration of correct keystrokes.

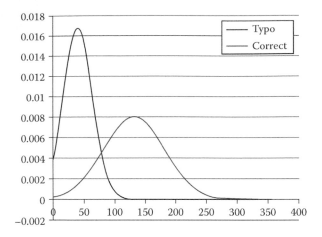

Step 2. Based on these data we can also calculate β_{OPT}:

$$\beta_{OPT} = \frac{P(S)}{P(N)} \times \frac{I(S)}{I(N)} = \frac{.6}{.4} = 1.5$$

Step 3. Now we need to find a value of X_C such that

$$\frac{P(X_C|N)}{P(X_C|S)} = \frac{1 - \varphi_N(X_C)}{\varphi_S(X_C)} = 1.5$$

Using Microsoft Excel, we find that if $X_C = 0.65$,

$$\frac{1 - INVDIST(65, 40, 23.80, TRUE)}{INVDIST(65, 131.56, 49.60, TRUE)} = 1.63$$

which is close enough to 1.5 for us.

Step 4 (optional). We can plot the ROC to examine the trade-off between different values for X_C.

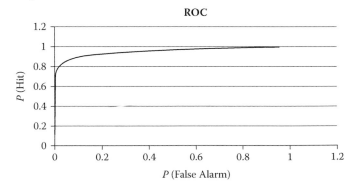

Step 5 (optional). We can also examine how different values for X_C will affect text entry rate. For this client, there was an average of 1.18 seconds between keystrokes.

First, calculate the average number of correct keystrokes, typos, and total keystrokes:

$$K_{cor} = P(S) \times \frac{60}{T_M + \mu_S} = .6 \times \frac{60}{1.18 + .131} = 27.46$$

$$K_{typo} = P(N) \times \frac{60}{T_M + \mu_N} = .4 \times \frac{60}{1.18 + .04} = 19.67$$

$$K_{avg} = 27.46 + 19.67 = 47.13$$

Then, for each value of X_C, calculate the expected number of hits, misses, false alarms, and correct rejections:

$$K_{miss} = K_{cor} \times P(M) = K_{cor} \times \varphi_S(X_C)$$

$$K_{hit} = K_{cor} \times P(H) = K_{cor} \times \left(1 - \varphi_S(X_C)\right)$$

$$K_{FA} = K_{typo} \times P(FA) = K_{typo} \times \left(1 - \varphi_N(X_C)\right)$$

$$K_{CR} = K_{typo} \times P(CR) = K_{typo} \times \varphi_N(X_C)$$

Next, calculate the average number of keystrokes that will be accepted each minute:

$$K_{acc} = K_{hit} + K_{FA}$$

Finally, calculate the net number of keystrokes per minute:

$$K_{net} = K_{acc} - 2 \times K_{FA} - K_{miss}$$

Here is a plot of K_{net} for different values of X_C.

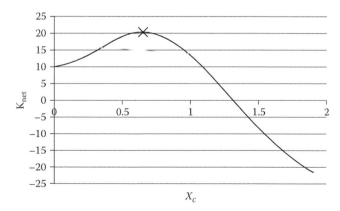

As you can see, K_{net} is maximized at $X_C = 0.65$.

EXAMPLE 5.2

Let's consider the same client, with one difference: the probability of a typo is much smaller:

	Mean Keystroke Duration (ms)	Standard Deviation	Frequency
Typos	40.00	23.80	0.10
Correct keystrokes	131.56	49.60	0.90

The only thing that has changed in the above table is the frequency of typos and correct keystrokes.

Step 1. Since there was no change in the mean or standard deviation of typos or correct keystrokes, the frequency distribution of the durations does not change.

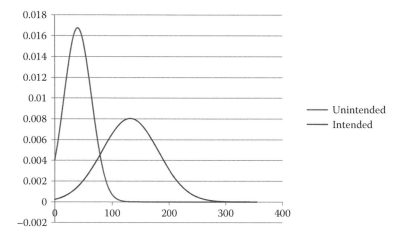

Step 2. Based on these data we can also calculate β_{OPT}:

$$\beta_{OPT} = \frac{P(S)}{P(N)} \times \frac{I(S)}{I(N)} = \frac{.9}{.1} = 9.0$$

Step 3. Now we need to find a value of X_C such that

$$\frac{P(X_C|N)}{P(X_C|S)} = \frac{1 - \varphi_N(X_C)}{\varphi_S(X_C)} = 9.0$$

Using Microsoft Excel, we can find that

$$\frac{1 - INVDIST(46,40,23.80,TRUE)}{INVDIST(46,131.56,49.60,TRUE)} = 9.5$$

Step 4. Because there was no change in the frequency distributions, there is no change in the ROC curve.

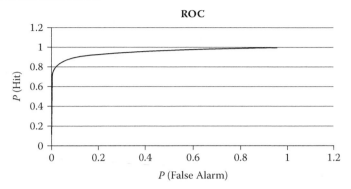

Step 5. Something interesting occurs when we look at the effect on text entry rate, however.

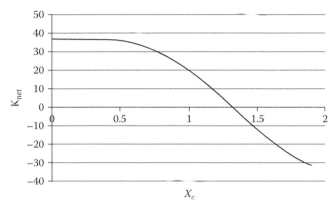

In this case, because errors are so infrequent, the client may be better off not using Slow Keys at all.

EXAMPLE 5.3

In the real world, we would expect the client to change his behavior as we changed the value of X_C to minimize rejections of correct keystrokes. In other words, the client would change μ_s to minimize misses and maximize hits. The results do not change much when we update the model to accommodate this.

Let's start with the original example, with $P(S) = 0.6$ and $P(N) = 0.4$, and assume that (whatever X_C is set to) the user changes his behavior such that only 2.5% of intentional keystrokes get rejected. That means

$$P\big(H\big) = P\big(x \geq X_C \big| S\big) = 1 - \Phi_s\big(X_C\big) = .975$$

$$P\big(M\big) = P\big(x \leq X_C \big| S\big) = \Phi_s\big(X_C\big) = .025$$

for all values of X_C.

Step 1. The frequency distribution does not change.

Step 2. β_{OPT} has not changed:

$$\beta_{OPT} = \frac{P(S)}{P(N)} \times \frac{I(S)}{I(N)} = \frac{.6}{.4} = 1.5$$

Step 3. Now we need to find a value of X_C such that

$$\frac{P(X_C|N)}{P(X_C|S)} = \frac{1-\varphi_N(X_C)}{\varphi_S(X_C)} = 1.5$$

Note that $\varphi_S(X_C)$ *has* changed, and is fixed at 0.025. So, we want a value of X_C such that

$$\frac{P(X_C|N)}{P(X_C|S)} = \frac{1-\varphi_N(X_C)}{.025} = 1.5$$

Using Microsoft Excel, we can find that

$$\frac{P(X_C|N)}{P(X_C|S)} = \frac{1-\varphi_N(X_C)}{.025} = 1.5$$

Step 4. Because we've fixed the probability of a hit at 0.95, the ROC looks a lot different.

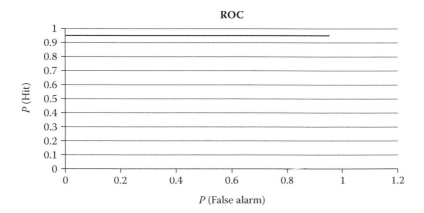

Step 5. The text entry rate estimate changes some, but not a whole lot. We are assuming that $\varphi_S(X_C)$ will change based on X_C.

We are going to assume that the standard deviation of the duration of correct keystrokes (σ_s) hasn't changed. Then, if we set μ_s to two standard deviations greater than X_C, 97.5% of correct keystrokes will be accepted:

$$\mu_s = X_C + 2\sigma_s$$

This results in the following plot:

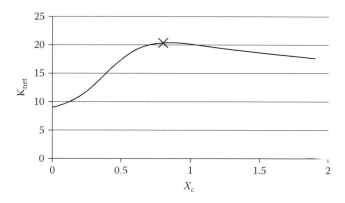

Once again, our chosen value of X_C maximizes our predicted text entry rate.

REFERENCES

1. Anson, D.K. 1997. *Alternative computer access: A guide to selection*. 1st ed. Philadelphia: F.A. Davis Company, p. 280.
2. King, T.W. 1999. *Assistive technology: Essential human factors*. Boston: Allyn and Bacon, p. 305.
3. King, T.W. 1999. *Assistive technology: Essential human factors*. Boston: Allyn and Bacon, p. 303.
4. Norman, D.A. 2002. *The design of everyday things*. New York: Basic Books.
5. Wickens, C.D., and J.G. Hollands. 2000. *Engineering psychology and human performance*. 3rd ed. Upper Saddle River, NJ: Prentice Hall, p. 573.
6. Keyboard—Single handed use. 2006, London: AbilityNet.
7. Kroemer, K.H.E. 2001. Keyboards and keying: An annotated bibliography of the literature from 1878 to 1999. *Universal Access in the Information Society* 1(2): 98–160.
8. Grant, C. 2009. Ergonomics of alternative keyboards. Available from http://office-ergo.com/ergonomic_seating.htm (accessed April 27, 2009).
9. Computer keyboard design. 2009. Available from http://ergo.human.cornell.edu/AHTutorials/ckd.htm.
10. One-handed keyboards. 2001. Atlanta, GA: Tech Connections.
11. Lau, C., and S. O'Leary. 1993. Comparison of computer interface devices for persons with severe physical disabilities. *American Journal of Occupational Therapy* 47(11): 1022–1030.
12. Trewin, S. 2002. Extending keyboard adaptability: An investigation. *Universal Access in the Information Society* 2(1): 44–55.
13. Trewin, S., and H. Pain. 1999. Keyboard and mouse errors due to motor disabilities. *International Journal of Human-Computer Studies* 50(2): 109–144.

14. Trewin, S., and H. Pain. 1999. A model of keyboard configuration requirements. *Behaviour and Information Technology* 18(1): 27–35.
15. Colven, D. 2002. *Using a keyboard to access windows*. Oxford, UK: ACE Centre Advisory Trust, p. 17.
16. Colven, D., and S. Judge. 2006. *Switch access to technology: A comprehensive guide*. Oxford, UK: ACE Centre Advisory Trust.
17. Johansen, A.S., and J.P. Hansen. 2006. Augmentative and alternative communication: The future of text on the move. *Universal Access in the Information Society* 5(2): 125–149.
18. Lesher, G.W., B.J. Moulton, and D.J. Higginbotham. 1998. Optimal character arrangements for ambiguous keyboards. *IEEE Transactions on Rehabilitation Engineering* 6(4): 415–423.
19. Arnott, J.L., and M. Javed. 1992. Probabilistic character disambiguation for reduced keyboards using small text samples. *Augmentative and Alternative Communication* 8(3): 215–223.
20. Zhai, S., M. Hunter, and B.A. Smith. 2002. Performance optimization of virtual keyboards. *Human-Computer Interaction* 17(2/3): 229–269.
21. Anson, D.K. et al. 2001. Efficiency of the Chubon versus the QWERTY keyboard. *Assistive Technology* 13(1): 40–45.
22. Soukoreff, R.W., and I.S. MacKenzie. 1995. Theoretical upper and lower bounds on typing speed using a stylus and soft keyboard. *Behaviour and Information Technology* 14: 370–379.
23. Sears, A. et al. 2001. The role of visual search in the design of effective soft keyboards. *Behaviour and Information Technology* 20(3): 159–166.
24. Wiklund, M.E., J.S. Dumas, and L.R. Hoffman. 1987. Optimizing a portable terminal keyboard for combined one-handed and two-handed use. In *Human Factors and Ergonomics Society Annual Meeting*. New York: HFES, pp. 585–589.
25. Matias, E., I.S. MacKenzie, and W. Buxton. 1996. One-handed touch typing on a QWERTY keyboard. *Human-Computer Interaction* 11(1): 1–27.
26. Keyboard—Dvorak layout. 2005. London: AbilityNet.
27. Gopher, D., and D. Raij. 1988. Typing with a two-hand chord keyboard: Will the QWERTY become obsolete. *IEEE Transactions on Systems, Man and Cybernetics* 18(4): 601–609.
28. Goettl, J.S., A.W. Brugh, and B.A. Julstrom. 2005. Call me e-mail: Arranging the keyboard with a permutation-coded genetic algorithm. In *Proceedings of the 2005 ACM Symposium on Applied Computing*. Santa Fe, NM: ACM Press.
29. Soukoreff, R.W., and I.S. MacKenzie. 2001. Measuring errors in text entry tasks: An application of the Levenshtein string distance statistic. In *CHI '01 extended abstracts on human factors in computing systems*, M.M. Tremaine, ed. Seattle, WA: ACM Press, pp. 319–320.
30. Tam, C. et al. 2002. Effects of word prediction and location of word prediction list on text entry with children with spina bifida and hydrocephalus. *Augmentative and Alternative Communication* 18(3): 147–162.
31. Zordell, J. 1990. The use of word prediction and spelling correction software with mildly handicapped students. *Closing the Gap* 9(1): 10–11.
32. MacKenzie, I.S., and R.W. Soukoreff. 2002. A character-level error analysis technique for evaluating text entry methods. In *Proceedings of the Second Nordic Conference on Human-Computer Interaction*, O.W. Bertelsen, ed. Aarhus, Denmark: ACM Press, pp. 243–246.
33. Soukoreff, R.W., and I.S. MacKenzie. 2003. Metrics for text entry research: An evaluation of MSD and KSPC, and a new unified error metric. In *Proceedings of the SIGCHI Conference on Human Factors in Computing Systems*, G. Cockton and P. Korhonen, eds. Ft. Lauderdale, FL: ACM Press, pp. 113–120.

34. Soukoreff, R.W., and I.S. MacKenzie. 2004. Recent developments in text-entry error rate measurement. In *CHI '04 extended abstracts on human factors in computing systems*. Vienna, Austria: ACM Press.
35. Wobbrock, J.O., and B.A. Myers. 2006. Analyzing the input stream for character-level errors in unconstrained text entry evaluations. *ACM Transactions on Computer-Human Interaction* 13(4): 458–489.
36. Smith, J., and R.C. Simpson. 2010. Analyzing performance with computer access technology using an unconstrained text entry protocol. *Journal of Rehabiliation Research and Development* 46(8): 1059–1068.

6 Techniques for Increasing Text Entry Efficiency

6.1 INTRODUCTION

Several techniques have been developed to increase text entry *efficiency*. These methods are similar in that they decrease the number of physical actions (e.g., keystrokes, switch activations) needed to generate text. Increasing text entry efficiency may increase text entry *rate*, but that is not guaranteed [1–4]. A frequent consequence of reducing the motor requirements associated with text entry is to increase the cognitive and perceptual load on the user, which can actually reduce text entry rate [5].

Techniques for increasing text entry efficiency rely on certain characteristics of the English language:

- Some characters are more common than others.
- Some words are more common than others.
- Some character sequences are very common.
- Some character sequences are very rare.
- Grammar dictates word order and combination.

Unfortunately, another characteristic of the English language is that normal word usage is dominated by a (surprisingly) small number of short words. For most English speakers, a set of 100 words would account for approximately 60% of all words used, 200 words would account for 70%, and 400 words would account for 80% [6]. Because most of these words have less than four characters, it is difficult to actually reduce the number of keystrokes or switch activations required to generate them.

6.2 WORD PREDICTION/COMPLETION (WPC)

6.2.1 WHAT IS WORD PREDICTION/COMPLETION?

Word prediction/completion (WPC) software presents the user with a list of the most likely words the user is currently typing (completion) or will type next (prediction) based on the text the user has already entered [7] (see Figures 6.1 and 6.2). If the desired word is in the list, the user can select the word (typically by pressing the corresponding number key) to have it automatically entered. WPC definitely reduces the number of keystrokes required to produce text, but does not necessarily increase text entry rate [1, 5, 8, 9]. WPC can also be used to help with spelling, which is discussed further in the chapter on cognitive and literacy impairments.

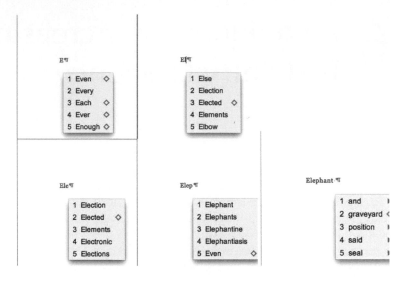

FIGURE 6.1   Word prediction/completion.

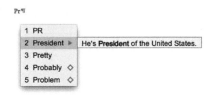

FIGURE 6.2   Word prediction/completion program. This shows a feature that demonstrates how the listed word is used in a sentence to help users select the correct one.

WPC can be deceptively taxing cognitively. Users need to be able to spell at least the first few letters of a word and distinguish words that look similar. In addition, users must be able to flexibly shift their attention back and forth between the input device and the WPC list [7], which can be very difficult for people with poor visual scanning skills.

6.2.2   THE LEXICON

WPC software requires a database of words, a *lexicon*, from which it draws its predictions. It is possible to have multiple topic-specific lexicons [7] or a base lexicon supplemented with smaller topic-specific lexicons.

An important design decision for the lexicon is the amount of information that needs to be stored with each word. A lexicon that includes lots of information about each word (e.g., parts of speech, frequency of use, recency of use) can potentially use this information to increase the accuracy of its predictions. All this additional information will increase the size of the lexicon, however. Although the size of the dictionary isn't that big of a deal for computers, it can be a concern for handheld devices with limited storage and processing power. In addition, the more information that is stored with each word, the more difficult it is for the user to add words to the lexicon [7].

Words can be added to the lexicon automatically, whenever the user enters a word that is not already in the lexicon. One obvious problem with adding words automatically is the possibility of adding misspelled words [7]. The alternative is to add words manually, either by using a hotkey as soon as the word is entered or after the fact through a separate lexicon maintenance interface. The manual approach provides much greater control over the lexicon but requires additional effort on the part of the user.

6.2.3   WPC Performance Measures

There are several measures for evaluating the performance of a WPC system. The most common measure is keystroke savings (k_{sav}) [7], which is the ratio of keystrokes *not entered* to total characters generated:

$$k_{sav} = \frac{(\text{total characters}) - (\text{total keystrokes})}{\text{total characters}}$$

For example, if 10 total characters are generated from 3 keystrokes, then

$$k_{sav} = (10 - 3)/10 = 0.7$$

Keystroke savings is a composite measure of both the user's performance and the WPC system's performance.

Hit ratio measures the likelihood that a desired word will appear in the WPC list. The hit ratio is the ratio of the number of times the desired word appears in the WPC list and the total number of written words [7]:

$$H = \frac{\text{words appearing in WPC list}}{\text{total words generated}}$$

The hit ratio improves as the number of words in the WPC list grows [7].

6.2.4   Configuring WPC Software

There are a surprising number of configuration options for WPC systems. Of course, few programs provide all of these configuration options.

6.2.4.1   WPC and Scanning

A configuration option unique to scanning interfaces determines how the WPC list is integrated into the scan pattern. Among the common ways to access the list are [4] (Figure 6.3)

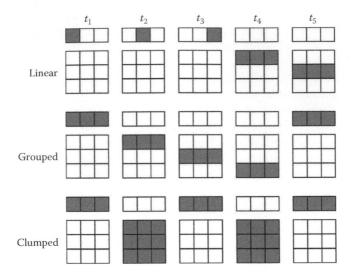

FIGURE 6.3 Accessing the WPC list while scanning. (Based on Lesher, G.W., B.J. Moulton, and D.J. Higginbotham, *Augmentative and Alternative Communication,* 14(2), 81–101, 1998 [4].)

- Linear list access: The system scans through each item in the list before initiating the normal scan pattern.
- Grouped list access: The WPC list is treated as a single group that is integrated into the group scanning pattern.
- Clumped list access: The system scans between the WPC list and the regular matrix; this option requires an extra switch press to select either the WPC list or the character matrix.

6.2.4.2 Maximum Number of Words in WPC List

The maximum number of words in the WPC list presents a trade-off between the likelihood that the desired word will appear in the list and the time required to search the list. The larger the number of words in the WPC list, the more likely it is that the desired word will appear. However, a long list of words will increase the time and cognitive effort required to find the desired word within the list [7, 10, 11]. Koester and Levine found that each additional word in the WPC list adds 150 ms to the time required to search the word prediction list [9]. Venkatogiri observed keystroke savings of about 31, 38, and 44% with maximum list sizes of 5, 10, and 15 words, respectively [10]. In a simulation study, Lesher et al. found that a list with seven words provided the greatest keystroke savings [4].

6.2.4.3 List Location and Orientation

A small number of WPC systems allow the user to choose where the WPC list is displayed on the screen and whether the list is displayed horizontally or vertically. Options for list position include the four corners of the screen, a user-determined fixed position, and floating (i.e., following the cursor). There is no empirical evidence indicating an advantage to any single list position [12]. In general, a vertical orientation is better than a horizontal orientation, as the perceptual effort required to process vertical lists is lower [7].

6.2.4.4   Keystrokes before List Is Displayed

This is another speed vs. accuracy trade-off. One line of reasoning goes like this: the WPC list is much more likely to contain the desired word after one or two letters have been entered, so it makes sense to enter a few keystrokes before looking at the list to avoid unnecessary list searches. Furthermore, after a few keystrokes, the WPC list may be shorter because there aren't enough words to fill up the entire list, which further decreases the time spent searching the list. The alternative line of reasoning is: there's always the chance that the desired word will show up right away, so not searching the list causes unnecessary keystrokes.

The right answer depends on how quickly the user can enter keystrokes, how quickly the user can search the WPC list, and how quickly the desired word tends to show up in the WPC list. In the absence of good information about the user or system configuration, Koester and Levine recommend requiring one keystroke before the WPC list is displayed [9].

6.2.4.5   Minimum Number of Characters in Each Word

The issue here is that WPC provides the most keystroke savings on long words, but short words are used much more frequently. Limiting the word completion list to words that are longer than four or five characters eliminates (shorter) common words like *the* and *and*. This setting also interacts with the setting for the number of keystrokes before the list is displayed. Word prediction lists often display a number of frequently used short words. Other programs opt to show some short words along with the most likely words that might follow the word just chosen.

6.2.4.6   Choosing and Ordering Words for the WPC List

Over the years, several approaches have been tried for choosing which words should go into the WPC list (Table 6.1). The simplest approach is to choose the words that have been used most recently, and display the words from most recently to least recently used [7]. If there is space for additional words in the WPC list, and there are more words in the lexicon that match the user's input, then these words are typically ordered either alphabetically or by length. WPC software that uses recency can have a very simple lexicon, which makes it easy to add words. On the other hand, the recency information needs to be built up over time, which can cause performance to suffer initially. In addition, the use of recency data causes the contents and order of the WPC list to change over time, which prevents users from learning where and when words will appear. In other words, *el3* can produce *elephant* one day and *elevator* the next.

Another relatively common approach is to choose and order words based on the frequency with which they are used [7]. The frequency data can come from generic English language usage, text entered by the user, or both. As with systems that use recency data, selecting and ordering words based on the user's frequency of use will cause the contents and order of the WPC list to fluctuate, interfering with learning. Another challenge with frequency data is that a small number of words (typically

TABLE 6.1

Options for Selecting and Ordering Words within WPC List

Method	Advantages	Disadvantages	Good When
Recency	Easy to add words to lexicon; predictions customized to user's writing	Takes time to accumulate data from user; contents of WPC list constantly changing	The user wants to add lots of words; keystroke time is much slower than list search time
Frequency of use	Predictions customized to user's writing	Contents and order of WPC list constantly changing; takes time to accumulate frequency of use data	The user has a consistent vocabulary and won't be adding lots of words; keystroke time is much slower than list search time
Frequency in English language	More accurate predictions; WPC list order stays constant	Hard to integrate new words; most words have a near-zero frequency	Keystroke time is not significantly slower than list search time
Syntax/grammar	Choices are grammatically appropriate; verbs can be conjugated automatically	Increases complexity of adding items to lexicon; doesn't provide much of a boost in performance	User struggles with writing skills

200 to 400) have very high frequency of use, and the remaining words have nearly identical nearly zero frequency of use.

Investigators have also explored the use of syntax and grammar to choose and order words. These systems consider everything from the beginning of the sentence in addition to the partial word fragment entered by the user [7]. As anyone who has used the grammar checker in Microsoft Word can attest, computers are still limited in their ability to parse sentences. In practice, the added cost of considering syntax and grammar outweighs the potential gain in accuracy.

When examining prediction methods, it is worthwhile to consider how well people can perform the same task. In a study by Lesher et al. [13], people acted as the WPC software to generate WPC lists of six words based on simulated input. Even when people were provided with a supplemental list of words generated and sorted using frequency information, the average keystroke savings was only 59%. In comparison, existing WPC software was able to generate keystroke savings of 54%.

6.2.5 Modeling Performance with Word Prediction/Completion

Koester and Levine used a keystroke-level model [14] of WPC to examine how changes in user behavior and interface configuration interacted to affect performance (Figure 6.4). The average time to generate each character is expressed as [8]

$$T_{wpc} = (S)(t_s) + (1 - k_{sav})t_k$$

where:

- S is the number of list searches per character
- t_s is the average time spent each time the user searches the WPC list (whether or not the word is in the list)
- k_{sav} is the number of key presses saved per character
- t_k is the average key press time during word prediction use
- T_{wpc} is expressed in seconds per character

The text generation rate (measured in characters per minute) is then simply [8]

$$60/T_{wp}$$

The key factors represented by model are the behavior of the user (t_s, t_k), the configuration of the word prediction system (S, k_{sav}), and the strategy used to search the WPC list [9]. From the model, and subsequent validation studies, Koester and Levine concluded that the factors with the greatest influence on performance [9] with WPC are [9]

- The delay in key press time caused by the increased cognitive load of WPC
- The keystroke savings achieved with WPC
- The strategy of use

Koester and Levine's model can also be used to understand why WPC is not guaranteed to increase text entry rate. Let us assume that we have a really good WPC system that always displays the desired word after the first letter has been entered. In this case, the sequence of actions to enter a single word would be

1. Enter one letter.
2. Find the desired word in the WPC list.
3. Press a key to select the desired word from the WPC list.

The user only searches the WPC list once per letter, so if we assume five letters per word:

$$S = 1/5 = 0.2$$

The user has to press two keys per word (one for the first letter, one to select the word from the WPC list):

$$k_{sav} = 3/5 = 0.6$$

$$T_{wpc} = (S)(t_s) + (1 - k_{sav})t_k = 0.2t_s + 0.4t_k$$

Since the average time per keystroke without WPC (T_{lo}) is t_k, when should someone use WPC? When T_{lo} is greater than T_{wpc}:

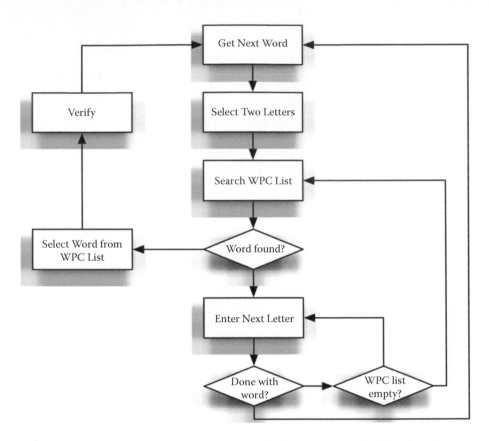

FIGURE 6.4   Koester and Levine's word prediction/completion model. (Based on Koester, H.H., and S.P. Levine, *Augmentative and Alternative Communication,* 13(4), 239–257, 1997 [8].)

$$T_{lo} > T_{wpc}$$

$$t_k > 0.2t_s + 0.4t_k$$

$$3t_k > t_s$$

$$t_k > t_s/3$$

What the model tells us is, even in the best possible world, the relationship between search time and keystroke time dictates whether someone should use WPC. This is why skilled typists do not use WPC: their keystroke time is much faster than their list search time (Figure 6.4).

6.2.6   IN THE CLINIC

As noted above, there is a distinction between efficiency and text entry rate. The importance of efficiency increases with the effort required for an individual user to generate each keystroke. For instance, for a client with cerebral palsy and difficulty hitting a key or switch, reducing overall effort may be primary. For someone else who types with little effort but is limited to typing with one finger or a head pointer, text entry rate may be the more important goal. However, the need to shift focus between the keyboard and the screen can actually reduce the entry rate of a slow but steady typist to a point where WPC would not be an appropriate solution. While this can only be determined by evaluating user performance and preferences with these tools, a common rule of thumb is that WPC is probably not of value for someone who can type faster than five words per minute without undue fatigue.

For writers with learning disabilities or poor spelling skills, the need to correctly enter the first few letters of a word can diminish the value of WPC. Several companies have been addressing this by entering lists of "confusables" in their lexicon. For instance, typing *sk* will generate a word list that includes *school*. For clients who have difficulty identifying the correct word choice from the presented list—especially homophones—some programs offer examples of a word used in the context of a sample sentence. Others also provide text-to-speech functionality to read back each word in a synthesized voice.

In some situations, word prediction can be problematic. Users may tend to just select from the choices in the prediction list to build sentences rather than using their own vocabulary and grammar skills to create a novel sentence. In these instances, the teacher or trainer will typically turn off the program's word prediction option but keep word completion active.

6.3   CHARACTER PREDICTION

An alternative (or complement) to word prediction is character prediction [4, 7]. Character prediction is more common on communication devices than on-screen keyboards and is most appropriate for clients who use a switch scanning interface. Because the problem is simpler (there are much fewer characters than words), character prediction is much more accurate than WPC. For the first letter in a word, the five most probable characters account for 46% of the actual selections and accuracy quickly rises toward 100% as the user enters additional letters. By comparison, after the first letter in a word is entered, the five most probable word prediction choices are selected only 17% of the time [4] (Table 6.2).

6.4   ABBREVIATION EXPANSION

6.4.1   WHAT IS ABBREVIATION EXPANSION?

Abbreviation expansion uses short sequences of keystrokes to trigger replacement by larger blocks of text. For example, an abbreviation of *ty* could be replaced by *thank you*. Abbreviation expansion is really a simplified form of macros used for quickly generating frequently used text. Abbreviation expansion reduces the total number of keystrokes required to enter text but imposes a high cognitive load because users must remember each abbreviation (and must remember to *use* the abbreviations when the opportunity presents itself).

TABLE 6.2
Frequency of English Letters

Letter	Frequency	Letter	Frequency	Letter	Frequency	Letter	Frequency
A	7.78	H	5.95	O	8.07	V	1.12
B	1.41	I	6.67	P	2.23	W	1.76
C	2.96	J	0.51	Q	0.08	X	0.27
D	4.02	K	0.74	R	6.51	Y	1.96
E	12.77	L	3.72	S	6.22	Z	0.17
F	1.97	M	2.88	T	8.55		
G	1.74	N	6.86	U	3.08		

Source: Reformatted from Garay-Vitoria, N., and J. Abascal, *Universal Access in the Information Society* 4(3): 188–203, 2006.
Note: Space isn't counted.

Abbreviation expansion can *theoretically* save a significant number of keystrokes. Lesher and Moulton optimized abbreviation-word pairings across 57,000 unique words and found a keystroke savings of 56.7% [15]. Of course, no one is going to memorize 57,000 abbreviations. In one study, able-bodied subjects were able to memorize 177 out of 200 codes after three training sessions [16]. On a more long-term basis, some teenagers have learned hundreds of abbreviations for instant messaging. Realistically, the number of abbreviations a person can effectively remember and use depends on their cognitive skills and the type of text they enter. The more repetitive the text, the more it lends itself to abbreviation expansion.

6.4.2 Defining Abbreviations

There are several options for defining abbreviations [6]. If only a few abbreviations are used, then the user can choose each individually to facilitate recall. It becomes more difficult to create unique and meaningful abbreviations, however, as the number of abbreviation expansions increases. Collisions (when the same abbreviation would be useful for more than one word) occur in all abbreviation expansion routines. One also has to be careful to avoid using abbreviations that occur in ordinary usage, such as *ms*, *mr*, or *cd*.

Abbreviations can also be chosen arbitrarily to minimize abbreviation length [15]. This technique has the advantage of achieving maximum motor efficiency by using minimum length abbreviations. It has a disadvantage due to the extreme difficulty of learning totally arbitrary codes for any large number of words, thus requiring extensive practice.

Another alternative is to generate abbreviations based on one or more rules [17]. Examples of rule-based abbreviation strategies include

- Contraction: Abbreviations are formed using first and last letters in a word.
- Truncation: The beginning of the word is used.

TABLE 6.3

Abbreviation Expansion Techniques

Technique	Abbreviation	Expansion
Automatic	th	there
Manual	th.	there
10-Branch	th8	there

With rule-generated abbreviation strategies, the individual does not have to remember the code, since he or she can construct the code by thinking about the target word. These approaches have the disadvantage of tending to create longer abbreviations, which significantly reduces the efficiency. There is also a problem with multiple words having the same abbreviation.

6.4.3 TRIGGERING ABBREVIATION EXPANSION

There are several approaches to expanding an abbreviation once it is entered (Table 6.3). Abbreviations can be expanded automatically, as soon as they are entered [6]. After each keystroke, the system looks up the currently accumulated sequence of keystrokes to see whether it matches any stored abbreviations. If a match is found, then the sequence is removed from the screen and replaced by the expansion (word, phrase, or sentence). This approach is the most efficient, but creates the possibility of a poorly chosen abbreviation being expanded unintentionally.

The alternative approach is to end each abbreviation with a special character or hotkey that triggers abbreviation expansion, frequently a separator such as a space, period, or other punctuation key [6]. With this technique, any set of characters can be used as the abbreviation without concern for collision with other words or abbreviations. This technique has the disadvantage, however, of requiring an extra keystroke for each abbreviation. Since the most frequently used words are short to begin with, this additional keystroke significantly reduces the efficiency of abbreviation expansion.

A variation on using a special character or hotkey is the 10-Branch technique, in which all abbreviations consist of a series of letters followed by a number [6]. Since it uses ten different termination characters rather than one (as with the manual expansion strategies above), an increased number of shorter codes is possible. This increases the efficiency of abbreviation expansion but introduces additional cognitive load. Of course, when the abbreviation completions are displayed on the screen, 10-Branch is identical to word prediction.

In addition to abbreviation expansion, some systems also provide an *unexpand* key that reverts text back to the originally entered letters. This is particularly useful when automatic expansion is used.

6.4.4 AUTOCORRECT AS ABBREVIATION EXPANSION

A powerful version of abbreviation expansion is available in word processors such as Microsoft Office and WordPerfect. In Microsoft Office, it is called AutoCorrect and is designed to automatically replace common typing or spelling mistakes with the correctly spelled word. In reality, any "mistake" can be replaced with text of any length, or a graphic or table. While this is an easy way to explore the value of abbreviation expansion, it is limited to Microsoft Office and won't work elsewhere.

Fortunately, there are a number of stand-alone utilities that provide this functionality in any application, monitoring keystrokes and triggering the expansions. Additionally, many programs that provide WPC allow the inclusion of abbreviation expansion sequences in their prediction lists or as a separate feature option. Ultimately, abbreviation expansion provides the only rate enhancement option for those who can generate text too fast to benefit from WPC but are not able to use speech recognition technology.

REFERENCES

1. Koester, H.H., and S.P. Levine. 1996. Effect of a word prediction feature on user performance. *Augmentative and Alternative Communication* 12(3): 155–168.
2. Venkatagiri, H.S. 1993. Efficiency of lexical prediction as a communication acceleration technique. *Augmentative and Alternative Communication* 9(3): 161–167.
3. Tumlin, J., and K. Wolff-Heller. 2004. Using word prediction software to increase typing fluency with students with physical disabilities. *Journal of Special Education Technology* 19(3).
4. Lesher, G.W., B.J. Moulton, and D.J. Higginbotham. 1998. Techniques for augmenting scanning communication. *Augmentative and Alternative Communication* 14(2): 81–101.
5. Koester, H., and S.P. Levine. 1994. Modeling the speed of text entry with a word prediction interface. *IEEE Transactions on Rehabilitation Engineering* 2(3): 177–187.
6. Vanderheiden, G.C., and D.P. Kelso. 1987. Comparative analysis of fixed-vocabulary communication acceleration techniques. *Augmentative and Alternative Communication* 3(4): 196–206.
7. Garay-Vitoria, N., and J. Abascal. 2006. Text prediction systems: A survey. *Universal Access in the Information Society* 4(3): 188–203.
8. Koester, H.H., and S.P. Levine. 1997. Keystroke-level models for user performance with word prediction. *Augmentative and Alternative Communication* 13(4): 239–257.
9. Koester, H.H., and S.P. Levine. 1998. Model simulations of user performance with word prediction. *Augmentative and Alternative Communication* 14(1): 25–36.
10. Venkatagiri, H.S. 1994. Effect of window size on rate of communication in a lexical prediction AAC system. *Augmentative and Alternative Communication* 10(2): 105–112.
11. Johansen, A.S., and J.P. Hansen. 2006. Augmentative and alternative communication: The future of text on the move. *Universal Access in the Information Society* 5(2): 125–149.
12. Tam, C. et al. 2002. Effects of word prediction and location of word prediction list on text entry with children with spina bifida and hydrocephalus. *Augmentative and Alternative Communication* 18(3): 147–162.
13. Lesher, G.W. et al. 2002. Limits of human word prediction performance. Presented at Technology and Persons with Disabilities Conference, Los Angeles.
14. Card, S.K., T.P. Moran, and A. Newell. 1980. The keystroke-level model for user performance time with interactive systems. *Communications of the ACM* 23(7): 396–410.
15. Lesher, G.W., and B.J. Moulton. 2005. An introduction to the theoretical limits of abbreviation expansion performance. In *28th Annual RESNA Conference*. Atlanta, GA: RESNA Press.

16. Gregory, E. et al. 2006. AAC menu interface: Effectiveness of active versus passive learning to master abbreviation-expansion codes. *Augmentative and Alternative Communication* 22(2): 77–84.
17. Barrett, J.A., and M. Grems. 1960. Abbreviating words systematically. *Communications of the ACM* 3(5): 323–234.

7 Automatic Speech Recognition

7.1 INTRODUCTION

Automatic speech recognition (ASR) defies categorical statements, even more than most computer access technologies, because of the rapid pace of change in the marketplace. Commercially available software is introduced, updated, and discontinued at a frantic pace, making published research results obsolete in short order. On the other hand, there are some fundamental truths of human performance that will always apply.

7.1.1 SPEECH RECOGNITION VS. VOICE RECOGNITION

The term *automatic speech recognition* refers to recognizing what a person said [1]. This distinguishes *speech recognition* from *voice recognition* or *speaker recognition*, which refers to using voice as a biometric identification method (i.e., the problem of who said it) [2].

7.1.2 DISCRETE VS. CONTINUOUS

ASR software is designed to work with either *discrete* or *continuous* speech. Discrete speech ASR requires the user to pause between each word [1]. The earliest ASR products were all discrete speech systems. Continuous speech ASR, on the other hand, allows the user to talk in multiword phrases. Affordable continuous speech systems for consumer use were introduced in 1997 and are the type of ASR system consumers expect to use.

This is not to say, however, that discrete ASR systems are no longer relevant or not worth considering. Discrete ASR products still exist, often in the form of systems for issuing voice commands (i.e., *command and control*). Discrete ASR is also useful for some clients with trouble speaking clearly or consistently [2]:

- Individuals who make involuntary sounds can often train a discrete ASR system to ignore these sounds [3].
- Users with dysarthria or on ventilators may experience better recognition accuracy because discrete ASR forces them to speak slowly with a distinct pause between each word [2].
- The word-by-word structure can also benefit individuals with cognitive or language impairments [2]. Discrete ASR also allows these individuals to take extra time for language processing and word retrieval [3].

7.1.3 DICTATION VS. COMMAND AND CONTROL

Users tend to think of using ASR exclusively for dictating text [4]. Command and control ASR systems, including the ASR interface built into the Mac OS X operating system, are used to access menu items and controls within dialog boxes, instead. Command and control ASR interfaces have much smaller vocabularies, consisting of command words and phrases. Because they use a small vocabulary, not all command and control ASR systems require the user to train the system to recognize the user's voice prior to use [4]. Also note that most dictation systems provide command and control functions in addition to dictation.

7.2 HOW ASR WORKS

Interpreting human speech is a daunting challenge for a computer. An average college-educated adult has a working vocabulary of about 7,000 words and can recognize up to 30,000 words [5]. Humans have the added advantage of context, syntax, and semantics to assist them in recognizing what a conversation partner said.

A computer, on the other hand, relies almost entirely on signal processing to recognize speech. A great deal of the ease we take for granted in verbal communication goes away when the listener doesn't understand the meaning of what we say [6]. One implication of this lack of understanding is that an ASR system needs to be told when to listen and when not to, because it cannot distinguish between dictation directed toward itself or someone else. A second implication is that ASR may insert wildly inappropriate text into a document.

As the processing power and speed of modern computers have increased, ASR software has been able to spend more of its recognition time (the time by which it has to send the results to the page) analyzing context—what other words are preceding and following the word in question. While this has improved recognition rates, it has also made it more problematic for those who can only speak one word at time.

ASR is a multistep process (Figure 7.1). Once the user speaks into the microphone, the speech signal is "preprocessed" to convert it into a digital form suitable for computational analysis. The processed speech input is then compared to a model of the user's voice to determine what was said. Finally, the identified speech is transmitted to the computer's operating system or active application [7].

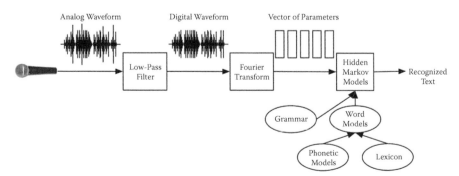

FIGURE 7.1   How ASR works. (Based on Fellbaum, K., and G. Koroupetroglou, *Technology and Disability,* 20(1), 55–85, 2008 [4]; Rosen, K., and S. Yampolsky, *Augmentative and Alternative Communication,* 16(1), 48–60, 2000 [7].)

7.2.1 SIGNAL PREPROCESSING

Preprocessing consists of several phases [4, 7]:

1. The user's raw speech, in the form of an analog wave signal, is captured by a microphone.
2. A low-pass filter is used to remove high-frequency components from the speech signal.
3. The analog signal is converted to a digital signal by sampling the signal at a fixed rate (typically every 10 to 30 ms).
4. The amount of data used to represent the signal is reduced through spectral analysis by converting each sample into a sequence of discrete features (or vectors of parameters).

The low-frequency portion of human speech consists of frequencies that a human with normal hearing needs to differentiate (phonemes), while the high-frequency portion is needed for voice identification and emotion detection [7]. The low-pass filter removes high-frequency sounds (in the sense of Fourier transforms). Note that women's voices cover a higher range than men's, so a low-pass filter will eliminate more of their voice signal.

Fourier analysis breaks down a signal into the sum of multiple sine waves of different frequencies [8]. A time-varying signal can be broken down into a series of separate sine waves, each with different frequencies that, when added, re-create the signal. This is known as Fourier analysis. Once the signal has been broken down into individual sine waves, the signal can be represented by the frequency and amplitude of each sine wave. This is what the bars on your stereo tuner are showing [8] (Figure 7.2).

7.2.2 RECOGNITION

The two greatest challenges to accurate speech recognition are the *invariance problem* and the *segmentation problem*. The invariance problem increases the difficulty

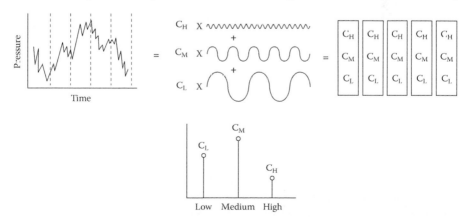

FIGURE 7.2 Fourier analysis. (Based on Wickens, C.D., and J.G. Hollands, *Engineering Psychology and Human Performance,* 3rd ed., Prentice Hall, Upper Saddle River, NJ, 2000, p. 573 [8].)

of matching speech signals with phonemes. Spoken English has 38 phonemes, and the physical form of each phoneme is highly dependent on the context in which it appears. For example, the auditory signal generated by pronouncing the phoneme *k* is quite different in *kid* than in *lick* [8].

The segmentation problem makes it difficult to identify the breaks between words in continuous speech. In a spectograph of continuous speech, breaks in the signal have little correspondence to breaks between words. For example, "She uses st*and*ard oil" would show two pauses marked by *, neither of which corresponds to a gap between words [4, 8].

Many recognition techniques have been reported in the literature [7]. The recognition technique that is used in most commercially available continuous speech ASR systems is hidden Markov models (HMMs) [7]. HMMs match segments of the speech signal to allophones, which combine to form phonemes that can be combined into words [7]. Other approaches include neural networks and template matching [7]. Template matching is most commonly used for discrete speech ASR.

7.3 BENEFITS OF ASR

ASR offers several benefits to individuals with disabilities. For those who need it (and have a sufficiently strong and consistent voice and the necessary skills), ASR can provide completely hands-free operation of the computer. ASR is also less physically demanding than other access methods, which can be valuable to users who are prone to fatigue [3]. Using ASR also allows a person to maintain a better working posture [9] and allows users to work in postures that otherwise would not be effective for computer use (e.g., reclined in a chair or bed).

ASR can also be very helpful for people with literacy impairments, such as individuals who have significant difficulty with spelling to the point where it interferes with their writing. Some people who have trouble writing grammatically correct sentences can do much better when speaking them.

For some users, dictating a command is much faster than navigating menus or dialog boxes by keyboard or mouse—especially if the user is not sure where the command is located in the menu structure.

7.4 LIMITS OF ASR

7.4.1 Error Correction and Navigation Take Longer

This is an aspect of ASR that has the potential to change as ASR software continues to evolve. Quantitative results from research are therefore of less interest than qualitative observations. In previous studies of ASR, users have spent a lot more time on navigation and error correction than text generation [9–12]. Critically, the average *number* of corrections when using ASR has been about the same as when using a keyboard and mouse, but the *number of steps per correction* was much higher for ASR [6]. In other words, the same number of typos were observed in these studies for the keyboard and ASR, but each typo took much longer to correct with ASR [2]. One reason for this disparity is that a keyboard error usually results in a single incorrect character, but an ASR error can result in multiple incorrect words [13]. In addition, ASR errors within the error correction process itself can further compound the difficulty [2, 11].

7.4.2   SOME TASKS ARE INAPPROPRIATE FOR ASR

ASR obviously requires speaking out loud, so it's not good for entering sensitive information, working in shared office environments, or taking notes in class [5, 14]. In addition, ASR is faster for text entry than mouse operations. Tasks that do not involve text entry can be significantly slower with speech than without for users who can also use a keyboard or mouse [11].

7.4.3   INCREASED COGNITIVE OVERHEAD

Using ASR software requires more than just talking [3, 14], including composing text and problem solving, all of which happens in the verbal part of working memory. This means that speech input/output interferes with problem solving in a way that physical input/output does not [14]. In other words, it may be easier to type and think than to talk and think [2]. Speaking and composing text requires frequent shifts between thinking about what to say, saying it, and problem solving to make corrections. If you forget what you wanted to say because you're busy talking or problem solving, what you wanted to say is lost and needs to be reconstructed [14]. Another source of overhead is the need to include commands for punctuation when using ASR [5].

7.4.4   ERRORS ARE HARDER TO SPOT WITH ASR

ASR errors are different from keyboard errors. Keyboard errors can often be "felt," but speech errors must be identified by looking at the display [2, 15]. It is difficult for users to develop an accurate internal model of when a recognition error will occur. When a user presses a key, he or she can be certain of the result. When ASR fails to recognize what the user said, the output can seem almost random. Imagine if a keyboard occasionally generated random characters when you pressed the keys [6]. Even worse, when a recognition error occurs, it's definitely going to be spelled correctly and may even be a homonym for the correct text, so being able to proofread carefully to identify errors is really important.

7.5   TEXT ENTRY RATE WITH ASR

Users are often disappointed at the text entry rate they can achieve with ASR [16]. In normal conversation, people speak at an average rate of 125 to 150 words per minute (wpm) [10]. Modern ASR products have no difficulty interpreting bursts of continuous speech spoken at 100 wpm, but users are unlikely to actually speak at this rate for long when composing (as opposed to transcribing) text.

Obviously, the text entry rate observed with older versions of ASR software may not be representative of what can be achieved with current ASR software. However, even with a perfect ASR system simulated by dictating to another human being, text entry rate was well below 20 wpm for composition tasks once formatting and thinking were taken into account [2, 17, 18]. Simply put, when composing (as opposed to transcribing) text, it takes time to figure out what to say. When composing or transcribing text, selecting and formatting text, editing text, and correcting errors when the ASR system misrecognizes one or more words is a slow process by voice.

7.6   ASR COMMANDS

There are four types of ASR commands [2]:

- Special words needed for dictation (e.g., punctuation marks, numbers, dates, military alphabet)
- Special words needed for editing (e.g., capitalization, tabs, blank lines, cursor navigation, insertion, deletion, cutting, pasting)
- Spoken equivalents to application or operating system commands (e.g., launching applications, opening windows, file manipulation, menu and button commands)
- Commands needed to operate the ASR system itself (e.g., turning the microphone on/off, correcting errors, playing back dictation)

The choice of command name has an effect on a user's ability to recall the command and the ASR system's ability to recognize the command. Short commands may match button and menu labels, but are less easily recognized by ASR software than longer commands. Longer commands are harder to memorize, and represent a second set of application commands to learn [2].

7.6.1   NAVIGATION COMMANDS

Navigation commands consist of the commands an ASR system makes available to move the text cursor. In other words, navigation commands are equivalent to the home, end, page up, page down, and arrow keys on the keyboard. There are two types of navigation commands in ASR systems: *target based* and *direction based*.

Direction-based navigation means giving directional commands (e.g., "move up," "end of document") [13]. Target-based navigation means moving the cursor to a target by saying the name of that target [13]. Target-based navigation is often used when navigating to a word that was incorrectly recognized (e.g., "select boo") [13].

A key aspect of improvement with ASR is learning when to use target-based and direction-based commands [19] and how to recover when commands are misrecognized by the software. When navigation commands fail, the cursor can be moved to the wrong location or text can be added or deleted from the document [10] and result in errors that require a lot of effort to fix [13].

7.6.2   ERROR CORRECTION COMMANDS

ASR systems typically offer multiple commands to correct recognition errors [2, 6]. There is typically a "scratch that" or undo command (which Koester referred to as a

SCRUNDO command [2]) that erases the last text entered. Users also have the option of selecting the erroneous text (with voice commands, the keyboard, or the mouse) and then redictating the desired text. Finally, most ASR systems include a command to activate a correction dialog box, into which the desired text can be entered.

While all three of these methods appear to produce the same results, they are actually very different under the surface. This is not the same as using a keyboard, in which all error correction methods are equivalent. SCRUNDO makes the ASR software forget that the utterance ever happened—no learning occurs at all, so it does not improve its performance. Select and redictate does not notify the software that a mistake was made, so no learning happens in this case either. Using the correction dialog box notifies the ASR software that it did something wrong *and lets it know what the right thing was*—so positive learning occurs, which leads to improved performance. Using the correction dialog box is critical for improving recognition accuracy over time [2].

7.6.3 Mouse/Pointing

There are several ways to move the mouse cursor using voice commands. Voice commands can be used to move the mouse cursor up, down, left, or right either in *discrete steps* (e.g., 5 pixels up, 2 inches left) or in a *continuous movement*. For continuous movement, one command (e.g., "move left") causes the cursor to start moving and another command stops the cursor (e.g., "stop" or "click"). Depending on the system, the cursor may move at a single fixed speed or the user may be able to vary the speed at which the cursor moves [4]. The *mouse grid* approach divides the screen into a series of blocks, which are selected and subdivided until the cursor is positioned on the target (Figure 7.3).

7.7 MICROPHONES

7.7.1 Types of Microphones

Headset microphones work best for ASR [5] because they place the microphone element close to the speaker's mouth, increasing the signal-to-noise ratio. The downside to a headset microphone is the need to put it on and take it off [5]. A headset may therefore be a poor choice for a client with limited manual dexterity who wants to be able to work at the computer without any assistance.

Array microphones allow high-quality reception at a distance of up to 2 feet. An array microphone consists of two to eight microphone elements that pick up both the user's voice and ambient noise. Digital signal processing then eliminates the noise without distorting the speech. Array microphones allow a user to move about and turn his or her head, but recognition is not as good as a headset microphone [20], and it is more susceptible to other noises in the environment. Desktop-mounted microphones can be more accurate but require a person to position himself or herself closer to the device (4–12 inches). Wireless microphones, including those using Bluetooth technology, allow for the option of a headset-style microphone that can be left in place while allowing the user to move about and attend to other tasks.

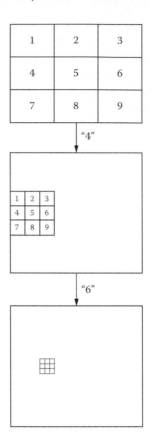

FIGURE 7.3   Mouse grid.

7.7.2   NOISE CANCELLATION

Pressure gradient noise cancelation is most common and uses one microphone with two openings, one in front and one in back. Background sounds enter both sides of the microphone and the sound waves cancel each other out, whereas the speaker's voice only enters one side and is unaffected [20].

Active noise cancellation uses two microphones facing in opposite directions. The signal from the outward microphone (assumed to be noise) is electronically processed and used to cancel out the same sound coming from the microphone facing the user's mouth.

7.7.3   USB MICROPHONES

USB microphones have their own sound card and send the signal in digital form direct to the ASR software through the USB bus. USB microphones are not necessarily better than a good analog microphone and sound card but can be extremely useful when trying to isolate problems with ASR performance [20].

7.7.4 Choosing a Microphone

Most users are going to be better off using a better microphone than whatever is included in the box with their ASR software. For basic needs, all the higher-end models appear to be reasonably good. Some low-cost models have good recognition, but can be flimsier, less flexible, and have shorter cords [20].

What to look for in a microphone [20]:

- Excellent high-frequency response and minimal bass response
- Noise cancelation (either active or pressure gradient)
- A microphone boom that can be easily adjusted to fit the person
- A headband and ear pieces that are tolerable to wear for long periods
- Long cables with strain relief

7.8 ASR AND SPECIAL POPULATIONS

7.8.1 Dysarthric Speech

Dysarthric speech can result in decreased intelligibility, affecting the pronunciation of consonants, vowels, or both [7]. However, ASR can work in spite of dysarthric speech because vocal inconsistencies that are perceived by humans may not affect ASR [7]. Disfluencies such as pauses, prolongations, stutters, and hesitations can also cause recognition errors but are more difficult for ASR to interpret because they are less consistent [7]. Consumers with severe dysarthria may be more successful with a command and control system that utilizes discrete ASR with a limited vocabulary [7].

An individual with dysarthric speech may also have a limited phonemic repertoire. An ASR system can be trained to recognize the way the user speaks certain words as alternative pronunciations [7]. Recognition accuracy will then depend more on distinctiveness and consistency between phonemes than whether the phonemes sound normal [7].

A reduced speech rate may cause ASR software to perceive extra gaps within words or commands [7]. Using a discrete ASR system may help the user concentrate on pronouncing each individual word more quickly and fluidly. Some systems also allow the user to increase the pause time between words [7].

Involuntary sounds such as audible exhalations, fillers (e.g., *uh*, *um*), and lip smacking may reduce accuracy, but modern ASR software is often able to ignore these [7]. Low vocal intensity may reduce recognition accuracy by lowering the signal-to-noise ratio [7], but a high-quality noise-canceling microphone can often compensate for a soft voice [7].

7.8.2 Low Vision

It is possible to use ASR if the user has impaired vision or is blind. For clients who have poor vision but can still read large print, decreasing the screen resolution or using a screen magnifier may be sufficient. For clients who are blind, the ASR software must be used in conjunction with a screen reader, along with additional software that links the ASR and screen reader together.

7.8.3 LITERACY IMPAIRMENTS

Using ASR requires adequate reading skills to identify errors [7]. When ASR makes a recognition error, you don't know what text it's going to generate, but you do know that it's going to be spelled correctly. That means that spell checkers are unlikely to identify errors. If the user is a poor speller or reader, he or she will have trouble identifying when a mistake is made. Poor spelling or reading will also make it difficult to train the system, because the client may not know how to pronounce some words, or type in the desired word when making a correction.

On the other hand, ASR can be very helpful for people who have dyslexia or significant difficulty with spelling to the point where it interferes with their writing because these individuals often forget what they are trying to write by the time they figure out how to spell or type a word. Using ASR allows them to "leap frog" over such obstacles. Other people who have trouble with writing (dysgraphia, motor planning) or who make many grammatical errors with written text can do much better when dictating if they have good verbal skills.

If a client has trouble with visual processing of text—a cognitive impairment unrelated to the ability/inability to spell or read—but does not have difficulty processing text that he or she hears, then ASR can be combined with speech output for identifying recognition errors. However, this is not always sufficient, as many words sound similar when using speech output. In this and similar situations, it is helpful for the person to get additional assistance with proofreading before submitting the final written product.

7.8.4 CHILDREN

Younger children with physical or learning disabilities are often suggested as candidates for ASR. There are particular concerns for those with an exceptionally high-pitched voice, as the system might not respond well.

7.9 VOICE ERGONOMICS

Users of ASR may tend to speak at a constant pitch, volume, and inflection, which can keep the vocal musculature tensed and in a fixed position [3, 9, 14, 21]. While there were growing concerns about reports of a number of voice problems being generated by ASR, these were more commonly associated with discrete speech tools where a hard stop was generated after each word. Nevertheless, speaking for long periods of time can be hard on the vocal cords.

Some problems that have been encountered after using ASR include [3]

- Sore throat
- Coughing
- Increased mucus
- Throat problems (itchiness, dryness, pain)
- Decreased vocal volume
- Hoarseness
- Vocal fatigue

Long-term problems with ASR use can include [3]

* Monotone speech
* Inappropriately low pitch
* Uncontrollable coughing bouts
* Chronic hoarseness
* Inability to modulate voice volume
* Weak, barely audible voice

Some users of ASR have reported problems with their voices, such as frequent hoarseness, loss of voice, sore throats, or discomfort when speaking [3, 20]. Users should be seated comfortably and maintain good posture when using ASR. Tilting one's head up to look at the computer screen can cause neck strain and affect both breathing and speech [3, 20]. Users should also focus on breathing in through the nose and exhaling deeply from the abdomen, rather than from the top of the chest.

Users should also speak in a relaxed manner, close to their normal way of speaking. Users should not whisper, speak in a loud or strained voice, or put extra emphasis on words. Users should also vary their intonation when speaking (i.e., adopt a sing-song pattern on the word at the start and in the middle of each line of text) rather than adopting a monotone voice. This will prevent the vocal musculature from remaining in a fixed position [3, 20].

Users should build up their use of ASR gradually, starting at 30 minutes a day, and slowly increasing the length of ASR sessions to a maximum of 2 hours. Users should alternate work tasks to avoid dictating for extended periods. Users should also take a break every 30 to 60 minutes, or more often if required. After speaking for 1 hour there is usually edema (redness around the vocal folds). After about 10 minutes this area usually returns to normal [3, 20]. Users should limit their use of ASR when tired or ill, as this strains your voice and also reduces recognition accuracy [3, 20].

Users need to keep their vocal cords moist. A user should begin drinking fluids before work, because it takes several hours for water to build up mucous around the vocal cords. Avoid caffeine, coffee, antihistamines, and acidic juices, if possible. Ensure that the environment in which you are speaking is not too dry. Use a humidifier to keep the room at a relative humidity of 35–40% [3, 20].

Users should be encouraged to limit throat clearing and coughing. Clearing one's throat or coughing causes the vocal folds to bang together. Many people are not aware that they frequently clear their throat when talking. When a client needs to clear his or her throat, encourage him or her to take a drink of water and swallow hard. If coughing is unavoidable, cough as gently as possible. ASR should be used in a room that is free of smoke and dust, which can irritate the vocal folds [3, 20].

7.10 MAXIMIZING PERFORMANCE WITH ASR

7.10.1 MAXIMIZE ACCURACY

In prior research, text entry rate has been strongly related to recognition accuracy [11]. Recognition accuracy has also been more important for user satisfaction [1, 11].

Anecdotally, 95% accuracy has been reported to be the threshold of user acceptance and successful use [2]. Only highly motivated individuals (including people with disabilities for whom other text entry methods are slower or more frustrating) use ASR with less than 95% accuracy [3].

When using ASR, the user should talk at a conversational pace (approximately 100 words per minute). Talking too quickly or too slowly will degrade recognition accuracy [20]. Clients should work on enunciating small words (e.g., *and, it, is, a*). ASR software has more trouble understanding small words than longer ones because multisyllable words have more verbal clues [20].

A client using continuous speech ASR should also talk in phrases and sentences, instead of using individual words. Continuous speech ASR recognizes longer utterances much better than shorter ones [20]. The client must learn to think ahead about what he or she is going to say before he or she says it [20].

Correct and consistent microphone placement is essential for high accuracy. The microphone should be approximately one thumb width (one-half to three-quarters of an inch) from the corner of the user's mouth. The microphone should be positioned so that it does not pick up the noise of breathing from your mouth or nostrils [20]. If the ASR software consistently adds extra small words (e.g., *to* and *a*), this may mean the microphone is in the path of the air stream and should be positioned a little higher or off the corner of the user's mouth [20].

If a client's voice varies over the course of the day, create more than one voice file [5] (e.g., one for the morning and one for the afternoon).

7.10.2   MULTIMODAL ERROR CORRECTION

Many experienced ASR users who have the requisite physical abilities use a multimodal (keyboard, mouse, and speech) error correction strategy that is much more efficient than relying entirely on speech. Using the keyboard and mouse also reduces the number of error cascades (where attempting to correct one error leads to subsequent errors) that occur [22]. Clients should experiment to see if error correction is faster by voice or using the mouse and keyboard. Some ASR users find that it is useful to get the rough text on the screen using speech, and then fix the document using the keyboard and mouse or other method [20].

7.10.3   TEXT ENTRY FIRST, PROOFREAD SECOND

There are two approaches to searching for errors [2]. With the in-line correction approach, the user identifies and corrects errors while the desired text is still fresh in the user's mind. This approach reduces the navigation distance to the error and makes it easier for the user to remember the desired text. However, this approach can also distract the user from the main task of entering text and may even cause the user to forget what he or she intended to say subsequently [2, 10].

In the proofreading approach, the user completes an entire thought before reviewing the text for errors. Proofreading is correlated with greater ASR expertise. Proofreading requires less task switching, which means the user does not have to split resources between text creation and editing. Some ASR software supports the proofreading approach by replaying the user's voice so the user can figure out what was actually said [2].

7.10.4 GET A POWERFUL COMPUTER

ASR requires a powerful computer. The minimum requirements listed by manufacturers significantly underestimate what is necessary for acceptable performance [2]. Fortunately, due to the advances in computing power, today's standard computer configurations are generally fine for speech recognition as long as plenty of RAM memory is provided.

7.10.5 MILITARY ALPHABET

Speech recognition systems still respond to the military alphabet, and it can be very useful when spelling out a word since the single-syllable letters can be difficult to recognize accurately, and similar sounding ones such as *b* and *d* can be confused by the software (Table 7.1).

7.11 IN THE CLINIC

7.11.1 ASSESSMENT

When performing a computer access assessment for a client who may be a good candidate for ASR, begin by assessing their ability to access the computer by other means [20]. Every client should have a method other than ASR for computer access, even if it is just as a backup for the (inevitable) occasions when the ASR software crashes.

When presenting ASR to the client, it is important to manage their expectations. ASR can be disappointing for clients who can type faster than 30 words per minute. ASR is also difficult to learn, especially if someone is not already computer literate. Determine the client's level of computer proficiency and his or her motivation.

TABLE 7.1
The Military Alphabet

A	Alpha	J	Juliet	S	Sierra
B	Bravo	K	Kilo	T	Tango
C	Charlie	L	Lima	U	Uniform
D	Delta	M	Mike	V	Victor
E	Echo	N	November	W	Whiskey
F	Foxtrot	O	Oscar	X	X-ray
G	Golf	P	Papa	Y	Yankee
H	Hotel	Q	Quebec	Z	Zulu
I	India	R	Romeo		

Questions to discuss with the client include [20]

- What computing tasks and software will the client be using?
- Are local training and support available?
- What is the client's level of computer expertise?
- What is the client's reading level?
- What is the client's ability and desire to learn?

Successful ASR use depends on several cognitive skills. The user must have good auditory and visual attending skills. Kinesthetic learners may be less successful than auditory and visual learners. The user must also have good problem-solving skills and must be able to learn the commands required to interact with the ASR software (e.g., navigating, correcting errors, interacting with the operating system). The user should be able to read at a fifth-grade level and be able to spell well enough to identify at least the first two or three letters of a word [20]. An ASR user must also be able to monitor and evaluate his or her performance and make changes when necessary to achieve his or her goals. ASR users must be able to reflect on and modify their speech patterns and articulation of words [20].

Successful ASR use also depends on developing oral communication skills that are more associated with public speaking than conversational speech. In addition, an ASR user must understand the differences in style between conversational and written language. An ASR user must be able to translate ideas into organized and sequenced speech without the pauses, backtracking, and repetition that characterizes conversation [20].

Ultimately, successful ASR use is about more than just learning to use some new software. The user must be prepared to change the way he or she talks, thinks, and behaves. This requires a high tolerance for frustration and a willingness to persevere in spite of inevitable difficulties. Motivation is therefore critical [20].

7.11.2 TRAINING

Good training up front (particularly developing good dictation and correction habits) makes chances of success and long-term use more likely. Clinicians should emphasize proper correction strategies, including when SCRUNDO is or is not appropriate [23]. Start with in-line correction and increasingly move toward the proofreading approach.

7.11.3 EVALUATING PERFORMANCE

7.11.3.1 What Do I Say?

One of the hardest things about introducing speech recognition to a client is coming up with something for the client to say. You want some text that doesn't have lots of proper nouns, which makes it difficult to use stories from the newspaper.
Suggestions:

- What did you have for breakfast?
- What's in your bedroom?
- What's your neighborhood like?

7.11.3.2   QuickMap Method

The QuickMap assessment method [24] consists of a dictation phase and a correction phase. In the dictation phase, the client dictates a short paragraph from hardcopy into a word processing program but does not correct any recognition errors. This allows the clinician to measure recognition accuracy and provides an upper limit of text entry rate if there were no recognition errors. In the correction phase, the client makes corrections to the output of the dictation phase (using any method desired), until it matches the transcription text as closely as possible. This allows the clinician to measure the client's true text generation rate when the time required to correct recognition errors is taken into account.

The QuickMap method uses three measures of performance. Dictation speed is the number of words dictated (spoken, not what shows up on screen), divided by the time required for the dictation phase:

$$\text{Dictation speed} = \text{\# of words dictated/time for dictation}$$

Net text entry rate is the number of correct words in the final output divided by the total time required for both the dictation and correction phases:

$$\text{Net TER} = \text{\# of correct words in final output/time for dictation and correction}$$

Recognition accuracy is the ratio of correct words to total words in text:

$$\text{Recognition accuracy} = \text{\# of correct words in dictated output/\# of words in the text}$$

7.11.3.3   Quick Accuracy Test

Have the user repeat the same text four to six times. If there is a plateau in recognition accuracy before the desired level of accuracy, then ASR is unlikely to work well [7].

7.11.3.4   Word Error Rate

One commonly used measure is word error rate (WER), also used in machine translation evaluation [4].

$$WER = 100\% \times \frac{\text{Substitions} + \text{Deletions} + \text{Insertions}}{Number.of.words.in.the.correct.sentence}$$

where [4]:

- A substitution is when an incorrect word substitutes for the correct word.
- A deletion is when a correct word is omitted from the recognized sentence.
- An insertion is when an extra word is added in the recognized sentence.

REFERENCES

1. Rebman, C.M., M.W. Aiken, and C.G. Cegielski. 2003. Speech recognition in the human-computer interface. *Information and Management* 40(6): 509–519.
2. Koester, H.H. 2001. User performance with speech recognition systems: A literature review. *Assistive Technology* 13(2): 116–130.
3. Kotler, A.-L., and C. Tam. 2002. Effectiveness of using discrete utterance speech recognition software. *Augmentative and Alternative Communication* 18(3): 137–146.
4. Fellbaum, K., and G. Koroupetroglou. 2008. Principles of electronic speech processing with applications for people with disabilities. *Technology and Disability* 20(1): 55–85.
5. Anson, D.K. 1997. *Alternative computer access: A guide to selection.* 1st ed. Philadelphia: F.A. Davis Company, p. 280.
6. Karat, C.-M. et al. 1999. Patterns of entry and correction in large vocabulary continuous speech recognition systems. In *Conference on Human Factors in Computing Systems (CHI '99).* Pittsburgh, PA: ACM Press.
7. Rosen, K., and S. Yampolsky. 2000. Automatic speech recognition and a review of its functioning with dysarthric speech. *Augmentative and Alternative Communication* 16(1): 48–60.
8. Wickens, C.D., and J.G. Hollands. 2000. *Engineering psychology and human performance.* 3rd ed. Upper Saddle River, NJ: Prentice Hall, p. 573.
9. de Korte, E.M., and P. van Lingen. 2006. The effect of speech recognition on working postures, productivity and the perception of user friendliness. *Applied Ergonomics* 37(3): 341–347.
10. Feng, J., and A. Sears. 2004. Are we speaking slower than we type? Exploring the gap between natural speech, typing and speech-based dictation. *ACM SIGACCESS Accessibility and Computing* (79): 6–9.
11. Koester, H.H. 2004. Usage, performance, and satisfaction outcomes for experienced users of automatic speech recognition. *Journal of Rehabiliation Research and Development* 41(5): 739–754.
12. Sears, A. et al. 2001. Productivity, satisfaction, and interaction strategies of individuals with spinal cord injuries and traditional users interacting with speech recognition software. *Universal Access in the Information Society* 1(1): 4–15.
13. Feng, J., and A. Sears. 2004. Using confidence scores to improve hands-free speech based navigation in continuous dictation systems. *ACM Transactions on Computer-Human Interaction* 11(4): 329–356.
14. Shneiderman, B. 2000. The limits of speech recognition. *Communications of the ACM* 43(9): 63–65.
15. Sears, A. et al. 2003. Hands-free, speech-based navigation during dictation: Difficulties, consequences, and solutions. *Human-Computer Interaction* 18(3): 229–257.
16. Koester, H.H. 2003. Abandonment of speech recognition by new users. In *RESNA 26th International Annual Conference.* Atlanta, GA: RESNA Press.
17. Gould, J.D., J. Conti, and T. Hovanyecz. 1983. Composing letters with a simulated typewriter. *Communications of the ACM* 26(4): 295–308.
18. Newell, A.F. et al. 1990. Listening typewriter simulation studies. *International Journal of Man-Machine Studies* 33(1): 1–19.
19. Feng, J., C.-M. Karat, and A. Sears. 2005. How productivity improves in hands-free continuous dictation tasks: Lessons learned from a longitudinal study. *Interacting with Computers* 17(3): 265–289.
20. Grott, R., and P. Schwartz. 2009. Speech recognition resource guide. In *International Conference on Rehabilitation Engineering and Assistive Technology.* Washington, DC: RESNA Press.
21. Williams, N.R. 2003. Voice recognition products—An occupational risk for users with ULDs? *Occupational Medicine* 53(7): 452–455.

22. Karat, J. et al. 2000. Overcoming unusability: Developing efficient strategies in speech recognition systems. In *Conference on Human Factors in Computing Systems (CHI '00)*. The Hague, The Netherlands: ACM Press.
23. Koester, H.H. 2006. Factors that influence the performance of experienced speech recognition users. *Assistive Technology* 18(1): 56–76.
24. Koester, H.H. 2002. A method for measuring client performance with speech recognition. In *25th Annual RESNA Conference*. Minneapolis: RESNA Press.

8 Hearing Impairment

8.1 HEARING LOSS

Hearing involves several skills beyond detecting and discriminating between sounds [1]. *Auditory attention* refers to the ability to focus on a single sound source to the exclusion of other competing sounds in the environment. *Oral comprehension* is the ability to understand spoken language. These abilities can be compromised by either a sensory (i.e., between the ear and the brain) or cognitive (within the brain) impairment. A *conductive hearing loss* is caused by damage or blockage of the moving parts in the outer or middle ear. A conductive hearing loss typically interferes with the ability to hear low-volume sounds [1, 2]. A *sensorineural hearing loss* results from damage to the inner ear (cochlea) or auditory (eighth) cranial nerve [1, 2]. Depending on the extent and location of the damage, a sensorineural hearing loss can prevent all auditory information from reaching the brain or a subset of auditory information within a specific frequency range [1, 2]. One of the most common forms of hearing impairment, particularly in older adults, is presbycusis. Presbycusis is a sensorineural impairment affecting the sound receptors in the cochlea that respond to high-pitched sounds [1].

As with vision, hearing loss is measured on a spectrum [1, 2] (Table 8.1):

- An individual with *mild hearing loss* has difficulty hearing sounds below 25 decibels (dB). Mild hearing loss can make it difficult to understand speech, especially in the presence of background noise.
- An individual with moderate hearing loss is unable to hear sounds below 40 dB.
- An individual with severe hearing loss cannot hear sounds below 65 dB.
- An individual who has profound hearing loss cannot hear sounds below 95 dB.
- An individual who is deaf cannot hear any sounds.

8.2 COMPUTER ACCESS INTERVENTIONS FOR HEARING LOSS

Hearing impairment is often not considered an obstacle to using a computer [3–5]. However, the growing use of audio and video on the web is increasing the impact of a hearing impairment on one's ability to use a computer. Unfortunately, there are limited interventions available to users and clinicians. It is possible to increase the volume, or even use an external speaker or headphones with an amplifier to provide additional volume. Some system sounds (such as error beeps) can be remapped to different frequencies. Several operating systems also offer the ability to provide simultaneous visual and auditory feedback for system sounds (Figure 8.1).

TABLE 8.1
Effects of Hearing Loss

Threshold Level of Noise Perception	Category	Hearing Ability
0–15 dB	Normal hearing	All (or most) speech sounds can be heard
15–25 dB	Slight hearing loss	Vowel sounds can be heard clearly but unvoiced consonant sounds may be missed
25–40 dB	Mild hearing loss	Speech sounds that are voiced loudly can be heard
40–65 dB	Moderate hearing loss	Most speech sounds voiced at normal conversational level are not heard
65–95 dB	Severe hearing loss	No speech sounds voiced at normal conversational level are heard
More than 95 dB	Profound hearing loss	No sounds (speech or otherwise) are heard

Source: Jacko, J.A., and H.S. Vitense, *Universal Access in the Information Society,* 1(1), 56–76, 2001 [1].

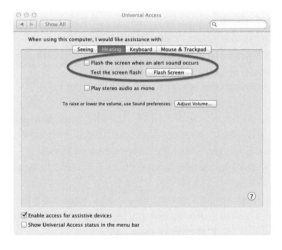

FIGURE 8.1   Some operating systems will provide visual feedback in addition to auditory prompts.

The bigger challenge is captioning. Captioning is necessary for individuals with hearing impairments, but has other advantages too [6]. As with captioning for television broadcasts, captions are potentially useful for able-bodied individuals watching video in noisy environments or in a foreign language. On the Internet, captions allow audio and video files to be searched and indexed, increasing their visibility to search engines. Unfortunately, very little of the audio content on the web is captioned [5], and that is unlikely to change anytime soon. Adding captioning to an audio or video file is time-consuming and somebody posting a 30-second clip on YouTube is unlikely to bother. There also isn't any reliable way to add captions to a file automatically (Figure 8.1).

REFERENCES

1. Jacko, J.A., and H.S. Vitense. 2001. A review and reappraisal of information technologies within a conceptual framework for individuals with disabilities. *Universal Access in the Information Society* 1(1): 56–76.
2. WebAIM. 2010. Auditory disabilities. Available from http://www.webaim.org/articles/auditory/ (accessed December 22, 2010).
3. Curran, K., N. Walters, and D. Robinson. 2007. Investigating the problems faced by older adults and people with disabilities in online environments. *Behaviour and Information Technology* 26(6): 447–453.
4. Hanson, V.L. 2001. Web access for elderly citizens. In *2001 EC/NSF Workshop on Universal Accessibility of Ubiquitous Computing: Providing for the Elderly*, R. Heller, ed. Alcacer do Sal, Portugal: ACM Press, pp. 14–18.
5. Hanson, V.L. 2009. Age and web access: The next generation. In *2009 International Cross-Disciplinary Conference on Web Accessibililty (W4A)*, D. Sloan, ed. Madrid: ACM Press, pp. 7–15.
6. Schroeder, P. 1998. *Access to multimedia technology by people with sensory disabilities*. Washington, DC: National Council on Disability.

9 Visual Impairment

9.1 INTRODUCTION

Computer use and Internet access can make a tremendous difference in the lives of individuals with visual impairments by providing educational and employment opportunities, supporting social networks, and facilitating independence [1, 4, 5]. However, individuals with visual impairments are much less likely to use computers than are sighted individuals [4].

9.2 VISUAL IMPAIRMENTS

9.2.1 COLOR BLINDNESS

A *trichromat* can perceive short-, medium-, and long-wavelength regions of the color spectrum [6]. A *dichromat* is a person who can only perceive light in two of the wavelength regions. [6]. The most common form of color blindness is red-green color blindness. Individuals with red-green color blindness are likely to be able to see reds and greens, but they have a harder time differentiating between them [3].

9.2.2 PRESBYOPIA

Presbyopia (farsightedness) is characterized by a decrease in the ability of the eye to change its focal length to keep close objects in focus [2]. Our eyes are optimized for viewing objects at least 6 meters away. As an object is brought nearer to our eyes, the crystalline lens in the eye has to bend into a more convex shape to keep the object in focus [2].

9.2.3 LOW VISION

Low vision is defined as a condition in which a person's vision cannot be fully corrected by glasses. Low vision can occur in individuals of any age as a result of such conditions as macular degeneration, glaucoma, diabetic retinopathy, or cataracts [3].

9.2.3.1 Diabetic Retinopathy

Diabetes can cause the retinal blood vessels to leak, resulting in dark patches in the field of vision where the leaks occur. Text can appear blurred or distorted in these regions [3] (Figure 9.1).

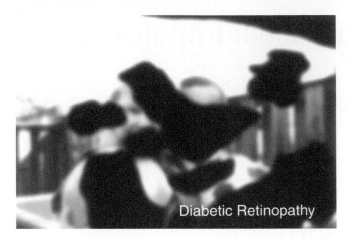

FIGURE 9.1 (See color insert.) Diabetic retinopathy. (From National Eye Institute, National Institutes of Health [NEI/NIH].)

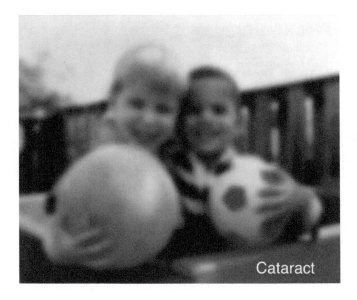

FIGURE 9.2 (See color insert.) Cataract. (From National Eye Institute, National Institutes of Health [NEI/NIH].)

9.2.3.2 Cataract

Individuals with cataract have opaque regions in the lenses of their eyes that cause a blurred or hazy effect, especially in bright light. Cataract can cause text to fade into the background. A high-contrast display is very important for people with advanced cataract [3] (Figure 9.2).

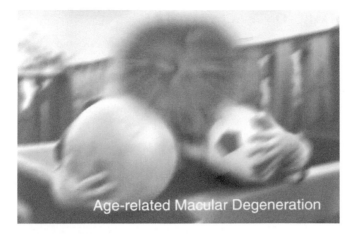

FIGURE 9.3 (See color insert.) Macular degeneration. (From National Eye Institute, National Institutes of Health [NEI/NIH].)

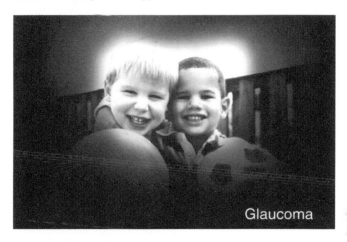

FIGURE 9.4 (See color insert.) Glaucoma. (From National Eye Institute, National Institutes of Health [NEI/NIH].)

9.2.3.3 Macular Degeneration

The aging process and the thinning of the tissues of the macula cause dry macular degeneration, resulting in a gradual loss of vision. Wet macular degeneration occurs when blood vessels in the back of the eye begin to leak fluid or blood, resulting in rapid loss of vision. In either form, the person's central area of sight is affected the most, making it difficult to see objects that the person is looking at directly [3] (Figure 9.3).

9.2.3.4 Glaucoma

Glaucoma is caused by damage to the optic nerve due to an increase in pressure inside the eye. The result is often the opposite of macular degeneration: the loss of peripheral vision and a blurry central area of vision. Reading can be particularly difficult because text seems faded as well as blurry [3] (Figure 9.4).

9.3   KEYBOARD-ONLY ACCESS

As visual impairment becomes more severe, the mouse becomes less and less useful. People with visual impairments may be able to move a mouse and operate the buttons, but they don't know where to move it or when to click, since they can't see what's on the screen [3]. However, even clients with slightly impaired vision might benefit from keyboard access as a way of reducing the need for visual search.

9.4   INTERVENTIONS FOR POOR VISION

9.4.1   AMBIENT LIGHTING

The uniformity of the light in a room can make self-luminous displays like computer monitors less visible in two ways. First, ambient light reflected from the screen reduces the contrast between items on the display and makes the colors on the display less intense. Second, light reflected from the front surface of the screen produces an image of the room, because the screen acts as a low-reflectance mirror. To compensate [10]:

- Pay attention to the position and orientation of the monitor. Make sure the monitor is not in direct light and is not tilted too far toward the ceiling.
- Use lighting that spreads light over a limited area

9.4.2   ANTIGLARE FILTERS

Screen filters can eliminate glare from overhead lighting. Much like the black louvers on the rear window of sports cars, a screen mesh will shade the screen from overhead lights, while providing a view of the display directly through the mesh [11]. Screen filters are effective in certain instances, but should be evaluated before purchase. Some screens reduce glare by 99%, but even that may not be enough in very bright environments [12]. In addition, filters will not block light from sources directly in line with the screen because, like the user, the light has a direct view of the screen through the filter [11]. In addition, screen filters can attract dust, which reduces the quality of the screen image [11, 13]. Once a screen filter is installed, increase the brightness of the monitor as necessary to compensate for any darkening caused by the filter itself [14].

Screens with matte finishes diffuse light from overhead lights and from windows. This reduces the brightness of the reflected image and equalizes the light reflected in any given direction. In addition, it reduces the perception of glare by eliminating well-defined edges in reflected images. The matte finish does reduce the quality of electronically generated images to a small extent, but the visual advantages often outweigh the disadvantages [11].

9.4.3   SCREEN RESOLUTION

Lowering the screen resolution reduces the total number of pixels on screen, which makes each pixel bigger and increases the size of everything drawn on the screen.

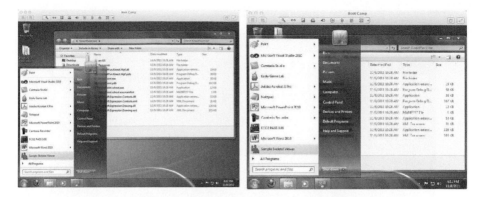

FIGURE 9.5 The same display in (a) high screen resolution and (b) low resolution.

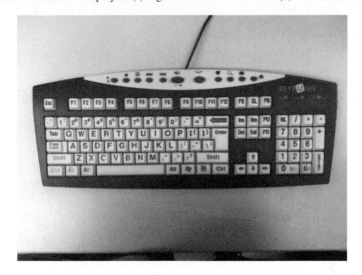

FIGURE 9.6 (**See color insert.**) Keyboard with large-print, high-contrast labels.

The trade-off when lowering the screen resolution is that fewer things can fit on the screen at one time (Figure 9.5).

9.4.4 KEYBOARD MODIFICATIONS

If a client has problems seeing the labels on the keyboard, stickers can be used to provide a larger, high-contrast label. There are also Braille dot stickers that can provide tactile feedback for locating keys (Figure 9.6).

9.4.5 OPERATING SYSTEM CHANGES

9.4.5.1 Screen Contrast

Light scattering within the eye can reduce the contrast between foreground and background objects within the image that reaches the retina. One way to reduce

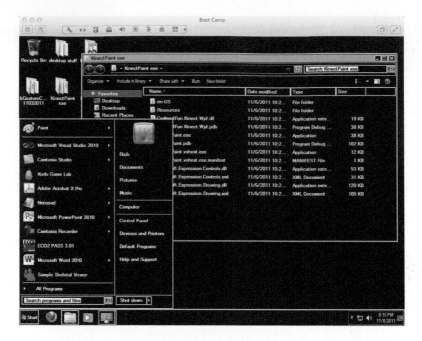

FIGURE 9.7   (**See color insert.**) Screen capture of a high-contrast color scheme.

the amount of scatter is to reduce the light intensity of the background area. For example, people with cataracts can read white letters against a black background much more easily than black letters against a white background [10]. It is possible to choose a color scheme at the operating system level that increases the contrast of the text in relation to the background. Common settings are a black background with white or yellow text, or a white or yellow background with black text, but many different combinations are possible [3, 15] (Figure 9.7).

9.4.5.2   Size of Screen Objects and Text

Individuals with visual impairments can have difficulty recognizing fine details of screen objects like icons, buttons, and toolbars [7, 16]. The size of all of these objects can be increased. Keep in mind, however, that software originally designed for the default size of screen objects may not easily accommodate larger objects (Figure 9.8).

In addition to screen objects, it is also possible to increase the size of text used in menus and labels. Enlarged text can make it possible for someone with vision impairment to see the computer screen [8, 9, 17].

9.4.5.3   Mouse Cursor

Individuals with visual impairments can have difficulty recognizing fine details of the small and dynamic pointers used in graphical user interfaces (GUIs) [7]. It is possible to choose larger mouse cursors or high-contrast mouse cursors (Figure 9.9).

Another option that is available is pointer trails. When pointer trails are active and the mouse is moving, the system allows images of the mouse cursor to persist

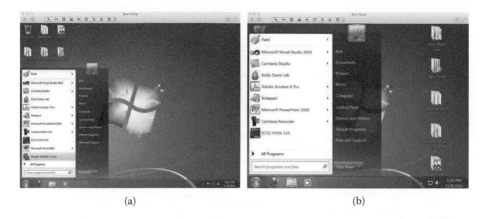

(a)   (b)

FIGURE 9.8   Screen capture of (a) default screen objects and (b) enlarged screen objects.

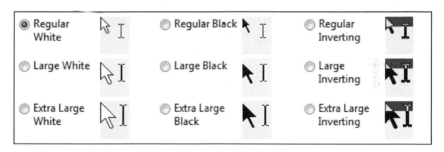

FIGURE 9.9   **(See color insert.)** Large and high-contrast mouse cursors.

in its previous location on the screen, resulting in a trail of ghostly mouse cursors that follow the actual mouse cursor. When the user stops moving the mouse, the trail disappears (Figure 9.10).

A final option is the mouse radar feature, which draws a series of increasingly larger concentric circles around the mouse cursor when a hotkey is pressed. This feature can help the user find the cursor on the screen.

9.4.6   SETTINGS AT THE OPERATING SYSTEM LEVEL VS. WITHIN INDIVIDUAL PROGRAMS

Some applications provide their own configuration options. For example, Microsoft Word has a zoom setting that allows the user to increase the magnification of the document. Many web browsers allow the user to choose a default font or high-contrast color scheme for web pages. The advantage of making changes within individual programs is that the changes can be narrowly targeted to specific tasks. More importantly, some applications either ignore or override changes made at the operating system level, so they must be set within the application. The primary disadvantage of within-application changes is that the changes need to be implemented within every program the client uses.

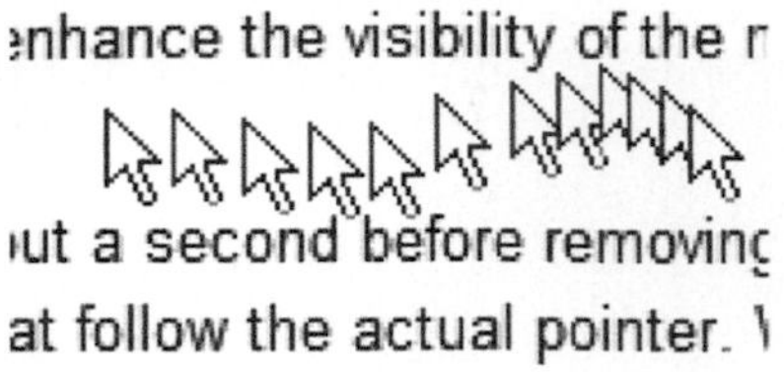

:nhance the visibility of the r

ıut a second before removinç

at follow the actual pointer. \

FIGURE 9.10   Pointer trails.
(From http://en.wikipedia.org/wiki/Cursor_%28computers%29.)

9.5   SCREEN MAGNIFIERS

9.5.1   Software Screen Magnifiers

A software screen magnifier is a program that enlarges a small area of the screen, allowing people with low vision to see it more clearly [3]. The magnification ratio is typically in the range from 2:1 to 16:1, but may be set as high as 32:1 [18]. The advantages of a software screen magnifier include that it magnifies all the contents of the screen at once, the magnification level can be changed easily, and it works across all applications. The principal disadvantages include that a software screen reader can only display a portion of the display at one time, and a software screen reader, being software, can crash.

Screen magnifier software can magnify the contents of the screen in several different ways. Many programs allow the user to choose between several different options. The different magnification methods are described in the following subsections.

9.5.1.1   Lens Magnifier

Lens magnifiers are analogous to a handheld magnifying glass. The user moves a cursor (generally the mouse cursor) around the screen and the area immediately around the cursor is enlarged and presented to the user in a separate window [18] (Figure 9.11).

9.5.1.2   Part-Screen Magnifiers

Part-screen magnifiers work in a way similar to that of lens magnifiers in that the area around the current position of the cursor is enlarged. However, rather than present the enlarged area in the same area of the screen as the cursor, it is displayed in a dedicated screen area, typically the top or the bottom of the screen [18] (Figure 9.12).

9.5.1.3   Full-Screen Magnifiers

Full-screen magnifiers enlarge the entire screen. The center of the magnified image typically corresponds to the cursor position. Of course, full screen magnification can only present a portion of the full computer screen at any one time [18] (Figure 9.13).

9.5.2   Physical Screen Magnifiers

The original screen magnifiers were literally magnifying glasses, attached to the computer monitor. These products are still available and offer several advantages. Unlike a software screen magnifier, a physical screen magnifier requires almost no

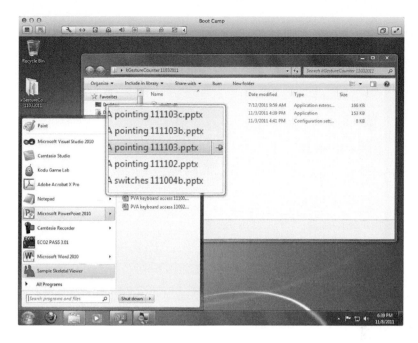

FIGURE 9.11 Lens magnifier.

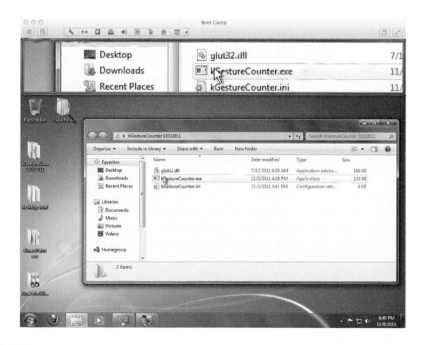

FIGURE 9.12 Part-screen magnifier.

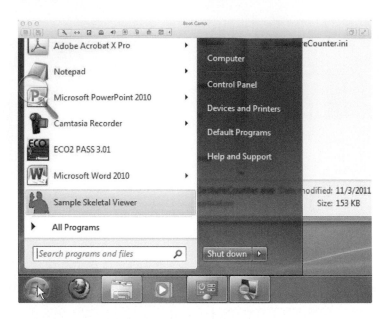

FIGURE 9.13   Full-screen magnifier.

learning to use, is easy to install and operate, and won't conflict with any software on the computer. Some physical screen magnifiers also provide antiglare features. On the other hand, physical screen magnifiers provide a fixed magnification level, which is much lower than the magnification that can be provided by a software screen magnifier, and may distort the screen image at the edges [19].

9.6   SCREEN READER

A sighted person tends to think of user interfaces and web pages in terms of blocks of information organized visually. For example, most web pages have navigation features either at the top or side of the page and may use graphics to attract your attention to important elements like new content [5, 23]. Visual representations of applications, files, or other objects allow users to locate and identify desired items rapidly [5]. Additional visual information includes text formatting (font size, color, and type, as well as typesetting like bold and italics) and simple or complex text structures (e.g., tables, hierarchical lists, scientific formulas, and layout such as columns, borders, and boxes) along with diagrams, drawings, charts, figures, logos, and photos [20].

Computer users with little or no functional vision are likely to use a screen reader [9]. Screen readers provide an auditory interface to the contents of the computer screen [3, 20, 21]. Screen readers do not read text like human beings do. The voice does not vary its speed or tone, making it sound robotic. Experienced users will often speed up the reading rate to 300 words per minute or more, which is faster than an inexperienced listener can easily understand. In fact, when many people hear a screen reader for the first time, at the normal rate of about 180 words per minute, they complain that it reads too quickly [21].

Graphical user interfaces present information on a two-dimensional screen, facilitating layout and organization. Spoken text, on the other hand, is inherently one-dimensional. The listener can move forward and backward within an audio stream, but there's no such thing as side to side. *Linearization* (or *serialization*) refers to the act of converting a two-dimensional interface (a computer display) into a one-dimensional interface [5]. Graphics and image-based text also pose problems for screen reader users [1, 5]. Screen readers cannot describe images. If there is no alternative text associated with the image, then the screen reader cannot accurately convey the meaning of an image [3, 20].

Sighted computer users are accustomed to visually scanning a page in all directions almost simultaneously, comprehending the overall layout and other macro-level aspects of an interface [3, 5, 20, 21, 23]. Screen reader users cannot perceive these macro-level aspects as quickly. The linear progression of an interface presented through speech is somewhat like automated telephone menu systems, which do not reveal all of the options at once. Users must progress through the interface in a stepwise manner [21].

Screen readers can be difficult to use, especially at first [22] because they impose a huge cognitive load on users. Users must construct and maintain a mental image of the contents of the computer screen. In addition, because blind users rely entirely on keyboard access, screen readers require the use of keyboard shortcuts, most of which the user has to memorize [23].

9.7   BRAILLE DISPLAY

Braille displays have small pins that can be raised or lowered to form Braille characters that the user can feel [3]. Braille displays typically provide one to four lines of Braille cells, with 40 to 80 cells per line. Braille displays do not support text formatting or images (Figure 9.14).

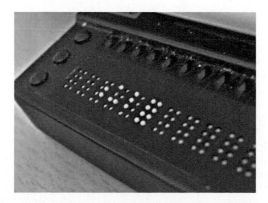

FIGURE 9.14   Refreshable Braille display. (From http://en.wikipedia.org/wiki/File: Refreshable_Braille_display.jpg.)

REFERENCES

1. Strobel, W. et al. 2006. Technology for access to text and graphics for people with visual impairments and blindness in vocational settings. *Journal of Vocational Rehabilitation.* 24: 87–95.
2. Nunes, F., P.A. Silva, and F. Abrantes. 2010. Human-computer interaction and the older adult: An example using user research and personas. In *PETRA '10: The 3rd International Conference on Pervasive Technologies Related to Assistive Environments,* F. Makedon, I. Maglogiannis, and S. Kapidakis, eds. Samos, Greece: ACM.
3. WebAIM. 2010. Visual disabilities. Available from http://www.webaim.org/articles/visual/ (accessed December 22, 2010).
4. Gerber, E. 2003. The benefits of and barriers to computer use for individuals who are visually impaired. *Journal of Visual Impairment and Blindness* 536–550.
5. Ratanasit, D., and M.M. Moore. 2005. Representing graphical user interfaces with sound: A review of approaches. *Journal of Visual Impairment and Blindness* 69–85.
6. Meyer, G.W., and D.P. Greenberg. 1988. Color-defective vision and computer graphics displays. *IEEE Computer Graphics and Applications* 8(5): 28–40.
7. Taveira, A.D., and S.D. Choi. 2009. Review study of computer input devices and older users. *International Journal of Human-Computer Interaction* 25(5): 455–474.
8. Rogers, W.A., A.J. Stronge, and A.D. Fisk. 2005. Technology and aging. *Reviews of Human Factors and Ergonomics* 1(1): 130–171.
9. Curran, K., N. Walters, and D. Robinson. 2007. Investigating the problems faced by older adults and people with disabilities in online environments. *Behaviour and Information Technology* 26(6): 447–453.
10. Boyce, P. 2003. Lighting for the elderly. *Technology and Disability* 15(3): 165–180.
11. Rea, M. 1991. Solving the problem of VDT reflections. In *Progressive architecture* (pp. 35–40). New York: Penton Media.
12. Grant, C. 2009. Visual ergonomics in the workplace. Available from http://www.office-ergo.com/setting.htm (accessed April 27, 2009).
13. HealthyComputing. 2009. The truth about "ergonomic" products. Available from http://www.healthycomputing.com/articles/publish/news/The_Truth_about_Ergonomic_Products.shtml (accessed 2009).
14. Grant, C. 2009. Pros and cons of ergonomic office equipment. Available from: http://office-ergo.com/pros-cons.htm (accessed April 27, 2009).
15. WebAIM. 2010. Fonts. Available from http://webaim.org/techniques/fonts/ (accessed December 27, 2010).
16. Scott, I.U., W.J. Feuer, and J. Jacko. 2002. Impact of graphical user interface screen features on computer task accuracy and speed in a cohort of patients with age-related macular degeneration. *American Journal of Opthalmology* 134(6): 857–862.
17. Mann, W.C. et al. 2005. Computer use by middle-aged and older adults with disabilities. *Technology and Disability* 17(1): 1–9.
18. Blenkhorn, P.L., D.G. Evans, and A. Baude. 2002. Full-screen magnification for Windows using DirectX overlays. *IEEE Transactions on Neural Systems and Rehabilitation Engineering* 10(4): 225–231.
19. Anson, D.K. 1997. *Alternative computer access: A guide to selection.* 1st ed. Philadelphia: F.A. Davis Company, p. 280.
20. Freitas, D., and G. Kouroupetroglou. 2008. Speech technologies for blind and low vision persons. *Technology and Disability* 20: 135–156.
21. WebAIM. 2007. Designing for screen reader compatibility. Available from http://webaim.org/techniques/screenreader/ (accessed December 30, 2010).

22. WebAIM. 2010. Planning, evaluation, repair and maintenance. Available from http://webaim.org/articles/process/ (accessed December 30, 2010).
23. WebAIM. 2010. Testing with screen readers: Questions and answers. Available from http://webaim.org/articles/screenreader_testing/ (accessed December 30, 2010).

10 Cognitive Impairment

10.1 LEARNING DISABILITIES

10.1.1 Literacy Impairment

Common forms of literacy impairment include dysgraphia, dysnomia, dyspraxia, and dyslexia. Dysgraphia causes difficulty writing quickly and legibly. Dysnomia is characterized by difficulty remembering words. Dyspraxia results in difficulty performing fine motor movements, like writing or typing [1]. Dyslexia causes visual distortions, resulting in problems with visual memory, keeping track of one's position in a document, and letter confusions and reversals [2]. As a result, people with dyslexia can experience difficulty with reading, writing, spelling, listening, speaking, and math [1]. Dyslexia can also lead to difficulties executing sequences of actions [2].

Many of the approaches that are useful for individuals with visual impairments are also useful for individuals with literacy impairments [3]. Presenting text in a large (at least 10-point size), bolded, sans serif font can make it easier to read [4–7]. Increasing the space between words and lines, and increasing the size of a document's margins (which decreases the length of each line) has also been shown to improve reading performance [2, 3, 6, 7]. The amount of space between lines should generally be no less than half the character height [6]. Avoid fully justified text, as it results in variable spacing between words and can result in distracting patterns of white spaces that flow downward through the text [6]. The use of color to distinguish letters or words has also been shown to improve reading performance [2].

Text-to-speech software is a common intervention for individuals with literacy impairments. Reading using text-to-speech software can be faster for some individuals [4, 8–10]. Text-to-speech software for individuals with literacy impairments can also act as a complement to visual input [3]. However, text-to-speech software can be more difficult to understand than human speech, because it lacks prosodic cues [11]. Text-to-speech software also does not address issues caused by problems with oral comprehension [12] or attention deficit disorder [10].

Several technologies developed for individuals with mobility impairments have also proven useful as writing aids for individuals with literacy impairments. Automatic speech recognition (ASR) software can be helpful to an individual whose oral language ability exceeds his or her writing ability (e.g., dysgraphia or dyspraxia) [8, 13]. However, the cognitive challenges involved in learning and using ASR should not be underestimated [12]. Word prediction/completion software can also help individuals who struggle with spelling, grammar, and word recall [8, 13]. Alternative keyboards that limit the number of keys, group similar keys by color or location, or use pictures to aid comprehension can also improve performance [13].

Literacy software is also available that combines multiple features into a single package. These products typically combine writing aids like speech recognition, word prediction, concept mapping tools, and sophisticated spelling and grammar tools with reading aids like text to speech and optical character recognition. The primary advantage of these products is that they offer multiple integrated capabilities with a consistent interface. These products are often adopted across an entire school or school system, which makes support more widely available and easy to obtain.

Keep in mind that technology, by itself, can compensate for an impairment but is unlikely to address the underlying problem [8]. While these tools make it easier to read and generate text, these tools do not help with originality, creativity, or fluency of ideas [12].

10.1.2 DYSCALCULIA

Dyscalculia refers to difficulty learning the rules and procedures for performing calculations or solving word problems [1, 14]. The types of problems students with dyscalculia can experience when performing mathematical calculations include [14]

- Identifying and interpreting mathematical symbols
- Recalling simple sums, differences, products, and divisions
- Solving multidigit operations that require borrowing or carrying
- Misaligning numbers or ignoring decimal points
- Forgetting steps within a multistep procedure

The types of problems students with dyscalculia can experience when solving word problems include [14]

- Reading and comprehending the word problem
- Identifying important and extraneous information
- Developing and executing a plan for solving the problem

Dyscalculia can be caused by problems with memory, visual-spatial skills, or cognitive development [14]. Memory problems can interfere with a student's ability to recall basic mathematical facts or the steps in a multistep procedure [14]. Visual-spatial problems can result in difficulty with misaligning numbers when performing a calculation and challenges when interpreting maps or learning geometry [14]. Delayed cognitive development can cause difficulty in understanding relationships between numbers and solving word problems [14].

Interventions for clients with dyscalculia include software for formatting mathematical equations and literacy software for interpreting word problems.

10.2 DEVELOPMENTAL DISABILITIES AND ACQUIRED BRAIN INJURY

There are a number of cognitive processes that are critical for computer access, and impairments in any of them can interfere with successful operation of a computer

[15]. Memory is a very general term for a collection of constructs and skills. Memory is divided between short-term (also called working) memory and long-term memory [5, 12]. Working memory is our mental "scratch pad" where information is stored for manipulation. Items are stored temporarily in working memory and are forgotten if not rehearsed though conscious mental effort.

What we refer to as learning is the process of encoding information in long-term memory. The encoding process works by linking new information to existing information. The more mental links that are created between new information and existing information, the easier that information will be to retrieve in the future.

We store several different types of information in long-term memory:

• Declarative knowledge: Factual statements, pieces of information (e.g., "George Washington was the first President of the United States"; your social security number).
• Procedural knowledge: Information on how to do things.
• Episodic knowledge: Memories of specific events.

There are two principal forms of reasoning that are relevant to computer access. *Deductive* reasoning refers to the ability to apply general rules to specific problems. Conversely, *inductive* reasoning is the ability to create general rules from separate pieces of information [12]. Individuals with cognitive impairments can have a variety of difficulties with reasoning and problem solving, including [12, 16]

• Identifying that a problem even exists
• Identifying the relevant aspects of the problem
• Determining whether an answer or conclusion makes sense

People with cognitive disabilities can have more difficulty solving technical problems with their equipment or maintaining security measures like antivirus software [16]. Individuals with cognitive impairments may have less resilience in the face of problems, and can choose to abandon a problem rather than trying to solve it [5].

There are two aspects of attention that are relevant to computer access. Selective attention is the ability to concentrate on one thing to the exclusion of all others [5, 12]. Selective attention is necessary to read the text on a web page without being distracted by the advertisements. Shared attention is the ability to divide one's attention across two or more tasks [12]. Shared attention is critical for someone who is using one or more computer access technologies to perform tasks on the computer.

Interventions for individuals with developmental disabilities or acquired brain injuries focus on simplifying tasks, through either training, task design, or interface design. Turning off system sounds can eliminate distractions [4, 6]. There are also programs designed to provide simplified interfaces. Software developed for young children can have simplified interfaces, but the content may be too childish for adult users.

Another alternative is to use a tablet (e.g., iPad) or smart phone instead of a computer. Apps designed for mobile devices typically provide a more streamlined interface and reduced functionality, which could simplify training and operation.

REFERENCES

1. Baumel, J. 2009. Frequently used educational terms: Learning and attention problems. Available from http://www.greatschools.net/LD/identifying/educational-terms-learning-and-attention-defiicit.gs?content=670&page=all (accessed November 2, 2009).
2. Gregor, P., and A. Dickinson. 2007. Cognitive difficulties and access to information systems: An interaction design perspective. *Universal Access in the Information Society* 5(4): 393–400.
3. Richards, J.T., and V.L. Hanson. 2004. Web accessibility: A broader view. In *13th International Conference on the World Wide Web*, S. Feldman and M. Uretsky, eds. New York: ACM Press, pp. 72–79.
4. WebAIM. 2010. Cognitive disabilities part 1: We still know too little, and we do even less. Available from http://www.webaim.org/articles/cognitive/cognitive_too_little/ (accessed December 22, 2010).
5. WebAIM. 2007. Cognitive disabilities part 2: Conceptualizing design considerations. Available from http://www.webaim.org/articles/cognitive/conceptualize/ (accessed November 24, 2007).
6. WebAIM. 2010. Evaluating cognitive web accessibility. Available from http://webaim.org/articles/evaluatingcognitive/ (accessed December 22, 2010).
7. WebAIM. 2010. Overview of Steppingstones cognitive research. Available from http://webaim.org/projects/steppingstones/cognitiveresearch (accessed December 24, 2010).
8. Misunderstood minds. 2002. Available from http://www.pbs.org/wgbh/misunderstood-minds/index.html (accessed November 2, 2009).
9. Buning, M.E., and J. Hanzlik. 1993. Adaptive computer use for a person with visual impairment. *American Journal of Occupational Therapy* 47(11): 998–1008.
10. Mckenna, M.C., and S. Walpole. 2007. Assistive technology in the reading clinic: Its emerging potential. *Reading Research Quarterly* 42(1): 140–145.
11. Power, C., and H. Jurgensen. 2010. Accessible presentation of information for people with visual disabilities. *Universal Access in the Information Society* 9(2): 97–119.
12. Jacko, J.A., and H.S. Vitense. 2001. A review and reappraisal of information technologies within a conceptual framework for individuals with disabilities. *Universal Access in the Information Society* 1(1): 56–76.
13. Stanberry, K., and M. Raskind. 2009. Assistive technology tools: Writing. Available from http://www.greatschools.net/LD/assistive-technology/writing-tools.gs?content=960 (accessed November 2, 2009).
14. Bryant, D.P. 2009. Math disability in children: An overview. Available from http://www.greatschools.net/LD/identifying/math-disability-in-children-an-overview.gs?content=526&page=all (accessed November 2, 2009).
15. WebAIM. 2010. Cognitive disabilities. Available from http://www.webaim.org/articles/cognitive/ (accessed December 22, 2010).
16. Fox, L.E. et al. 2009. Public computing options for individuals with cognitive impairments: Survey outcomes. *Disability and Rehabilitation: Assistive Technology* 4(5): 311–320.

11 Computer Access for Older Adults

11.1 INCREASING NUMBER OF OLDER ADULTS ONLINE

Published research, statistics, design guidelines, and other literature typically define *old* as at least 65 years of age [1]. However, this isn't universally true, so care should be taken when reading. In this chapter, *older adult* will refer to someone 65 years of age or older, unless otherwise specified. The number of older adults is growing in many developed countries [2–6]. By 2030, more than 20% of the U.S. population is expected to be over the age of 65 [7]. The age-based digital divide is shrinking even as the number of older adults increases [8]. Estimates of computer use among older adults range from 36 to 55% [8–10]. The number of older adults online is increasing faster than any other age group [3, 8, 11 19], and the number of older adults using computers and the Internet is likely to grow dramatically as more adults who are accustomed to using computers at work reach the age of 65 [11, 20].

Older adults use computers and the Internet in the same ways as their younger counterparts, and find them equally indispensable for employment, community participation, and independent living [1, 3, 5, 18, 21–25]. Computer and Internet use can have a positive effect on older adults' health and well-being [21, 24, 26–29]. Psychological benefits of computer and Internet use include increased self-esteem, life satisfaction, and feelings of autonomy and decreased depression, stress, and loneliness [10, 24, 26, 28, 30]. Older adults also frequently use the Internet to find health information [3, 5, 8, 21, 28, 29].

An important use of computers and the Internet is communication, through email and social media [1, 3, 5, 10, 13, 21, 24, 25, 27–29]. Older adults also use computers and the Internet to seek information and obtain news [1, 5, 8, 10, 19, 21, 24–26, 29, 31]. Older adults use computers and the Internet to access online services like banking and shopping [1, 3, 5, 8, 10, 13, 18, 19, 21, 24–28, 30–33]. Computers and the Internet are used for entertainment, in the form of games, movies, and computers [1, 5, 8, 18, 19, 31].

11.2 OBSTACLES TO COMPUTER USE

Functional impairments (physical, perceptual, or cognitive) are a common impediment to computer and Internet use by older adults [8, 10, 13, 23, 24, 34]. The challenges posed by functional impairments associated with the aging process are magnified by older adults' lack of information about the accessibility options available to them [8, 11, 20–22] and the difficulty in accessing configuration options within software and operating systems [8, 11, 21, 22, 35]. Many older adults report that a lack of technical assistance is a barrier to computer and Internet use [8, 10, 21, 36]. Even if an older adult is aware of available computer access technology that might be appropriate, he or she may not have access to the technology [8, 20] or want the stigma of using assistive technology [22]. While some adults are financially secure, others may not have resources to devote to computer technology, Internet access, and assistive technology [8, 10, 37]. Finally, some older adults choose not to use a computer or the Internet because they do not perceive any personal benefits [8, 10, 13, 38–42].

11.3 EFFECTS OF AGING

The natural aging process brings with it changes in physical, perceptual, and cognitive skills [3, 22, 35, 43, 44] that can result in a combination of physical, cognitive, and perceptual impairments [1, 22, 45]. However, which impairments emerge and the rate with which abilities decline are unique to each individual. As a result, there is considerable variation among older people in terms of ability [9, 21]. An older adult whose impairments are a result of the natural aging process may not consider himself or herself disabled [2, 22, 46]. Older adults may also be reluctant to acknowledge age-related impairments [11].

11.3.1 VISUAL

Vision is the most common physiological change associated with aging [45], and aging also increases the likelihood of experiencing a pathological change in the eye [12, 23, 45, 51, 55]. Approximately one in three American adults will experience a vision-reducing eye condition by the age of 65 [23, 47]. Visual acuity is dependent on the ability of the lens of the eye to change shape. As we age, the crystalline lens becomes harder to bend, and older adults have more difficulty focusing on text close to the eye (i.e., near acuity) without the assistance of reading glasses or bifocals [3, 9, 45, 48–50]. The range of objects that can be brought to focus on the retina decreases with age. By 60 years of age, the eye is essentially a fixed-focus optical system [51]. Most people over the age of 70 must wear eyeglasses due to age-related declines in acuity [9, 48, 49].

The lens of the eye also yellows and thickens, which affects our colors perception and our contrast sensitivity. Older adults find it easier to see reds and yellows than blues and greens, and can find darker blues indistinguishable from black [1, 3, 9, 12, 16, 51–53]. These changes to the lens interfere with the light reaching the retina, resulting in a general decline in visual acuity [3, 9, 12, 16, 29, 45, 48, 49, 51, 54]. The maximum amount the pupil can open decreases with age. Older adults thus have difficulty compensating for low light levels [1, 3, 51]. At the same time, the ability of the pupil to close also decreases (meaning the pupil cannot become as small and thus admits more light), leading to increased sensitivity to glare and bright illumination [9]. With age, the visual field shrinks, which reduces peripheral vision [2, 45, 48, 51].

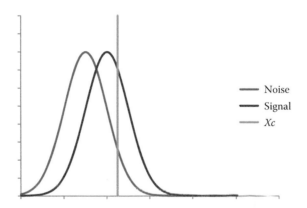

FIGURE 5.32 Graphical depiction of signal detection theory problem.

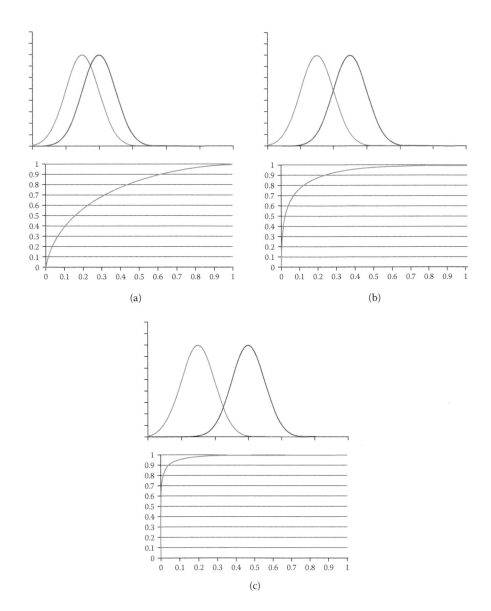

FIGURE 5.37 When sensitivity is (a) low, performance on the SDT task is poor; performance on the SDT task improves as sensitivity (b) increases; when sensitivity is (c) high, performance improves.

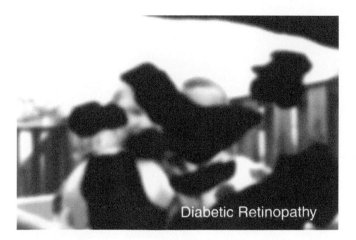

FIGURE 9.1 Diabetic retinopathy. (From National Eye Institute, National Institutes of Health [NEI/NIH].)

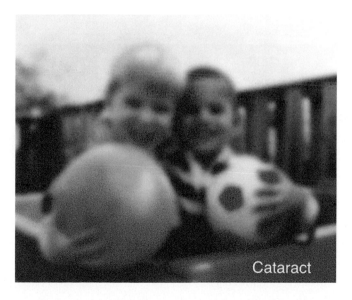

FIGURE 9.2 Cataract. (From National Eye Institute, National Institutes of Health [NEI/NIH].)

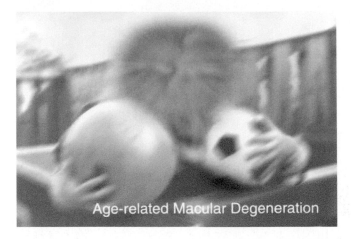

FIGURE 9.3   Macular degeneration. (From National Eye Institute, National Institutes of Health [NEI/NIH].)

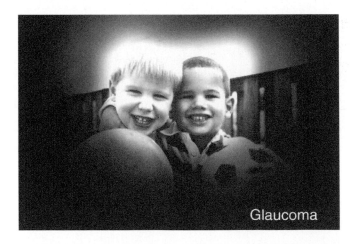

FIGURE 9.4   Glaucoma. (From National Eye Institute, National Institutes of Health [NEI/NIH].)

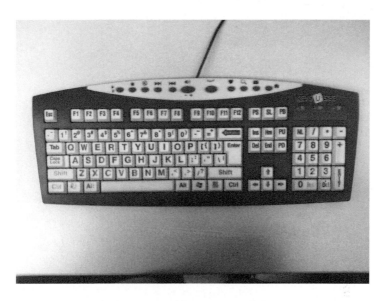

FIGURE 9.6 Keyboard with large-print, high-contrast labels.

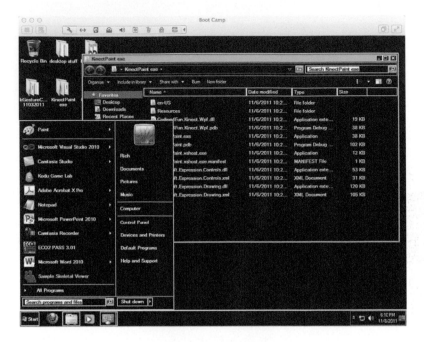

FIGURE 9.7   Screen capture of a high-contrast color scheme.

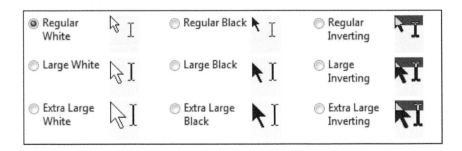

FIGURE 9.9   Large and high-contrast mouse cursors.

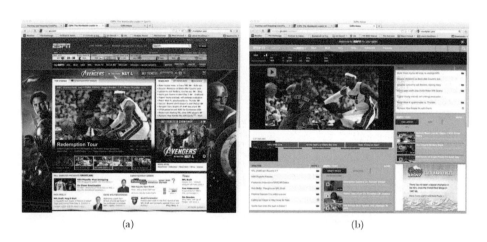

(a)　　　　　　　　　　　　　　　　　　　　　(b)

FIGURE 12.5　Picture of the same website accessed through (a) the traditional website and (b) the mobile version of the website, using Mozilla Firefox (v12.0).

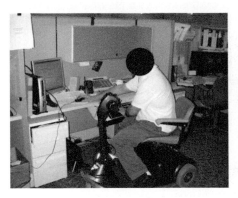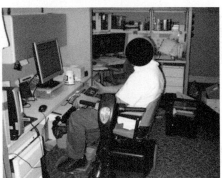

FIGURE 13.21 Case study.

11.3.2 Auditory

Hearing impairment is a common result of the aging process. Older adults typically experience a gradual reduction in their ability to hear sounds of low intensity or high pitch [1, 9, 11, 45, 48]. Older adults also have difficulty detecting small changes in sound frequency or intensity, which interferes with their ability to localize a sound or separate sounds within a noisy environment [9, 54].

11.3.3 Motor

As we age, physiological changes in our muscles and nervous system reduce our ability to perform motor tasks. Aging is also associated with increased incidence of arthritis and of neurological disorders such as tremor, essential tremor, and Parkinson's disease, all of which affect the ability to perform motor tasks [1, 11, 23, 31, 48].

Many aspects of behavior slow with age [13, 44, 57–59]. Older adults tend to emphasize accuracy over speed [60]. Older adults have slower reaction times and take longer to perform movements than younger adults, with lower peak velocities and a greater number of submovements [16, 23, 45, 48, 61, 62]. As a result, their movements are less smooth and less coordinated [3, 45, 48, 60, 63, 64].

Older adults have difficulty with fine motor coordination [9, 23, 31, 44, 48, 61, 64, 65]. Older adults have reduced strength and difficulty producing and maintaining consistent low levels of force and have an increased noise-to-force ratio [9, 23, 61]. Older adults also have reduced range of motion [23].

11.3.4 Cognitive

Processing speed declines with age. Older adults take longer to process, and respond to, incoming information [15, 21, 48]. Age-related declines are especially apparent when a task is complex or unfamiliar [9, 21]. The storage capacity of our working memory and our ability to manipulate information within it both decrease with age [3, 9, 15, 48, 66]. Our semantic memory, which consists of knowledge gained through education or experience, tends to remain stable throughout the life span [9, 21, 48, 67]. Other forms of memory, including prospective memory (the ability to remember to do something in the future), episodic memory (memory for specific events), and procedural memory (knowledge about how to perform specific tasks), also show declines with age [1, 21, 45, 48].

Older adults exhibit declines in selective attention, the ability to focus on something in the presence of distractions [9, 15, 22, 45, 48, 68, 69]. Older adults have difficulty dividing their attention between more than one task at the same time (i.e., multitasking) [9, 21, 48]. Fluid intelligence depends upon abilities that allow people to think quickly and reason abstractly, such as short-term memory and processing speed [16, 21]. As these underlying capabilities decline, so does fluid intelligence. As we age, our ability to comprehend written material declines [3, 12]. Older adults have difficulty with spatial reasoning tasks, such as mental manipulation of images or patterns and reasoning about spatial relationships [9, 14, 21, 35, 44].

Dementia is strongly associated with age. Symptoms of dementia include loss of memory, confusion, mood changes, and communication difficulties [1, 2, 17]. Many older adults who are not diagnosed with dementia or Alzheimer's disease may present with mild cognitive impairment (MCI). Symptoms of MCI include difficulty remembering names of people recently met, difficulty remembering the flow of a conversation, and a tendency to misplace things [1, 2]

11.4   COMPUTER ACCESS CHALLENGES

11.4.1   POINTING

Using a pointing device requires a combination of skills that are affected by age, including [23, 59, 60, 70–74]

- Performing fine motor tasks both rapidly and with precision
- Coordinating muscles in the eyes, shoulder, elbow, wrist, and hand
- Locating and tracking the cursor (i.e., visual search)
- Verifying that the cursor is on the target (i.e., visual acuity)
- Mapping coordinates in desk space to screen space (i.e., spatial reasoning)

The physical, perceptual, and cognitive effects of aging all contribute to difficulty performing tasks with pointing devices, including clicking on targets, double-clicking on targets, scrolling, navigating menus, and clicking and dragging. Older adults diagnosed with neuromuscular conditions (e.g., arthritis, tremors, Parkinson's disease) or visual impairments (e.g., age-related macular degeneration) are especially likely to have problems with pointing tasks [2, 3, 9, 11, 20, 22, 23, 32, 48, 59]. Older adults are at risk for developing musculoskeletal disorders, particularly from adopting an awkward posture while using the mouse [23, 63].

Double-clicking on items can be difficult for older adults, because of the need to rapidly press the mouse button twice without moving the mouse cursor [44, 59]. Click-and-drag (or drag-and-drop) tasks are challenging for older adults because of the need to position the cursor on two separate targets (the start and end of the drag) and the need to maintain pressure on the mouse button during the drag movement [22, 23, 32, 75]. Older adults can have difficulty with scrolling due to its visual and motor demands. Scrolling requires the user to locate and click on a small target, then hold down the mouse button while moving the mouse smoothly in the desired direction [1, 9, 22, 76]. Older adults can have problems navigating multilevel menu structures because of the underlying spatial reasoning requirements and the need to move the mouse cursor on a straight line within narrow confines [1, 20].

Older adults typically perform point-and-click tasks with the same accuracy as younger adults, but they require more time and effort to do so [9, 23, 44, 58–61, 63, 65, 70, 71, 74, 75, 77, 78]. Submovement analysis has shown that the movement strategies used by older adults are different from those used by younger adults. Older adults perform pointing tasks with a lower peak velocity, more submovements, a longer deceleration phase, and more frequent pauses [9, 16, 60, 65, 70, 71, 74, 77, 78]. Older adults are more affected than younger adults by increases in task difficulty, by either reducing the target size, increasing the distance to the target, or limiting the time available to complete the task [3, 23, 59–61, 71, 74, 79].

11.4.2 TEXT ENTRY

As with the mouse, older adults typically type more slowly than younger adults, but with no loss in accuracy [23, 80–82]. Age-related impairments in hand mobility can cause typing difficulties such as releasing a key before repeated keystrokes are registered or pressing two or more keys simultaneously [9, 11, 22, 76].

11.4.3 VISION

Due to reduced visual acuity, older adults can have trouble locating small targets like the mouse cursor or text caret, particularly when the targets are located outside of central vision [23, 55, 83]. Decreases in visual acuity, color perception, and contrast discrimination can also lead to difficulties in reading text printed in a font that is small or complex or text printed on a white background [16, 45]. Older adults also have difficulty reading text that is closely surrounded by other visual elements [16, 48].

Older adults can have problems seeing information at the top of the screen because they wear bifocals (which are designed to accommodate close vision in the lower half of the visual field) or due to conditions like ptosis (drooping eyelids) [22, 29, 83].

11.4.4 AUDITORY

Age-related hearing impairment can interfere with an older adult's ability to access audio and video files [2]. Older adults also have trouble understanding computer-generated voices [20].

11.4.5 COGNITIVE

Older adults take longer to learn new concepts or skills [21, 83]. Older learners can become confused when presented with more than one method for performing a task [83]. Older adults also have difficulty learning multistep tasks [21, 83]. Declines in the ability to share attention between multiple stimuli can make it difficult to switch attention between different information sources or process multiple forms of information (e.g., text and speech) simultaneously [21].

11.4.6 WEB BROWSING

Older adults have difficulty with several aspects of searching for information on the Internet [6, 9, 11, 16, 29, 50]. Overall, older adults tend to be slower and less efficient than younger adults [11, 16, 57, 84, 85]. Cognitive changes associated with aging, such as decreased working memory, decreased processing speed, and impaired spatial reasoning, can all impact the ability to navigate across web pages or between websites or recover after an error [1, 14, 16, 29, 57, 85]. Information overload is a common problem experienced by older adults. Older adults have more difficulty focusing attention, which can cause them to become easily distracted by irrelevant information and graphics on a web page or confused by poorly organized websites [2, 11, 14, 21, 49, 57].

Older adults also have difficulty detecting changes (e.g., minor updates) on a web page [3, 22]. Visual acuity, contrast discrimination, and color perception are all affected by the aging process, making it difficult to read text printed in a small font or against certain background colors, or distinguish text from a background image [2, 3, 22]. Decreasing motor coordination can make it difficult to scroll down a web page or click on a link [3, 16, 21, 49, 57].

11.5   INTERVENTIONS

11.5.1   KEYBOARD ACCESS

Encouraging older clients to use the keyboard for more tasks can help them be more efficient. Using the keyboard can also eliminate the need to click on small targets with the mouse cursor. However, many older adults are used to using the mouse and may have difficulty relearning how to perform tasks with the keyboard.

11.5.2   ALTERNATIVE POINTING DEVICE

It can be tempting to try a different pointing device, like a trackball or touch screen. However, investigators have observed varying (and conflicting) results when comparing older adults' performance across pointing devices and tasks [9, 10, 23, 31, 44, 60, 75, 83, 86, 87]. What seems clear is that, as with other populations, every older adult has a best pointing device, but no single pointing device is best for every older adult.

Some things to keep in mind:

- An older adult's problems with pointing may be physical (reduced manual dexterity), perceptual (difficulty seeing the target), or both.
- Cognitive changes associated with aging may make it difficult to learn to use a new device or strategy.
- Different devices may be appropriate for different tasks, depending on the precision required and the need to coordinate cursor movement with button activation [9, 44].
- Other concerns (some older adults don't see themselves as disabled, some older adults have a strong preference for a mouse or aversion to assistive technology) may outweigh the performance advantages of a new device.

Before trying a different pointing device:

- Will changes to the interface (control-display gain [9, 44, 60, 61], target size [1, 16, 56, 63, 71], double-click interval [48]) improve performance with the mouse?
- Will changes to strategy (more keyboard use) improve pointing performance?

TABLE 11.1

Guidelines for Training Older Adults to Use Computer Technology

- Minimize demands on working memory through the use of cues and aids.
- Provide feedback in a timely manner.
- Allow practice after each step.
- Provide extra time to read written instructions.
- Minimize distractions to allow people to focus on the training materials.
- Ensure optimal organization of training materials and provide a structure with clear identifiers, headings, and subheadings. Provide advance organizers such as overviews.
- Ensure that the reading level of all instructions and manuals matches the abilities of the user population.
- Use part-task training techniques such as simplification and segmentation.
- Present information explicitly to minimize need for inferences.
- Capitalize on the user's preexisting knowledge base (e.g., use analogies or metaphors).
- Model procedures to illustrate what the steps are.
- Allow extra time for training older adults (1.5 to 2 times the training time expected for young adults).
- Self-paced instruction enhances learning relative to fixed-paced instruction.
- Learning appears to be better when trainees are paired with a partner or taught in small groups, compared to learning alone or in large groups.

Source: Based on Rogers, W.A., A.J. Stronge, and A.D. Fisk, 2005; Fisk, A.D. et al., 2004; Jones, B.D., and U.J. Bayen, 1998; Morrell, R., and K. Echt, 1996; Morrell, R., and K. Echt, 1997 [9, 89–92].

11.5.3 TRAINING

Research has shown that computer training can be beneficial for older adults [9, 10, 16, 21, 44] as long as the training is designed with the needs of older adults in mind [9, 21, 88] (see Table 11.1). Older adults learn new skills more slowly than younger adults [9, 16, 21] and have more negative reactions to computer errors [9, 13, 24]. Begin training with a needs assessment to determine your client's needs [9].

11.5.4 ADDRESSING VISION PROBLEMS

Using a screen magnifier or screen reader may be too complicated for an older adult. Instead, try to use simpler options, like a bigger monitor with a low screen resolution [9, 22], a high-contrast color scheme [51], or changes in ambient lighting [48, 51]. Trade-offs to keep in mind:

- If you give someone a bigger display, but fill it with more stuff, you might actually decrease performance [60].
- Increasing the font size without increasing the display size may be counter-productive, because it will increase the amount of scrolling needed to read the same amount of text [20, 29].

11.5.5 TABLET COMPUTER

Another alternative is to use a tablet (e.g., an iPad) rather than a full-fledged computer. Tablets have a simplified user interface and can connect to an external monitor to provide a larger display. On the other hand, tablets rely on pointing and gesturing on a touch-sensitive screen, which can be difficult for older adults with poor aim or manual dexterity. An older adult may also be reluctant to give up the computer interface he or she is familiar with in order to relearn how to do everything on a tablet. Tablets also offer fewer accessibility options than a regular computer, so they are not accessible to all individuals.

REFERENCES

1. Arch, A. 2008, May 14. Web accessibility for older adults: A literature review. Available from http://www.w3.org/TR/wai-age-literature/ (accessed December 2, 2008).
2. Arch, A., S. Abou-Zahra, and S.L. Henry. 2009. Older users online: WAI guidelines address older users web experience. *User Experience Magazine* 8(1).
3. Becker, S.A. 2004. A study of web usability for older adults seeking online health resources. *ACM Transactions on Computer-Human Interaction* 11(4): 387–406.
4. Chadwick-Dias, A., M. McNulty, and T. Tullis. 2002. Web usability and age: How design changes can improve performance. In *ACM SIGCAPH Computers and the Physically Handicapped.* New York: ACM Press, pp. 30–37.
5. Eastman, J.K., and R. Iyer. 2004. The elderly's uses and attitudes towards the Internet. *Journal of Consumer Marketing* 21(3): 208–220.
6. Sharit, J. et al. 2008. Investigating the roles of knowledge and cognitive abilities in older adult information seeking on the web. *ACM Transactions on Computer-Human Interaction* 15(1): 1–25.
7. Federal Interagency Forum on Aging-Related Statistics. 2010. *Older Americans 2010: Key indicators of well-being.* Washington, DC: Federal Interagency Forum on Aging-Related Statistics.
8. Carpenter, B.D., and S. Buday. 2007. Computer use among older adults in a naturally occurring retirement community. *Computers in Human Behavior* 23: 3012–3024.
9. Rogers, W.A., A.J. Stronge, and A.D. Fisk. 2005. Technology and aging. *Reviews of Human Factors and Ergonomics* 1(1): 130–171.
10. Mann, W.C. et al. 2005. Computer use by middle-aged and older adults with disabilities. *Technology and Disability* 17(1): 1–9.
11. Arch, A. 2009. Web accessibility for older users: Successes and opportunities. In *2009 International Cross-Disciplinary Conference on Web Accessibililty (W4A)*, D. Sloan, ed. Madrid: ACM Press, pp. 1–6.
12. Hodes, R., and D. Lindberg. 2002. *Making your web site senior friendly.* National Institute on Aging and National Library of Medicine.
13. Wagner, N., K. Hassanein, and M. Head. 2010. Computer use by older adults: A multidisciplinary review. *Computers in Human Behavior* 26: 870–882.
14. Becker, S.A. 2005. E-Government usability for older adults. *Communications of the ACM* 48(2): 102–104.
15. Fairweather, P.G. 2008. How older and younger adults differ in their approach to problem solving on a complex website. In *10th International ACM SIGACCESS Conference on Computers and Accessibility (ASSETS '08)*, S. Harper, ed. Halifax, Canada: ACM Press, pp. 67–72.

16. Hanson, V.L. 2009. Age and web access: The next generation. In *2009 International Cross-Disciplinary Conference on Web Accessibililty (W4A)*, D. Sloan, ed. Madrid: ACM Press, pp. 7–15.

17. Jimison, H. et al. 2004. Unobtrusive monitoring of computer interactions to detect cognitive status in elders. *IEEE Transactions on Information Technology in Biomedicine* 8(3): 248–252.

18. Jones, S., and S. Fox. 2009. *Generations online in 2009*, P.I.A.L. Project, ed. Washington, DC: Pew Research Center.

19. Zickuhr, K. 2010. *Generations 2010*. Washington, DC: Pew Research Center.

20. Holt, B. 2000. *Creating senior-friendly web sites*. Washington, DC: Center for Medicare Education.

21. Czaja, S.J., and C.C. Lee. 2007. The impact of aging on access to technology. *Universal Access in the Information Society* 5(4): 341–349.

22. Hanson, V.L. 2001. Web access for elderly citizens. In *2001 EC/NSF Workshop on Universal Accessibility of Ubiquitous Computing: Providing for the Elderly*, R. Heller, ed. Alcacer do Sal, Portugal: ACM Press, pp. 14–18.

23. Taveira, A.D., and S.D. Choi. 2009. Review study of computer input devices and older users. *International Journal of Human-Computer Interaction* 25(5): 455–474.

24. Saunders, E.J. 2004. Maximizing computer use among the elderly in rural senior centers. *Educational Gerontology* 30(7): 573–585.

25. McMellon, C.A., and L.G. Schiffman. 2002. Cybersenior empowerment: How some older individuals are taking control of their lives. *Journal of Applied Gerontology* 21(2): 157–175.

26. Shapira, N., A. Barak, and I. Gal. 2007. Promoting older adults' well-being through Internet training and use. *Aging and Mental Health* 11(5): 477–484.

27. Fokkema, T., and K. Knipscheer. 2007. Escape loneliness by going digital: A quantitative and qualitative evaluation of a Dutch experiment in using ECT to overcome loneliness among older adults. *Aging and Mental Health* 11(5): 496–504.

28. Karavidas, M., N.K. Lim, and S.L. Katsikas. 2005. The effects of computers on older adult users. *Computers in Human Behavior* 21: 697–711.

29. Grahame, M., J. Laberge, and C.T. Scialfa. 2004. Age differences in search of web pages: The effects of link size, link number, and clutter. *Human Factors* 46(3): 385–398.

30. Billip, S. 2001. The psychosocial impact of interactive computer use within a vulnerable elderly population: A report on a randomized prospective trial in a home health care setting. *Public Health Nursing* 18(2): 138–145.

31. Wood, E. et al. 2005. Use of computer input devices by older adults. *Journal of Applied Gerontology* 24(5): 419–438.

32. Jacko, J.A. et al. 2004. Isolating the effects of visual impairment: Exploring the effect of AMD on the utility of multimodal feedback. In *SIGCHI Conference on Human Factors in Computing Systems*, E. Dykstra-Erickson and M. Tschcligi, eds. Vienna: ACM Press, pp. 311–318.

33. Vuori, S., and M. Holmlund-Rytkonen. 2005. 55+ people as Internet users. *Marketing Intelligence and Planning* 23(1): 58–76.

34. Hendrix, C. 2000. Computer use among elderly people. *Computers in Nursing* 18(2): 62–68.

35. Dickinson, A. et al. 2007. Approaches to web search and navigation for older computer novices. In SIGCHI Conference on Human Factors in Computing Systems, M.B. Rosson, ed. San Jose, CA: ACM Press, pp. 281–290.

36. Morrel, R., C. Mayhorn, and J. Bennett. 2000. A survey of World Wide Web use in middle-aged and older adults. *Human Factors* 42(2): 175–182.

37. Fisk, A.D., and W.A. Rogers. 2002. Psychology and aging: Enhancing the lives of an aging population. *Current Directions in Psychological Science* 11(3): 107–110.

38. Frissen, V. 2005. The myth of the digital divide. In *E-merging media: Communication and the media economy of the future*, A. Zerdick, et al., eds. Berlin: Springer, pp. 271–284.

39. Selwyn, N. et al. 2003. Older adults' use of information technology in everyday life. *Aging and Society* 23(5): 561–582.

40. Melenhorst, A., W.A. Rogers, and D. Bouwhuis. 2006. Older adults' motivated choice for technological innovation: Evidence for benefit-driven selectivity. *Psychology and Aging* 21(1): 190–195.

41. Morris, A., J. Goodman, and H. Brading. 2007. Internet use and non-use: Views of older users. *Universal Access in the Information Society* 6(1): 43–57.

42. Peacock, S., and H. Kunemund. 2007. Senior citizens and Internet technology: Reasons and correlates of access versus non-access in a European comparative perspective. *European Journal of Ageing* 4(4): 191–200.

43. Brajnik, G., Y. Yesilada, and S. Harper. 2009. Guideline aggregation: Web accessibility evaluation for older users. In *2009 International Cross-Disciplinary Conference on Web Accessibility (W4A)*, D. Sloan, ed. Madrid: ACM Press, pp. 127–135.

44. Charness, N. et al. 2004. Light pen use and practice minimize age and hand performance differences in pointing tasks. *Human Factors* 46(3): 373–384.

45. Zaphiris, P., S.H. Kurniawan, and M. Ghiawadwala. 2007. A systematic approach to the development of research-based web design guidelines for older people. *Universal Access in the Information Society* 6(1): 59–75.

46. Trewin, S. 2002. Extending keyboard adaptability: An investigation. *Universal Access in the Information Society* 2(1): 44–55.

47. Strobel, W. et al. 2006. Technology for access to text and graphics for people with visual impairments and blindness in vocational settings. *Journal of Vocational Rehabilitation* 24: 87–95.

48. Nunes, F., P.A. Silva, and F. Abrantes. 2010. Human-computer interaction and the older adult: An example using user research and personas. In *PETRA '10: The 3rd International Conference on Pervasive Technologies Related to Assistive Environments*, F. Makedon, I. Maglogiannis, and S. Kapidakis, eds. Samos, Greece: ACM Press.

49. Curran, K., N. Walters, and D. Robinson. 2007. Investigating the problems faced by older adults and people with disabilities in online environments. *Behaviour and Information Technology* 26(6): 447–453.

50. Arch, A. 2008. *Web accessibility for older users: A literature review*. Cambridge, MA: World Wide Web Consortium.

51. Boyce, P. 2003. Lighting for the elderly. *Technology and Disability* 15(3): 165–180.

52. Kline, D., and C.T. Scialfa. 1997. Sensory and perceptual functioning: Basic research and human factors implications. In *Handbook of human factors and the older adult*, A.D. Fisk and W.A. Rogers, eds. San Diego: Academic, pp. 27–54.

53. Fiorentini, A. et al. 1996. Visual ageing: Unspecific decline of the responses to luminance and color. *Vision Research* 36(21): 3557–3566.

54. Schieber, F. 2003. Human factors and aging: Identifying and compensating for age-related deficits in sensory and cognitive function. In *Impact of technology on successful aging*, N. Charness and K. Schaie, eds. New York: Springer, pp. 42–84.

55. Leonard, V.K., J.A. Jacko, and J.J. Pizzimenti. 2005. An exploratory investigation of handheld computer interaction for older adults with visual impairments. In *7th International ACM SIGACCESS Conference on Computers and Accessibility* A. Sears and E. Pontelli, eds. Baltimore: ACM Press, pp. 12–19.

56. Scott, I.U., W.J. Feuer, and J. Jacko. 2002. Impact of graphical user interface screen features on computer task accuracy and speed in a cohort of patients with age-related macular degeneration. *American Journal of Opthalmology* 134(6): 857–862.

57. Hart, T.A., B.S. Chaparro, and C.G. Halcomb. 2008. Evaluating websites for older adults: Adherence to "senior-friendly" guidelines and end-user performance. *Behaviour and Information Technology* 27(3): 191–199.
58. Hwang, F., H. Batson, and N. Williams. 2008. Bringing the target to the cursor: Proxy targets for older adults. In *CHI '08 extended abstracts on human factors in computing systems*, M. Czerwinski and A. Lund, eds. Florence, Italy: ACM Press, pp. 2775–2780.
59. Mahmud, M., and H. Kurniawan. 2005. Involving psychometric tests for input device evaluation with older people. In *17th Australia Conference on Computer-Human Interaction: Citizens Online: Considerations for Today and the Future*, A. Donaldson, ed. Canberra, Australia: ACM Press, pp. 1–10.
60. Hertzum, M., and K. Hornbaek. 2010. How age affects pointing with mouse and touch-pad: A comparison of young, adult, and elderly users. *International Journal of Human-Computer Interaction* 26(7): 703–734.
61. Sandfeld, J., and B. Jensen. 2005. Effect of computer mouse gain and visual demand on mouse clicking performance and muscle activation in a young and elderly group of experienced computer users. *Applied Ergonomics* 36(5): 547–555.
62. Fozard, J.L. et al. 1994. Age differences and changes in reaction time: The Baltimore longitudinal study of aging. *Journal of Gerontology* 49(4): 179–189.
63. Bohan, M., and D. Scarlett. 2003. Can expanding targets make object selection easier for older adults? *Usability News* 5(1).
64. Ketcham, C.J., and G.E. Stelmach. 2001. Age-related declines in motor control. In *Handbook of the psychology of aging*, J. Birren and K. Schaie, eds. San Diego: Academic, pp. 313–339.
65. Walker, N., D.A. Philbin, and A.D. Fisk. 1997. Age-related differences in move-ment control: Adjusting submovement structure to optimize performance. *Journal of Gerontology: Psychological Sciences* 52B(1): P40–P53.
66. Craik, F. 2000. Age-related changes in human memory. In *Cognitive aging: A primer*, D. Park and N. Schwartz, eds. Philadelphia: Taylor & Francis, pp. 75–92.
67. Zacks, R., L. Hasher, and K. Li. 2000. Human memory. In *The handbook of aging and cognition*, F. Craik and T. Salthouse, eds. Mahwah, NJ: Erlbaum, pp. 295–358.
68. Rogers, W.A., and A.D. Fisk. 2000. Human factors, applied cognition, and aging. In *The handbook of aging and cognition*, F. Craik and T. Salthouse, eds. Mahwah, NJ: Erlbaum, pp. 559–591.
69. Rogers, W.A., and A.D. Fisk. 2001. Understanding the role of attention in cognitive aging research. In *Handbook of the psychology of aging*, J. Birren and K. Schaie, eds. San Diego: Academic, pp. 267–287.
70. Keates, S., and S. Trewin. 2005. Effect of age and Parkinson's disease on cursor posi-tioning using a mouse. In *7th International ACM SIGACCESS Conference on Computers and Accessibility*, A. Sears and E. Pontelli, eds. Baltimore: ACM Press, pp. 68–75.
71. Lee, D., S. Kwon, and M.K. Chung. 2012. Effects of user age and target-expansion methods on target-acquisition tasks using a mouse. *Applied Ergonomics* 43(1): 166–175.
72. Laursen, B., B.R. Jensen, and A. Ratkevicius. 2001. Performance and muscle activity during computer mouse tasks in young and elderly adults. *European Journal of Applied Physiology* 84(4): 329–336.
73. Ranganathan, V.K. et al. 2001. Effects of aging on hand function. *Journal of the American Geriatrics Society* 49(11): 1478–1484.
74. Smith, M.W., J. Sharit, and S.J. Czaja. 1999. Aging, motor control, and the performance of computer mouse tasks. *Human Factors* 41(3): 389–396.
75. Chaparro, A. et al. 1999. Is the trackball a better input device for the older computer user? *Journal of Occupational Rehabilitation* 9(1): 33–43.

76. Richards, J.T., and V.L. Hanson. 2004. Web accessibility: A broader view. In *13th International Conference on the World Wide Web*, S. Feldman and M. Uretsky, eds. New York: ACM Press, pp. 72–79.

77. Iwase, H., and A. Murata. 2002. Comparison of mouse performance between young and elderly—Basic study for designing mouse proper for elderly. In *2002 IEEE International Conference on Systems, Man and Cybernetics*, A. El Kamel, K. Mellouli, and P. Borne, eds. Yasmine Hammamet, Tunisa: IEEE, pp. 246–251.

78. Ketcham, C.J. et al. 2002. Age-related kinematic differences as influenced by task difficulty, target size, and movement amplitude. *Journal of Gerontology: Psychological Sciences* 57B(1): P54–P64.

79. Riviere, C.N., and N.V. Thakor. 1996. Effects of age and disability on tracking tasks with a computer mouse: Accuracy and linearity. *Journal of Rehabilitation Research and Development* 33(1): 6–15.

80. Bosman, E.A. 1993. Age-related differences in the motoric aspects of transcription typing skill. *Psychology and Aging* 8(1): 87–102.

81. Bosman, E.A., and N. Charness. 1996. Age-related differences in skilled performance and skill acquisition. In *Perspectives on cognitive change in adulthood and aging*, F. Blamchard-Fields and T. Hess, eds. New York: McGraw-Hill, pp. 428–453.

82. Salthouse, T.A. 1984. Effects of age and skill in typing. *Journal of Experimental Psychology: General* 113(3): 345–371.

83. Dickinson, A., R. Eisma, and P. Gregor. 2011. The barriers that older novices encounter to computer use. *Universal Access in the Information Society* 10(3): 261–266.

84. Czaja, S.J. et al. 2001. Examining age differences in performance of a complex information search and retrieval task. *Psychology and Aging* 16(4): 564–579.

85. Mead, S.E. et al. 2000. Influences of general computer experience and age on library database search performance. *Behaviour and Information Technology* 19(2): 107–123.

86. Iwase, H., and A. Murata. 2003. Empirical study on the improvement of the usability of a touch panel for the elderly—Comparison of usability between a touch panel and a mouse. *IEICE Transactions on Information and Systems* E86-D(6): 1134–1138.

87. Murata, A. 2005. Usability of touch-panel interfaces for older adults. *Human Factors* 47(4): 767–776.

88. Rogers, W.A., R. Campbell, and R. Pak. 2001. A systems approach for training older adults to use technology. In *Communication, technology and aging: Opportunities and challenges for the future*, N. Charness and D. Park, eds. New York: Springer, pp. 187–208.

89. Fisk, A.D. et al. 2004. *Designing for older adults: Principles and creative human factors approaches*. Boca Raton, FL: CRC Press.

90. Jones, B.D., and U.J. Bayen. 1998. Teaching older adults to use computers: Recommendations based on cognitive aging research. *Educational Gerontology* 24(7): 675–689.

91. Morrell, R., and K. Echt. 1996. Instructional design for older computer users: The influence of cognitive factors. In *Aging and skilled performance: Advances in theory and application*, W.A. Rogers, A.D. Fisk, and N. Walker, eds. Mahwah, NJ: Erlbaum, pp. 241–265.

92. Morrell, R., and K. Echt. 1997. Designing written instructions for older adults: Learning to use computers. In *Handbook of human factors and the older adult*, A.D. Fisk and W.A. Rogers, eds. San Diego: Academic, pp. 335–361.

12 Web Accessibility

12.1 INTRODUCTION

Most clinicians and consumers think of themselves as web users rather than web programmers. However, anyone who creates a profile on Facebook or posts videos on YouTube is, in some sense, creating a web page. This chapter will focus on what users and clinicians can do to increase their access to existing websites. We will not focus on design guidelines or tools for website designers.

When someone is browsing the web, there are two interfaces that have to be negotiated: the web page and the browser. Some computer access technologies (especially things that are built in to the browser) only work on the web page. The advantage of computer access technology that is integrated with the web browser is that it typically has access to more information about the web page being displayed, including the underlying HTML that defines the web page. This is not always true, however. For example, the JAWS screen reader is tightly integrated with the Internet Explorer web browser, in spite of being a separate piece of software. The primary disadvantages of browser-specific tools are that they can't be used with applications outside the browser and they are not typically as sophisticated as general-purpose computer access technology.

12.2 WHY ARE WEBSITES INACCESSIBLE?

Intuitively, a website's accessibility is determined by the range of people who can successfully use that site [1]. A website that is highly accessible can be used by more people than a website that is not. In practice, no website of even moderate complexity can be completely accessible to all users [2, 3].

Of course, very few people intentionally set out to design an inaccessible website. The whole point of creating a website, after all, is to attract attention. So why have so many studies documented the prevalence of partially or completely inaccessible websites [1, 4, 5]?

Many developers don't know much about web accessibility standards [1, 5]. This is complicated by the existence of multiple standards. Developers also lack tools for evaluating their website against the standards. The largest websites are constantly being updated from multiple sources simultaneously, with some content (like advertisements) being provided by third parties. Constantly evaluating these websites for accessibility is a huge undertaking. In addition, most people who develop websites aren't assistive technology (AT) experts. Finally, even if a website developer wanted to test his or her website with AT and had access to AT, he or she would probably have problems because of his or her lack of familiarity with AT [6].

Websites are often developed using drag-and-drop authoring tools that automate many elements of website design. These tools greatly simplify the task of building a website, but they often don't support accessibility [5]. For example, many drag-and-drop website authoring software specifies the font to be used for each web page, interfering with a web browser's ability to substitute a font that is easier for the user to read [2].

12.3   MEASURING WEBSITE ACCESSIBILITY

People are always looking for a single number with which to compare things. We give ratings to movies, restaurants, wine, hotels, books, and all sorts of things. We accept that these single numbers aren't definitive, that they abstract away the nuances of the underlying experience, and that some people will inevitably disagree with subjective ratings. The danger with website accessibility ratings is that they are often presented as applying equally to all user populations, regardless of disability or access technology.

The accessibility of a website can't be boiled down to a single number, no matter how much we want it to be. A website's accessibility for someone who is blind and uses a screen reader and Braille display has little bearing on the same website's accessibility for someone with a spinal cord injury who uses a head-mounted mouse emulator. In some cases, design choices that enhance a website's accessibility for one population can decrease accessibility for another population [3]. For example, a website design with lots of graphics and icons may be useful for someone with a cognitive impairment but can be extremely inefficient for someone with a visual impairment.

Automated accessibility evaluation tools do not work very well [5, 6]. Automated tools can examine the structure of a website, but not its content. They are unable to determine whether the content of a website, including descriptive text associated with pictures, charts, and tables, is logical, understandable, or intuitive [5]. Automated accessibility evaluation tools fail to consider the interaction between multiple disabilities. Automated tools also don't consider the goal of the user [4]. Different people may use the same website for very different things.

Automated accessibility evaluation tools lack human judgment [6, 7]. Unfortunately, manually evaluating a website for accessibility is time-consuming. It also requires a significant amount of training to understand the needs of different user populations and the capabilities of different types of computer access technology [6].

12.4   INTERVENTIONS

Other chapters in this book have focused on general-purpose computer access technology. This chapter will focus on interventions that are implemented within the web browser itself. The interventions described below are going to be most useful for consumers who spend most of their computer time within the web browser.

12.4.1   CHANGES TO FONT OR COLOR SCHEME

Individuals who have difficulty reading text within a web page, due to either a visual or literacy impairment, may benefit from changes to the font with which text is displayed, including [8]

- Increasing the font size
- Choosing a sans serif font style
- Increasing the interletter spacing

Many web browsers offer the ability to choose a default font for displaying text. It is important to note, however, that the user must typically specify that the default font is to be used even if the website specifies a different font. Also keep in mind that a website that is designed for a specific font and font size may not display properly if a different font is used.

Individuals with visual or literacy impairments may also benefit from changes to the color scheme used by web pages. The same cautions about changing the font also apply to the color scheme. In addition, many web pages use a picture for their background, which will not be affected by a change to the color scheme (Figures 12.1 and 12.2).

12.4.2 Text to Speech

Individuals with cognitive or visual impairments may prefer to have the contents of a web page read out loud by the web browser, rather than having to read it themselves. Several web browsers offer extensions or plug-ins that provide text-to-speech capability. These plug-ins are typically much less sophisticated than a full-fledged screen reader. However, this simplicity can be an advantage for individuals who do not need (or cannot use) more complex software.

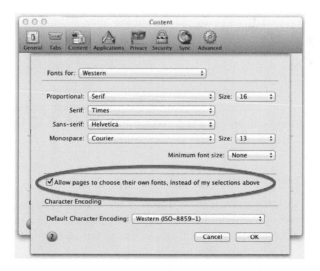

FIGURE 12.1   Dialog box for choosing the default font in Mozilla Firefox® (v12.0) web browser. Note the option for forcing websites to display text in the chosen font.

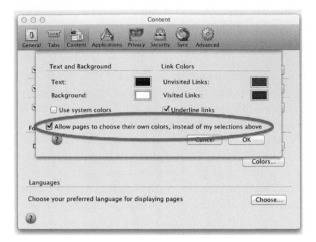

FIGURE 12.2   Dialog box for choosing the default colors in Mozilla Firefox (v12.0) web browser. Note the option for forcing websites to use the chosen color scheme.

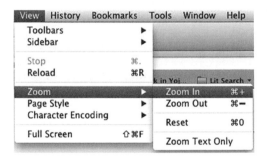

FIGURE 12.3   Menu option for increasing the magnification (zooming in) or decreasing the magnification (zooming out) of a web page within Mozilla Firefox (v12.0).

12.4.3   PAGE MAGNIFICATION

Many web browsers allow the user to magnify the contents of a web page [8]. This is different from using a screen magnifier in that only the web page itself is magnified, and not anything else on the screen (including the interface for the web browser itself) (Figure 12.3).

12.4.4   LINEARIZE CONTENT

Some web browsers allow the user to linearize the contents of a web page, either through the browser or a plug-in. Linearizing a web page reduces a multiple column format to a single column [8, 9], which can be useful for users with [8]

- Low vision who want to reduce screen clutter
- Cognitive limitations who similarly want to reduce screen clutter
- Limited manual dexterity who wish to reduce horizontal scrolling requirements

The downside to linearizing content is that the computer isn't going to be smart about how the content is modified, and text may be jumbled or displayed out of order.

12.4.5   ELIMINATE GRAPHICS

Most web browsers allow the user to prevent images from loading. This removes all pictures, backgrounds, and animations, leaving only text [8]. This option was originally intended for users downloading websites over slow network connections, but it is also useful for clients who use screen readers or text-to-speech software and clients with cognitive impairments who can become distracted or confused.

The principal limitation of this approach is that the only option available (typically) is to eliminate all images from every web page, without exception. While this approach is straightforward, some images are critical for understanding some web pages and eliminating all images can render them useless (Figure 12.4).

12.4.6   USE THE MOBILE VERSION OF A WEBSITE

Some websites (and the number is increasing) design separate web pages for the full-featured web browsers used on a computer and the stripped-down mobile web browsers used by handheld computing devices, like smart phones. By default, a web browser on a computer is steered to the full-featured web pages, but it is possible to access some mobile websites from desktop browsers. One downside to this approach is that some content on the full website may not be available on the mobile website. A second possible problem is that because mobile devices do not support nearly as much computer access technology as a computer, a mobile website may not be designed to work well with assistive technology (Figure 12.5).

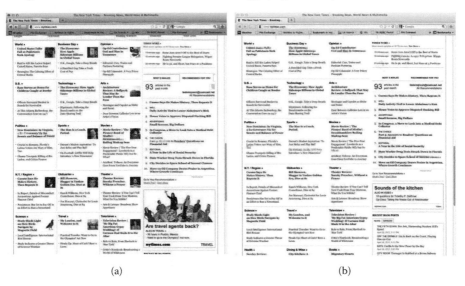

(a)   (b)

FIGURE 12.4   Picture of the same web page displayed (a) with and (b) without images using Mozilla Firefox (v12.0).

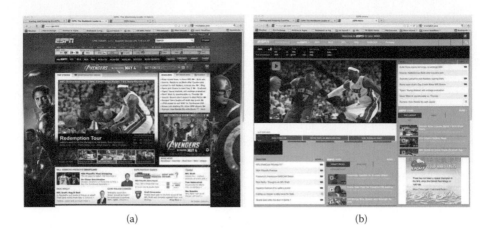

(a) (b)

FIGURE 12.5 **(See color insert.)** Picture of the same website accessed through (a) the traditional website and (b) the mobile version of the website, using Mozilla Firefox (v12.0).

12.4.7 CASCADING STYLE SHEETS

Cascading style sheets (CSS) allow you to modify how a web page looks [9]. A style sheet instructs the browser how to display the content of a web page. Every HTML tag is defined in a style sheet, which specifies the size, color, position, and other characteristics [9]. Style sheets are called cascading because there can be multiple places where styles are defined. The user's style sheet has the highest precedence. Styles defined by the user will override styles defined anywhere else within a website [9]. Keep in mind that using your own style sheet may make a website difficult to read or use. A style sheet also has no effect on the content of graphics within a web page.

REFERENCES

1. Curran, K., N. Walters, and D. Robinson. 2007. Investigating the problems faced by older adults and people with disabilities in online environments. *Behaviour and Information Technology* 26(6): 447–453.
2. Hanson, V.L. 2009. Age and web access: The next generation. In *2009 International Cross-Disciplinary Conference on Web Accessibililty (W4A)*, D. Sloan, ed. Madrid: ACM Press, pp. 7–15.
3. WebAIM. 2010. Design considerations—One size fits all? Available from http://www.webaim.org/articles/design/ (accessed December 22, 2010).
4. Hart, T.A., B.S. Chaparro, and C.G. Halcomb. 2008. Evaluating websites for older adults: Adherence to "senior-friendly" guidelines and end-user performance. *Behaviour and Information Technology* 27(3): 191–199.
5. Power, C., and H. Jurgensen. 2010. Accessible presentation of information for people with visual disabilities. *Universal Access in the Information Society* 9(2): 97–119.
6. WebAIM. 2010. Planning, evaluation, repair and maintenance. Available from http://webaim.org/articles/process/ (accessed December 30, 2010).
7. WebAIM. 2010. Evaluating cognitive web accessibility. Available from http://webaim.org/articles/evaluatingcognitive/ (accessed December 22, 2010).

8. Richards, J.T., and V.L. Hanson. 2004. Web accessibility: A broader view. In *13th International Conference on the World Wide Web*, S. Feldman and M. Uretsky, eds. New York: ACM Press, pp. 72–79.
9. WebAIM. 2010. Creating accessible CSS. Available from http://webaim.org/techniques/css/ (accessed December 30, 2010).

13 Ergonomics

13.1 INTRODUCTION

The word *ergonomics* derives from the Greek words *ergon* (work) and *nomos* (laws) to denote the science of work [1]. Ergonomics provides theoretical principles, empirical data, and design methods for optimizing human well-being and performance during work activities [1]. The goal of ergonomics is to fit the work environment to the person, which is a marked change in practice from previous decades, where it was the person who was made to fit. Ergonomics spans the physical, cognitive, and organizational aspects of work, but this chapter will focus exclusively on the aspects of ergonomics that directly relate to computer access.

Seating and positioning should be the first part of any computer access assessment. This is true for anyone who uses a computer, whether they have a physical or sensory impairment or represent the typical computer user. The success of almost any computer access intervention is going to depend on adequate seating and positioning of the client. Furthermore, you want to make sure your intervention isn't going to lead to new problems down the road through poor positioning.

13.2 MUSCULOSKELETAL DISORDERS

Our emphasis in this chapter is on the use of ergonomics to design computer access interventions that treat the onset or reduce the risk of musculoskeletal disorders (MSDs). MSD is the term adopted by Occupational Safety and Health Administration (OSHA) and is widely used in the United States, but there are many other names for these disorders that you might encounter, including [2]

- Cumulative trauma disorders
- Repetitive strain injuries (used in the United States and UK)
- Occupational cervicobrachial disorders (used in Scandinavian countries and Japan)
- Overuse syndromes (used in sports medicine)
- Regional musculoskeletal disorders (used by rheumatologists)
- Work-related disorders (used by the World Health Organization)
- Repeated trauma disorders (used by the Bureau of Labor Statistics)
- Work-related musculoskeletal disorders (used in ergonomics)

MSDs are regional impairments of muscles, tendons, tendon sheaths, ligaments, nerves, spinal discs, blood vessels, bursae, and joints associated with activity-related repetitive mechanical trauma [2–6]. Unlike strains and sprains, MSDs are not typically the result of a single event (such as a slip, trip, or fall) but reflect a more gradual or chronic development [2, 4]. These conditions result in pain and functional impairment and may affect the neck, shoulders, elbows, forearms, wrists, and hands [6].

13.3   RISK FACTORS

MSDs are caused by a complex interaction of factors having to do with job activities, individual physiology, the work environment, technology, management, and sociology, as well as nonwork activities and environments [2]. As a result, there are few definitive answers about what causes MSDs [7]. There is general agreement regarding what risk factors can contribute to developing an MSD, but much less consensus about which risk factors are most important or how these risk factors might interact.

13.3.1   REPETITIVE ACTIONS

The human body is not designed to perform highly repetitive tasks, even if the movements require very little force [8]. In particular, repetitive work is a risk factor for MSD when the frequency of repetition exceeds the ability of the soft tissues to recover from this exertion [9, 10]. Computer users who spend a significant amount of time typing are particularly at risk. Some research suggests that human tendons cannot tolerate more than 1,500 to 2,000 exertions per hour [2], but keyboard work can involve many thousands of finger movements [9, 11]. At 5 letters per word and 50 words per minute, a keyboardist performs 90,000 digit flexions, each followed by a digit extension, over 6 hours of work [3].

Some people with neuromuscular, orthopedic, or sensory impairments may be especially at risk because they use a smaller set of actions more often to access the computer. For example, a computer user who is blind will access the computer entirely through the keyboard, which increases the number of keystrokes he or she must enter compared to someone using both the keyboard and mouse. At the extreme, a single-switch user will use a single motion repeatedly to access the computer. To date, no research exists to determine how existing disabilities and the use of alternative computer access methods interact to increase the risk of MSDs.

13.3.2   EXCESSIVE FORCE OR EXERTION

People don't normally think of operating a computer as involving large amounts of force, but even small exertions can cause stress if small muscles are involved [12]. The repetitive nature of typing and pointing may result in enough cumulative fingertip force throughout the workday to contribute to MSDs such as carpal tunnel syndrome and tenosynovitis [13, 14]. In addition, some individuals with disabilities may have to use smaller/weaker muscles to access buttons, keys, or switches, or to operate a pointing device. Low-force switches and joysticks are available, but the long-term effects of using these devices are unknown. Finally, some individuals with disabilities, particularly those with tremors or spasticity, can have difficulty regulating the amount of force they apply or may have to work harder to access small targets.

Another source of excessive exertion can come from maintaining one's work posture. Unless support is provided, effort is required to keep the hands, arms, and trunk in their working positions [3], and this effort is physiologically equivalent to generating a force [15]. In fact, holding a position for a long time requires a longer recovery time than an equivalent period of equivalent repeated movements [2]. In addition, maintaining a static posture for an extended period of time reduces blood flow, depletes nutrients, and leads to a buildup of harmful metabolic wastes. This causes fatigue and, over a long period, can result in permanent damage [2].

13.3.3 WORK DURATION

Work duration refers to both the amount of computer use between breaks and the total amount of computer use per day. More than 25% of the workforce uses a computer for at least 4 hours per day [16], and there is a consistent association between keyboarding more than 4 hours per day and MSDs [11, 16–21]. Also keep in mind that some people with disabilities may use the computer extensively, for work, relaxation, augmentative communication, and environmental control.

13.3.4 AWKWARD/EXTREME POSTURES

Working with parts of the body in awkward, overextended, or unbalanced positions can lead to MSDs because awkward positions press on nerves, stretch tendons, or otherwise push and pull tissues beyond their normal capacity [2]. Any joint position significantly different from neutral is considered to be a risk factor for MSDs, where neutral is considered to be the position about halfway through the available range of motion for a joint [12]. Some things to look for when evaluating a client's workstation are

- Is the client able to access objects on the workstation without significant reaching, especially reaching that is held for long durations, is repetitive, or requires trunk/torso deviations [22]?
- Does the client frequently reach more than 15 inches forward or to the side [2]?
- Does the client frequently reach to shoulder height or above [2]?
- Does the client lean to one side for long periods [2]?

Some individuals with disabilities naturally adopt postures that would otherwise be considered awkward due to muscle weakness, spasticity, or orthopedic deformities (e.g., scoliosis, kyphosis, lordosis). Don't try to force clients to adopt neutral postures that they cannot maintain. Instead, find a solution that accommodates their posture and limits the risks it poses to their health. If this is beyond your skill set, refer the individual to an occupational or physical therapist knowledgeable about technologies for seating and postural control.

Similarly, some individuals are forced into awkward postures because of their assistive technologies. For example, a visually impaired computer may position a Braille display directly in front of the keyboard, requiring the user to reach over the Braille display to type. Positioning the Braille display on the work surface and the keyboard on a keyboard tray beneath the work surface can eliminate the need to reach.

13.3.5 STATIC POSTURES

Working in one unchanging position or static posture is associated with the development of MSDs [23]. Clients with mobility impairments may maintain a static posture because they have difficulty switching between positions. They may need external or technological assistance to shift position (e.g., wheelchairs with tilt or recline features) or to rearrange their workstation once they have shifted position (e.g., extending a keyboard tray, raising or lowering the work surface).

Clients with limited sensation (e.g., spinal cord injury [SCI]) may not perceive the buildup of pressure, moisture, or temperature that cue able-bodied individuals to shift position. Clients with cognitive impairments may not remember to shift position often enough. These individuals may benefit from software that cues them to change position periodically.

Remember that there is no one perfect posture, and that frequent posture changes are a good way to reduce stress and redistribute pressure related to maintaining a static posture for a long duration [22–25]. The ideal work environment supports frequent posture changes without requiring your client to adopt extreme positions [9, 26]. This is not the same as a workstation that forces the user to maintain 90° angles at the ankle, knee, hips, and elbows [23, 27]. Generally, people can only maintain a rigidly upright posture for a few minutes and will naturally shift to a slightly reclined posture, if given the opportunity [26, 28–30].

Voluntary posture change may be more important for computer users because using a computer requires little involuntary posture change. Increasingly, computer users are sending and receiving mail, filing, getting phone messages, and even attending meetings via their computers [10]. Voluntary postural changes should be encouraged when using the computer. Even postures that look awkward may be acceptable if they are used for short-term relief from the discomfort caused by sustained, fixed postures [12, 27, 31, 32].

The goal for designing a client's workstation should therefore be to support easy and frequent readjustment between many positions, rather than finding a single fixed position that will be kept for the entire day [33]. Unfortunately, most office furniture is not adjustable enough, and most adjustable office furniture does not make it quick or easy to switch among postures quickly [23]. Keep this in mind when selecting office furniture.

13.3.6 LOCALIZED PRESSURE

The main effect of a hard or sharp edge in direct contact with part of the body is to increase external pressure in that area [8]. Too much external pressure on muscles, blood vessels, nerves, and tendons can lead to inflammation, reduced blood flow, and paresthesia. Over time, constant pressure can cause MSDs [2, 9, 12]. Individuals with limited sensation (e.g., SCI) may be at particular risk because they do not perceive localized pressure on some parts of their body.

13.3.7 GLARE

Glare can be either direct or reflected. Direct glare is caused by a light source (artificial lights or windows) shining directly into the eyes [34]. Reflected glare, such as on computer screens, can sometimes cause eyestrain, but its worst effect may be causing a worker to change posture in order to see well [34].

13.3.8   PSYCHOSOCIAL RISK FACTORS

An often overlooked source of risk for MSDs is the psychosocial work environment [5, 6, 35]. The term *psychosocial* describes factors that fall within three separate domains: (1) the job and work environment, (2) the extra-work environment, and (3) the individual worker [5]. The effect of psychosocial factors on the development of MSDs is more modest than biomechanical factors, but is consistent [36]. Psychosocial factors that have been identified as risk factors for MSDs include [2, 5, 6, 8, 12, 16, 18, 36]

- Perceptions of intensified workload
- Limited task diversity
- Limited job control
- Low job clarity
- Lack of social support from colleagues and superiors
- Low decision latitude
- Time pressure
- Mental stress
- Job dissatisfaction
- Isolation
- Boredom
- Unclear rules
- Job insecurity
- Management-labor conflicts
- Major workplace changes

13.4   THE ERGONOMICS TOOLBOX

Approaches to MSD prevention include changes to the workspace, the tools used to perform the work, and the work itself. Other approaches include administrative controls, training, organized exercise, and using personal protective equipment to reduce exposures [37]. MSDs often cannot be adequately dealt with without using multiple approaches in combination [12].

13.4.1   CHAIRS

Office workers spend a lot of time sitting. Professional-level office workers spend about 70% of their time (up to 80,000 hours over a career) sitting [10, 33]. Some workers such as telephone operators, telemarketers, and data entry workers spend nearly 100% of their working time sitting [10]. Hence, choosing an appropriate office chair can go a long ways toward preventing MSDs.

13.4.1.1   Seat Pan

The seat pan is the "business end" of a seat, the one part that every seat has to have. The seat pan should be contoured to allow even weight distribution and it should be comfortable to sit on [38]. A seat pan that is too wide or too deep may prevent the sitter from taking advantage of the armrests and the backrest [39]. When your client sits in the chair, the seat pan should be at least 1 inch wider than his or her hips and thighs on either side [22, 38] and should have a curved or "waterfall" front edge to prevent pressure on the back of the knees [22, 28, 38]. The seat depth (the distance from the front of the seat pan to the back) should allow the back to be supported by the backrest while fully supporting the thighs and maintaining a gap between the back of the knees and the front of the seat [24, 28, 38, 40]. A seat pan that is too long will press against the sensitive back of the knees and encourage the user to slouch or slide forward or to sit further forward, losing the benefit of contact with the backrest. Some chairs allow the seat pan depth to be adjusted, either by an adjustment that moves the backrest or by a sliding seat pan [10, 41] (Figure 13.1).

Almost all office chairs include a mechanism for adjusting the seat pan height. Most chairs are pneumatically adjustable, but some chairs have a mechanical height adjustment (threaded or spinning) mechanism [38]. The pneumatic mechanisms are a better choice for someone who will be transferring into the chair from a wheelchair because the chair's height can be adjusted much more quickly.

The height of the seat pan should be adjusted so your client's thighs are approximately parallel to the floor and his or her feet can be placed flat on the floor [10, 22, 28, 29, 41, 42]. Seat pans that are so high that the feet dangle cause uncomfortable pressure on the backs of the thighs [10, 39]. Seats that are too low reduce pressure

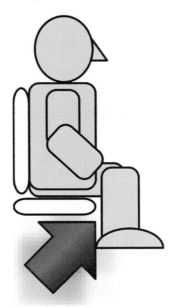

FIGURE 13.1   The seat pan should provide space between the edge of the seat and the knee and leave a gap between the seat and backrest.

distribution across the thighs but can increase pressure on the pelvic bones. People who sit forward in their seat tend to prefer to sit high, while people who recline often prefer to sit lower so their feet can remain on the floor when they recline [10]. Similarly, people in knee-tilt chairs tend to prefer higher positions than people with column-tilt chairs that lift the feet when reclining [10].

Some clients will need to keep their seat pan higher than would otherwise be recommended to facilitate getting into and out of the chair. These individuals may benefit from a footrest (see Section 13.4.3.3) to provide support while seated. Individuals who have trouble getting into and out of the chair may also benefit from a seat pan that doesn't spin.

13.4.1.2 Backrest

The whole point of a backrest is to allow the person sitting in the chair to lean back. A good backrest will allow its height and angle to be adjusted. The backrest should support both the lower and middle back, but leave a gap between the seat and backrest to accommodate the buttocks [28].

A backrest that allows the user to lean back or recline beyond 90° vertical, even if the seat pan remains horizontal, reduces the load on the back muscles and intervertebral discs [41, 43]. Most users prefer a backrest angle between 90 and 105° [42]. Keep in mind, however, that increasing the backrest angle also moves the person's upper body further away from the work surface, which may require the user to lean forward to type or use the mouse. One solution is to provide a tray that can move the keyboard and mouse outward as the user reclines (see Section 13.4.3.6).

Instead of reclining (where only the backrest changes orientation), some chairs tilt both the backrest and seat pan around a central pivot point. Chairs that pivot where the seat attaches to the chair's central post lift the knees while the back descends, and the user's feet may lift off the ground. Knee-tilt chairs that pivot nearer the knees can keep the feet on the floor, but the back and head descend toward the ground [10, 41] (Figure 13.2).

Some chair backrests provide additional padding for the lower (lumbar) back. When lumbar support is positioned correctly, the lower back muscles relax with less downward and forward slumping of the torso [10]. Research suggests that about 2 inches of contour at the level of the fourth and fifth lumbar vertebrae (about 6 to

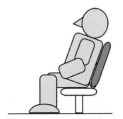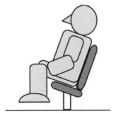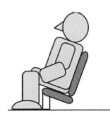

FIGURE 13.2 Common mechanisms for changing backrest angle: (a) recline mechanism, (b) tilt mechanism at central post, and (c) tilt mechanism at knees. (Redrawn from About Seat Mechanisms, 1998, available from http://www.officeorganix.com/ChairMechanism.htm [accessed May 5, 2010] [44].)

10 inches above the seat pan) produces optimal spinal curves in terms of minimizing disc pressure [10]. Remember that the degree and height of the lumbar curve vary significantly between individuals, so no one make or model of chair will be suitable for all users.

13.4.1.3   Armrest

The advantages and disadvantages of armrests are still being debated among therapists and ergonomics professionals. When used appropriately, the armrests on a chair support the arms and remove stress on the neck, shoulders, and lower back [10, 18, 20, 25, 45, 46]. A lack of arm support can result in a slumped posture as the weight of the arms pulls the upper trunk forward and downward [10]. Having armrests on a chair can also be helpful when getting into and out of the chair [26]. However, some clinicians argue that armrests encourage poor posture and reduce trunk muscle strength.

Users should be encouraged not to rest the elbows or forearms on the armrests while typing or using the mouse unless they need to for reasons such as reducing tremor. Using the armrests while typing can cause compression in the finger flexor muscles in the forearm or compression of the ulnar nerve at the elbow [25, 26]. Instead, the armrests should be used in between periods of typing to provide rest and support for the arms.

Armrests that are too high result in elevated shoulders and pressure on the undersides of the elbows and forearms, while armrests that are too low require the worker to slump or lean to one side to use them. Armrests that are too high can also interfere with typing, using the mouse, or other activities requiring free motion [10, 41] and can force the user into an awkward hand position as he or she reaches around the armrest.

Armrests that are too wide can encourage the user to adopt an awkward posture with splayed elbows and bent wrists while typing. Width-adjustable armrests let the sitter change the distance between armrests but can be problematic for clients who need to use the armrests to get into and out of the chair [10, 41] (Figure 13.3).

An alternative to armrests that are part of the chair are armrests that clamp to the work surface (see Section 13.4.3.1). These can be especially useful when armrests on the chair itself interfere with transferring into the chair from a wheelchair.

13.4.1.4   Materials

While no one wants to sit on a hard, unpadded seat, users should also avoid chairs with too much padding. Too much soft padding or seat contouring can put pressure on the sides of the buttocks, causing muscle pain. It can also put pressure on

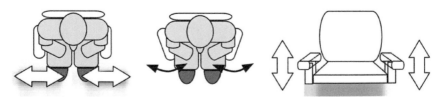

FIGURE 13.3   Armrest adjustments: (a) width adjustment, (b) angle adjustment, and (c) height adjustment.

the heads of the femur bones (the greater trochanter) and on the adjacent sciatic nerves [10]. Chairs can be covered in a variety of upholstery materials, each of which entails different trade-offs. Vinyl and vinyl-like coverings are easy to clean and spill resistant but do not "breathe," which can lead to the accumulation of uncomfortable amounts of moisture beneath the thighs or back. Cloth upholstery is more common, but is less resistant to spills and more difficult to clean. This can be an issue for clients who have issues with drooling or incontinence. A cloth-covered seat pan can also become warm and damp, and cloth-covered foam seat pans can harbor dust mites [38]. Leather is durable and can be treated to protect against spills, but is the most expensive covering material.

13.4.1.5 Choosing the Right Chair

The most important attributes of any office chair are that it (1) provide adequate support and (2) allow the user to change position frequently and easily [2, 32, 42]. The features that are most relevant or useful in this regard are

- Adequate back support with an ability to recline or tilt to 120° easily [10, 38, 42, 45, 47].
- A height-adjustable seat pan that allows the legs to assist in posture changes and allows different postures for the legs and feet [10, 45, 47].
- If a chair has armrests, they should be height and width adjustable [10].

Despite manufacturers' claims to the contrary, more adjustable features on an office chair are not necessarily better. People are more likely to get proper support from a chair that requires only minor adjustments to fine-tune the fit [32, 39]. The more adjustments provided, the more likely it is that a person will use the chair with inappropriate settings [32, 39]. A survey of 417 office workers who used adjustable office chairs found that while 69% adjusted the seat height, only one-third adjusted the back height and only 27% adjusted the tilt tension [42]. The study also found that more than half of those surveyed did not know how to tighten or loosen the tilt tension, 45% did not know how to adjust the back height, and 21% were unfamiliar with the seat height adjustment feature [42].

When working with a client to choose an office chair, there is really no substitute for actually sitting in the chairs under consideration [39]. Instead of having the client sit in several chairs and then decide amongst them, a more reliable approach is to use the optometrist's strategy of making a series of pairwise comparisons between chairs until a preferred choice emerges [47]. The memory of the biomechanical and proprioceptive states associated with sitting in an office chair last for only a few seconds. Pairwise comparisons allow your client to change chairs very quickly so he or she can better compare the present chair with the fading impression of the previous chair [47].

When comparing chairs it is not necessary, or even useful, to exhaustively sample every chair and configuration. People cannot perceive minor design changes in ergonomic variables [47]. For example, people cannot discriminate between changes in seat height that are smaller than 2 cm, or changes in seat back angle and seat pan angle that are smaller than 3° [47]. Instead, choose a range of chairs and configurations that provide distinct differences.

It is also desirable, though often not possible, to sit in an office chair for an extended period of time before purchase [10, 38]. Research has shown that comfort ratings after 5 minutes don't correspond to ratings after half an hour [10]. Many ergonomists suggest that chairs be evaluated for at least as long as users are expected to sit at one time, preferably over a week or more [10].

13.4.2 Work Surfaces

13.4.2.1 Adjustable Height

Most office workers would benefit from a height-adjustable desk because a single flat work surface cannot be set at an appropriate height for all of the tasks of office work [26]. For example, many people type and write at different heights and prefer a writing surface that is a little higher than the typical keyboard surface [25]. A height-adjustable work surface also allows the same workstation to accommodate different-size workers, or different postures for the same worker [25]. The height adjustment mechanism can be manual (e.g., a crank or pneumatic mechanism) or electronic [26, 48]. Electronic mechanisms require less effort but are significantly more expensive.

Work surfaces (and the equipment on them) should be at a height where the user can sit with his or her feet supported, type with neutral wrists, and read or write without either slumping forward too much or raising the arms or shoulders [10, 22, 25]. There may actually be three different "right" heights for a work surface: the right height for the forearms and shoulders, the right height for the eyes and head, and the right height for the legs [25]. One option is to use a split work surface design [26], while another option is to use work surface modifications like keyboard trays (see Section 13.4.3.6) and monitor arms (see Section 13.4.3.5).

Keep in mind that if only one person is going to use the workstation, and if the work surface will be staying at a fixed height, then a height-adjustable desk may not be necessary. Instead, consider using leg raisers if the work surface needs to be raised a few inches to accommodate a taller person or wheelchair user [48] (Figure 13.4).

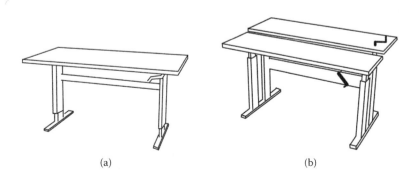

(a)   (b)

FIGURE 13.4   Height-adjustable desks: (a) a single-level height-adjustable desk and (b) a height-adjustable desk with two independently adjustable surfaces.

13.4.2.2 Sit-to-Stand Desks

Some height-adjustable desks provide a sufficient range of heights to accommodate working while sitting and while standing. These workstations are often recommended for people with back injuries who cannot tolerate sitting for more than a short period of time [2, 25], but there is limited evidence that sit-to-stand work surfaces have cost-effective benefits [33, 43]. The real benefit of sit-to-stand work surfaces may be that they encourage workers to change positions between sitting and standing. However, standing in a static posture is even more tiring than sitting in a static posture, so workers should be discouraged from standing for the entire workday [26].

An alternative to a sit-to-stand work surface is to purchase a monitor arm and keyboard tray that turns a standard workstation into one that can be used from a standing position [48]. Another way to obtain the benefits from sitting and standing is for people to work in a seated posture and occasionally stand and move around doing other things (e.g., filing papers, making phone calls) rather than trying to use the computer while standing [26].

13.4.2.3 Wheelchair-Compatible Desks

There are a few manufacturers whose workstations are designed specifically for people who use wheelchairs [48]. These workstations typically offer greater height adjustability than standard height-adjustable desks to accommodate the increased seating height of a wheelchair compared to a standard office chair and limited obstructions beneath the work surface to make it easier to pull the wheelchair in and out. Other features include work surfaces that tilt to accommodate mouthstick typists, and turntables (or lazy susans) to reduce the need to reach for items [48].

One drawback to desks designed for wheelchair use is the lack of storage. In order to provide additional room for the wheelchair, the desks typically eliminate all drawers beneath the work surface. Thus, a client who receives a wheelchair-compatible desk may also need additional storage for papers and office supplies.

13.4.2.4 Reclining Workstations

Some workstations allow individuals to work in a reclined or supine position, to relieve pain [48]. The simplest of these are lap desks. The needs of many clients can be met with inexpensive tiltable frames that can position a laptop or keyboard over a bed or reclining chair. Some of the more complex reclining workstations are self-contained units with an integrated seat and work surface.

13.4.3 WORK SURFACE MODIFICATIONS

13.4.3.1 Forearm Supports

Forearm supports are an alternative to armrests that are part of the office chair (see Section 13.4.1.3) (Figure 13.5). They are typically articulating arms that attach to either the front of the work surface or chair armrests [25]. Others are fixed, padded extensions from the work surface [25]. When positioned correctly, forearm supports should allow plenty of movement and should not immobilize the forearm so the wrist

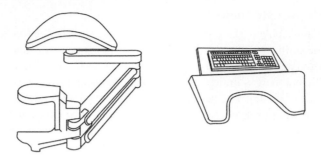

FIGURE 13.5   Forearm support: (a) articulating forearm support and (b) fixed forearm support.

is doing more sideways bending than before [25]. Forearm supports are not as strong as the armrests on a chair so they shouldn't be used for weight bearing when getting into and out of a chair. As an alternative to chair armrests or external forearm supports, wheelchair users can use their tray or wheelchair armrests [40], but be aware that positioning the wheelchair armrests for computer use may interfere with wheelchair use or other functions.

13.4.3.2 Wrist Supports

Wrist rests are intended to reduce arm and shoulder muscle work [9, 25] and soften the surface beneath the wrist [9, 25] (Figure 13.6). Wrist rests can also be used to provide forearm support in the absence of chair armrests [45, 49]. However, research has not shown that wrist rests provide significant benefits to users. In fact, a wrist rest can actually increase pressure on nerves and blood vessels inside the wrist by compressing the undersurface of the wrist [9, 16, 25, 26, 29, 31, 45]. If a wrist rest is used, clients should be encouraged to rest the heel of their palm on the wrist rest rather than their wrists [26].

Ergonomists recommend choosing a rest with a broad, flat, firm surface that distributes pressure over a large area [25, 26, 45]. A wrist rest that is less than 2 inches wide is probably too narrow [25]. The wrist rest should not have sharp edges and should not be so thick that it encourages forward wrist flexion [25]. Clients should avoid soft wrist rests that deform to contour to the wrist, because these are likely to restrict movement of the hands and encourage more lateral deviation of the wrist during typing and mouse use [2, 25, 26, 45]. The rest should be made from material that is either easy to clean or cheap enough to be discarded when soiled [25].

Most importantly, clients should be encouraged to float their hands over the wrist rest when typing or using the mouse and only use the wrist rest during pauses [9, 25, 26, 29, 31, 45, 49]. Research has shown that resting the hands on some kind of a surface during pauses is associated with reduced muscle activity in the arms and shoulders, straighter wrist postures, and increased comfort [9].

13.4.3.3 Footrests

Footrests are often used to compensate when more appropriate interventions, such as lowering the chair or work surface, are unavailable [25]. Footrests should be used as a last resort because they leave the feet with only one place to be, and limit possible

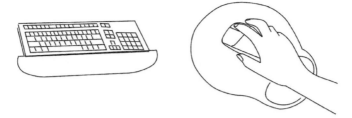

FIGURE 13.6 Wrist rests for (a) keyboard and (b) mouse.

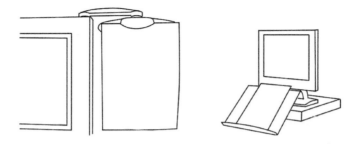

FIGURE 13.7 Document stands: (a) Attached to side of monitor. (From http://www.wellland.com.) (b) Positioned in front of monitor. (From http://www.ergodirect.com.)

leg postures [29]. If a footrest is needed, most clients would be best served by a support resting on the floor in front of the chair that allows the client to rest his or her feet out in front of the body in a comfortable manner [38, 50]. If the client's legs do not reach the ground when seated in the chair, however, then consider a chair-mounted footrest. Clients with limited knee or ankle flexibility should use a footrest that can be adjusted to accommodate their range of motion.

13.4.3.4 Document Stands
Document stands are used to position source documents close to the computer monitor to avoid craned necks and twisted torsos [2, 25] (Figure 13.7). Document stands can position the document to the side of the monitor or between the monitor and the keyboard [26]. Documents stands also reduce eyestrain by keeping the source document at approximately the same distance and angle as the screen [25].

13.4.3.5 Monitor Arms
Monitor arms allow users to easily reposition the monitor to reduce glare [2] and support posture changes [25]. Monitor arms can mount on the desk or wall (Figure 13.8).

There is no single best position for the monitor, but there are guidelines to follow. The computer monitor should be placed directly in front of the user to eliminate neck twisting [26]. Conventional wisdom dictates that the center of the monitor be placed at eye height. New evidence, however, shows that users are more comfortable when the monitor is between 15° and 50° below horizontal eye level [10, 26, 27, 29, 30, 50]. People see more visual field below the horizon than above, so your client will be able to see more of the screen if it is positioned lower. Looking downward also means

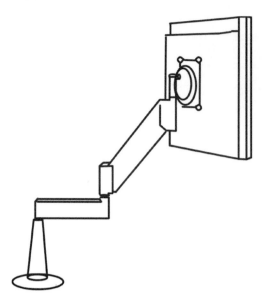

FIGURE 13.8 Monitor arm.

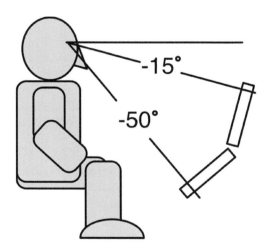

FIGURE 13.9 The monitor should be positioned between 15° and 50° below horizontal eye height. (Based on Grant, C., Visual Ergonomics in the Workplace, 2009, available from http:// www.office-ergo.com/setting.htm [accessed April 27, 2009] [27].)

more of the eye surface is covered by the eyelid and the eyes unconsciously blink more, producing more lubrication [27, 34]. Lowering the monitor also helps bifocal users avoid craned neck and twisted torsos [2].

The greatest challenge to positioning the monitor below horizontal eye level is that the work surface may prevent positioning the monitor more than a few degrees below horizontal. One solution to this is a split-level work surface (see Section 13.4.2.1) that allows the back section to be set at a lower height than the front section (Figure 13.9).

Conventional wisdom also dictated that the monitor should be positioned at an arm's length (about 18–24 inches) from the user [29]. Ergonomists currently recommend that the monitor be positioned as far away as possible while still being easy to read [27, 29, 34, 51]. It is usually better to make items on the screen larger than to bring the monitor closer [27, 51].

Bifocal wearers often experience sore necks and shoulders because they have to tip their heads back to see the computer screen [34]. If this is a problem, then lower the screen as much as possible. People should also consider other options besides bifocals, including [34]

- Computer glasses that focus at the right distance for the computer screen
- Wearing contact lenses corrected for computer or reading distance in one eye, and for far distance (if needed) in the other eye

13.4.3.6   Keyboard Trays and Arms

The terminology surrounding mounting/positioning hardware for keyboards varies by vendor. Often, the *arm* or *drawer* is the mechanism that moves to position the keyboard and the *tray* or *platform* is the actual surface on which the keyboard (and often the mouse) rests. Trays, drawers, and arms can be ordered independently or in combination as a complete package.

Keyboard arms can be used to adjust the height and angle of a keyboard in order to fit the user or allow posture changes [25] (Figure 13.10). Arms may also provide a better viewing arrangement by moving the user back from the screen or work surface [25]. At the same time, however, a major limitation of using keyboard arms is that these push the user back from all the other items on the work surface, increasing the reach required to access the telephone, notepads, documents, and other items that may be used frequently.

Keyboard arms may be in a fixed position on the desk or may slide in and out from beneath the desk. Keyboard arms that have multiple joints (i.e., are *articulated*) offer greater flexibility in terms of positioning, but the additional arm sections can take up more space than a keyboard drawer. Keyboard drawers slide in and out from beneath the desk, and offer limited flexibility in terms of changing the height or orientation of the keyboard.

Both keyboard arms and drawers can reduce vertical knee clearance beneath the work surface [25]. Further, the presence of a keyboard arm or drawers does not guarantee appropriate keyboard positioning. Keyboard arms and drawers can be adjusted too low, too high, or at the wrong angle [25]. Finally, some keyboard drawers and arms only provide enough room for the keyboard, forcing a long reach to use a mouse on top of the work surface [25].

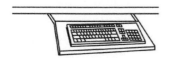 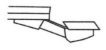 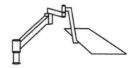

FIGURE 13.10   Keyboard arms and trays: (a) keyboard drawer, (b) under-desk keyboard arm, and (c) articulating keyboard arm that can be used from a standing position.

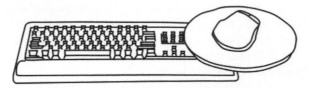

FIGURE 13.11   Mouse tray positioned above the number pad to reduce lateral reach.

Many ergonomists recommend positioning the keyboard such that it slopes away from the user (i.e., the number row at the back of the keyboard is actually lower than the space bar at the front of the keyboard), referred to as negative tilt, to reduce wrist extension [26, 29, 45, 52, 53]. However, a negatively tilted tray can reduce leg clearance and make it difficult to use the mouse. At an extreme negative tilt, users may be forced to bend their hands up and over the front of the keyboard [9].

Make sure that the user is centered on the part of the keyboard he or she will actually use. Most modern keyboards are asymmetrical in design (the alphanumeric keyboard is to the left and a numeric keypad to the right). If the outer edges of the keyboard are used as landmarks for centering the keyboard and monitor, the user's hands will be deviated because the alphanumeric keys will be to the left of the user's midline. Move the keyboard so that the center of the alphanumeric keys (the B key) is centered on the user's belly button [26, 49, 53].

When choosing a keyboard arm, look for a product that is height adjustable, allows the keyboard to be tilted away from the user (i.e., negative tilt), and allows the user to reach the mouse with upper arms relaxed and as close to the body as possible [26]. If mice are used often, the tray should hold the mouse as well as the keyboard [25]. The keyboard should be positioned at or below the height of the elbow [10, 20, 29].

13.4.3.7   Mouse Arms/Trays

A separate mouse tray can be used to compensate for a keyboard tray that is too small or negatively tilted [25] (Figure 13.11). A mouse tray can also be used to position the mouse independently of the keyboard to reduce the distance a user needs to reach [10, 29, 31, 49, 54, 55]. For example, a mouse tray can be positioned directly above the number pad of a keyboard (assuming the user doesn't use the number pad very often) to reduce the amount of lateral reach needed to use the mouse [26, 31].

13.4.4   Text Entry Devices

The existing research indicates that some users, some kinds of discomfort or injuries, and some tasks are probably appropriately served by some alternative keyboard features. The research does not support the idea that one keyboard works for everyone and every circumstance. Nor does the research say that alternative keyboards will not cause discomfort, productivity impairment, or worse [9].

Today's keyboard is ideal for people with arms coming out of their chest, and fingers all the same length [56].

This section covers variations on the traditional keyboard intended to reduce the risk of MSDs. There are also alternative keyboard designs that bear little resemblance to

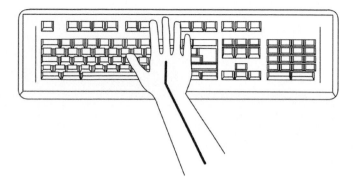

FIGURE 13.12   Ulnar deviation. (Based on NIOSH, ed., Alternative Keyboards, NIOSH, Washington, DC, 1997 [57].)

traditional keyboards. Alternative keyboard designs can be expensive, often result in slower typing, and can have significant learning curves. More importantly, there is no evidence that alternative keyboards actually reduce the risk of MSDs. A more complete discussion of alternative keyboards is provided in Chapter 5.

13.4.4.1   Split Keyboards

One concern with the design of conventional computer keyboards is that people bend their wrists to the side when they are typing on the keyboard. This lateral bending of the wrist toward the little finger is called ulnar deviation [53] (Figure 13.12). Ulnar deviation is a nonneutral position that has been shown to contribute to the fatigue of certain muscles, increase friction and pressure experienced by some tendons (particularly in the thumb area), and add pressure to two major nerves running through the wrist, which can increase the risks of developing problems such as carpal tunnel syndrome [9, 53].

People use ulnar deviation for a number of reasons when typing [9]:

- To align their hands with the rows of keys
- To align the left hand with the diagonal direction of columns of keys
- To reach the space bar with the right thumb

Split keyboards encourage users to adopt a straighter wrist by changing the orientation of the keys on the keyboard. Most split keyboards keep the two halves of the keyboard connected at the top, with each half of the keyboard aimed toward the elbows (Figure 13.13). These keyboards can be molded in one piece, with a fixed angle between the two halves, or can have a hinge or other adjustment that allows the user to set the angle. The fixed keyboards are typically less expensive than the adjustable ones, but offer less flexibility [9]. Some split keyboards, on the other hand, completely separate the two halves [9, 53]. Completely split keyboards can be expensive and are hard for hunt-and-peck typists to use [53].

It should be noted that there is no consistent research proving that split keyboards produce any postural benefits [26, 45]. However, research does support the idea that split keyboards can help relieve some postural stresses. In some studies,

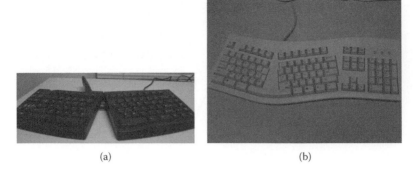

(a)   (b)

FIGURE 13.13   Split keyboards: (a) a Goldtouch split keyboard with adjustable angle and (b) a split keyboard with a fixed angle.

split keyboards reduced ulnar deviation and muscle activity. In other studies, users reported that split keyboards reduced discomfort and increased feelings of relaxation. These positive results have not always been found in studies of split keyboards, however, particularly with regard to discomfort among healthy users. And not all study participants prefer split keyboards over more traditional ones [9, 53].

13.4.4.2   Tented Keyboards

Tented keyboards address the problems caused by the wrist posture called pronation, which involves rotating the forearms to make the hands parallel with the work surface [9, 53] (Figures 13.14 and 13.15). Working with the palms parallel with the work surface twists and stretches the extensor muscles that lift the fingers while shortening the flexor muscles that curl the fingers, causing them to work less efficiently and therefore fatigue more easily than they would at their ideal length. Other muscles in the arm are affected as well, and some of them must contract constantly to maintain this position. The pronated position also twists and shifts tendons in the carpal tunnel, potentially pushing the vulnerable median nerve against the transverse ligament that forms one wall of the tunnel [9, 53].

Tented keyboards allow the user to work with the palms held in a more neutral position. Different keyboard designs have fixed or adjustable angles [9]. A few tented keyboards either fix the two halves or allow the user to adjust the two halves, to be perpendicular to the work surface [9, 53]. Studies of preference, comfort, and perceived fatigue have found that tented keyboards have moderate advantages over conventional keyboards for some people. In most studies, the best angle for both performance and preference measures varied dramatically from person to person [9]. Tented keyboards can be significantly taller than conventional keyboards and must be positioned lower, which can reduce leg clearance [9].

13.4.4.3   Negative Slope Keyboards

Conventional computer keyboards slope or step the keys at a positive angle, which can cause the user to bend his or her wrists backward (i.e., wrist extension) [49, 52]

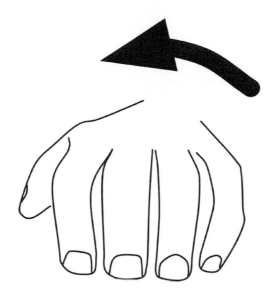

FIGURE 13.14   Wrist pronation.

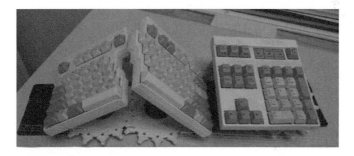

FIGURE 13.15   Tented keyboard.

(Figure 13.16). Excessive wrist extension has been shown to reduce the diameter of the carpal tunnel, potentially increasing pressure on the median nerve. In addition, it causes some forearm muscles to work in a shortened form, which is an inefficient work mode that increases susceptibility to muscle fatigue [9, 26, 45, 49, 53, 58]. Negatively sloped keyboards are either thicker in front (where the space bar is located) or have extendable legs at the front of the keyboard to create a backward slope [9, 58].

13.4.4.4   Key Stiffness

Although it's not clear why, people exert less force when typing on some keyboards than on others. This may happen because the keys depress more easily on these keyboards, or perhaps because the keys give clearer or quicker feedback through a tactile or audible click [2]. On the other hand, some researchers believe that soft keys may actually be *worse* than stiff keys. Softer keys may provide less tactile feedback to signal when peak contact force has been reached, resulting in excess typing force [13].

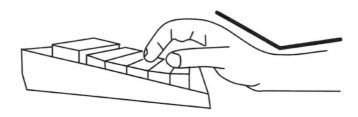

FIGURE 13.16   Wrist extension. (Based on NIOSH, ed., Alternative Keyboards, NIOSH, Washington, DC, 1997 [57].)

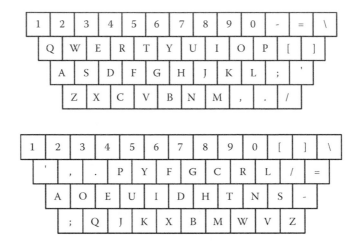

FIGURE 13.17   QWERTY and Dvorak keyboard layouts.

13.4.4.5   Key Layout

The reasoning behind the traditional QWERTY keyboard layout (named for the six letters in the upper left row of the keyboard) has never been definitively established [3]. Alternative keyboard layouts have been proposed with the goal of reducing the risk of MSDs by (1) limiting finger movement and (2) placing the most frequently used letters beneath the strongest fingers. The most popular alternative keyboard layout is the Dvorak layout, patented in 1936 [59] (Figure 13.17). There is no evidence, however, that the Dvorak keyboard (or any keyboard layout) reduces the incidence of MSDs [3].

13.4.4.6   Choosing the Right Text Entry Device

For most people, a regular keyboard design works just fine if it's put in the proper position and used appropriately [26]. If your client wants or needs an alternative or ergonomic keyboard, however, keep in mind that no single keyboard design is best for everyone [53]. Help your client identify a keyboard that is compatible with his or her existing computer technology and job requirements [9]. For example, determine whether the job requires use of the numeric keypad and specialized keys because some alternative keyboards eliminate or move these keys [9].

If possible, have your client try the keyboard prior to purchase. The trial period should be at least 2 days, because of the learning curve involved. If the keyboard design is adjustable, encourage the client to change the geometry gradually. Anticipate some frustration while your client gets accustomed to the new design due to reduced typing speed or accuracy [9].

Use the trial period to determine whether the keyboard fits within the client's existing workspace [9]. Some alternative keyboards are extra-wide, long, or high, and don't fit well on ordinary keyboard trays or may make it impossible to retract the tray under the work surface. Some keyboards, particularly the tented ones, require low placement, limiting leg clearance. Check whether the keyboard's shape will affect the placement of adjacent devices such as trackballs [9].

13.4.5 POINTING DEVICES

As a general rule, computer users spend one- to two-thirds of their computer work using the mouse [14]. There is no research that conclusively demonstrates that one type of pointing device (mouse, trackball, stylus, touchpad, joystick, etc.) is less likely to result in MSDs than any another [45]. The main problem is overuse regardless of device. The best approach (other than reducing pointing device use) may be to switch between limbs or different types of pointing devices to distribute effort across multiple parts of the body [25]. The best ergonomic mice, therefore, are designed to allow the user to vary posture while working with the mouse [31] (Figure 13.18). What is generally agreed upon is that all pointing devices should be used in a neutral position (arm relaxed, close to your body) [2, 45]. In addition, mouse movements should be made using the elbow as the pivot point, not the wrist [31]. Choose a mouse design that fits the client's hand but is as flat as possible to reduce wrist extension [31]. A more complete discussion of pointing devices is provided in Chapter 4.

13.4.6 MONITOR

13.4.6.1 Types of Monitors

The current standard monitors for computers are liquid crystal display (LCD) flat-panel monitors. Compared to the previous generation of cathode ray tube (CRT) monitors, LCD monitors are lighter, take up significantly less desk space, and generate significantly less heat.

It is possible to use a high-definition television (HDTV) as a computer monitor. Using an HDTV as a monitor and a TV can save money, but HDTVs are not optimized for computer use. HDTVs have lower resolution than comparably sized computer monitors and are intended to be viewed from several feet away. In addition, your client will need to switch between the TV input signal and the computer input signal to make use of both functions. If your client decides to use an HDTV, look for an HDTV with 1080 progressive scan (i.e., 1080p) vertical resolution and a dedicated PC video signal input.

Another alternative is a high-definition LCD projector. Most projectors provide significantly lower resolution than monitors (as low as 480p). Many projectors claim

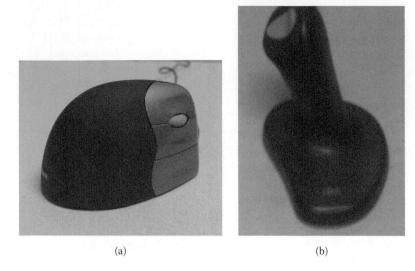

(a)   (b)

FIGURE 13.18   Ergonomic mice.

they support higher resolutions (720p, 1080i, 1808p) but convert the video signal to a lower resolution before displaying it. Projectors that actually display in 1080p are still extremely expensive. Bulbs are also expensive and last an average of 2,000 hours. Finally, the ambient environment must also be taken into account. A projector's image can be washed out by too much ambient light.

13.4.6.2   Screen Filters

Screen filters can eliminate glare from overhead lighting. Much like the black louvers on the rear window of sports cars, a screen mesh will shade the screen from overhead lights, while providing a view of the display directly through the mesh [60] (Figure 13.19). Screen filters are effective in certain instances, but should be evaluated before purchase. Some screens reduce glare by 99%, but even that may not be enough in very bright environments [27]. In addition, filters will not block light from sources directly in line with the screen because, like the user, the light has a direct view of the screen though the filter [60]. In addition, screen filters can attract dust, which reduces the quality of the screen image [45, 60]. Once a screen filter is installed, increase the brightness of the monitor as necessary to compensate for any darkening caused by the filter itself [25].

13.4.6.3   Matte Finishes

Screens with matte finishes diffuse light from overhead lights and from windows. This reduces the brightness of the reflected image and equalizes the light reflected in any given direction. In addition, it reduces the perception of glare by eliminating well-defined edges in reflected images. The matte finish does reduce the quality of electronically generated images to a small extent, but the visual advantages often outweigh the disadvantages [60].

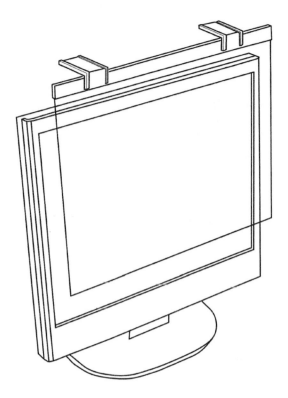

FIGURE 13.19 Monitor glare filter.

13.4.6.4 Choosing the Right Monitor

Most clients are going to get an LCD flat panel monitor. The more pertinent question is how large should the monitor be? Monitors are available that are 40 or even 50 inches in diagonal width. It is also possible to connect multiple monitors to the same computer, to produce truly huge displays. Research supports the notion that larger displays are better than smaller displays, but there are practical issues that can limit the benefits of extremely large displays [61]. For example, finding a small mouse cursor on a large display can be difficult.

Once a monitor is chosen, several steps can be taken to maximize its performance. The principal factors affecting the ability to see what is on a computer monitor are [34]

- Glare
- The luminance (brightness) difference between the monitor and its immediate environment
- The distance between the eye and the monitor
- The readability of the screen and document
- The client's vision and his or her corrective lenses

Reduce glare by changing or shielding the light source or rearranging the workstation, not by compromising the monitor's height, angle, or location [10].

13.4.7 LIGHTING

Lighting is often overlooked when designing a client's workstation, but appropriate lighting can have a significant impact on performance. The right amount of light depends on a number of factors. There should be plenty of light for easy reading, but too much light can cause eyestrain or glare [26, 34].

Because some tasks and workers require more light than others, it is best to keep the ambient light level low and allow workers to supplement it with individually controlled task lights (i.e., desk lamps) [27]. Task lighting reduces eyestrain by illuminating paperwork and reducing the need for bright ambient light that may cause screen glare [25]. However, poorly positioned task lights can cause glare on the computer screen, can shine directly into workers' eyes, or can illuminate the area around and behind the monitor too brightly [25]. The bulb within the task light should not be visible to the worker. If it is, shield the bulb or move the fixture [25].

Remember, because the front of the screen is glass, something is going to be reflected from it [27]. The guiding principle is to avoid very bright, high-contrast, sharp-edge reflections on the computer monitor [60]. Contrast reflected from the screen competes for the user's attention with the contrast on the screen. In some cases this can be an irritation, but in others it can make sections of the screen impossible to read [27].

Ceiling-mounted direct lighting should be avoided. Aside from absolute brightness, a big problem with direct ceiling lights is that they provide a high contrast with the rest of the ceiling. That contrast can reflect onto the computer screen. Many guidelines mistakenly specify only a luminance (brightness) value for ceilings and walls. While absolute intensity is important (a bright light reflecting off the screen will always cause problems), reducing the contrast is much more critical. Interrupting the ceiling with patches of bright light almost guarantees competing reflections on the screen [27]. Instead, the best solution for overall visual performance is ceiling-suspended, indirect lighting (sometimes referred to as uplighting) [27] (Figure 13.20).

In addition to overhead lights, reflected images from windows can be a big problem [60]. Locate the monitor in a position that eliminates reflections from windows [25, 60], generally by placing it perpendicular to the windows when possible, and use blinds and shades to control outside light [27, 60]. Also make sure that the computer monitor screen isn't backed to a bright window, which can make the screen look washed out [26] and can cause eyestrain from having too much contrast in your client's field of vision [25].

13.4.8 LAPTOPS

For sustained laptop use the client should use an external monitor, keyboard, and mouse [26, 62]. Some laptops are designed to connect to a port replicator or docking station that simplifies attaching and detaching peripherals. Research has shown that docking stations decrease subjective discomfort and increase productivity compared to a laptop used with its built-in keyboard, trackpad, and monitor [63].

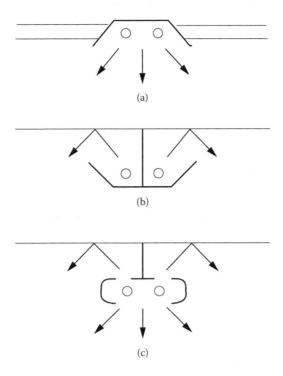

FIGURE 13.20 Lighting fixtures can provide (a) direct light, (b) indirect light, or (c) both.

If your client will be frequently transporting a laptop, think about the weight of the entire system, including accessories (e.g., power supply, spare battery, external disc drive, etc.). Many lightweight portables can become as heavy as regular laptops when you add the weight of all of the components together. If the laptop and its components collectively weigh more than 10 pounds, your client should consider using a laptop bag that is pulled rather than carried [62].

13.4.9 BREAKS

Ergonomists agree that it's a good idea to take brief rest breaks on a frequent basis [26]. Studies show that regular rest breaks, including stretching, are beneficial in reducing stress, back shoulder, neck, and wrist pain, low back discomfort, and eye-strain [2, 64]. In addition, rest breaks appear to enhance productivity and leave work-ers more physically and mentally refreshed [2, 64]. Breaks can be divided between micro-breaks, which last 30 seconds to 3 minutes, and more traditional rest breaks, which last 10 to 15 minutes.

Micro-breaks can be very effective but should not replace traditional rest breaks [2]. Micro-breaks should occur every 10 to 15 minutes [29]. A micro-break isn't nec-essarily a break from work, but it is a break from using the set of muscles that are doing most of the work (e.g., the finger flexors if you're doing a lot of typing). During a micro-break your client can briefly stretch, stand up, move around, or do a different work task (e.g., make a phone call) [12, 26]. Every 30 to 60 minutes your client should take a brief rest break. During this break your client should move around and do something else. This allows your client to exercise different muscles [26]. Looking at a computer screen for extended periods of time causes a person to blink less often and exposes more of the eye surface to the air. Every 15 minutes your client should briefly look away from the screen for a minute or two to a more distant scene, preferably something more that 20 feet away, to let the muscles inside the eye relax [26, 34].

Research suggests that when workers determine break length and frequency themselves, they tend to wait until they have begun to feel fatigued before taking breaks or resume work before recovery is complete. Individuals with cognitive impairments may not remember to take breaks. A better approach is to ask the client to follow a predetermined schedule of break times and lengths [2, 12, 64]. One option is to buy software that monitors computer use and prompts your client to take a rest break at appropriate intervals [26, 45].

13.4.10   STRESS MANAGEMENT

General stress reduction programs are common in large corporations, but smaller organizations may also benefit from introducing stress reduction practices. Stress reduction programs might include education about stress recognition, coping behaviors, relaxation methods, health behavior, and personality typing. Employee stress management programs can be powerfully effective when used in conjunction with an MSD management program [2].

13.4.11   WRIST BRACES

There is no consistent research evidence that wearing wrist supports during computer use actually helps reduce the risk of injury [26, 45]. There is some evidence, however, that wearing wrist supports during periods of *inactivity* can help relieve symptoms for those with carpal tunnel syndrome [26, 45].

13.5   ASSESSMENT ISSUES

13.5.1   HIERARCHICAL TASK ANALYSIS

Hierarchical task analysis (HTA) is a systematic approach to performing ergonomic assessments. HTA begins with very general descriptions of what your client does (e.g., job objectives and activities) and concludes with very detailed descriptions of how your client does those things (e.g., tools, displays, actions) [65]. Start by systematically examining every work-related task performed by your client [15]:

* What is being done?
* Why is it being done (purpose)?
* Where is it being done (place)?

- When is it being done (sequence)?
- Who is doing it (person)?
- How is it being done (means)?

When using this information to design your client's workstation, remember that designing for ergonomics requires understanding and consideration of [22]:

- The physical and psychological attributes of the person or population of people who will perform the job
- The tasks required to perform the job
- The design and arrangement of the workstation furniture, computer hardware, computer software, and other workstation accessories
- The work environment, including such things as noise and temperature, and also management and organizational methods and constraints

13.5.2 PUTTING IT ALL TOGETHER

No checklist can capture the interactions and complexities of all possible combinations of people, task, equipment, and work environment [22]. Additionally, the fact that a component cannot be adjusted does not mean that it is not appropriate for a given individual. Balancing what the research literature advocates with what is practical and affordable for a specific client is a skill that can only be obtained through experience.

It is unlikely that you will be presented with a completely blank slate in which to create an ergonomic work environment for your client. Some aspects of the job, the environment, or the workstation are going to be fixed. Your job, then, is to use the tools from the ergonomic toolbox to change what you can to create a functional work environment that limits the risk factors for developing an MSD. Keep in mind that there is often more than one way to achieve each goal and that every solution has trade-offs that can possibly make matters worse rather than better. The best way to evaluate ergonomic fixes is by considering all the ergonomic risk factors. For example, a wrist rest may force a straighter wrist (vertically) but may also put too much pressure on the underside of the wrist or make the individual bend the wrist sideways to reach some keys [12].

Starting from the bottom, the feet should be firmly supported to ensure stability, and maintenance of hip, knee, and ankle position [10, 24, 26, 40, 66]. Methods to accomplish this include lowering the seat pan (see Section 13.4.1.1) or providing a footrest (see Section 13.4.3.3). Lowering the seat pan raises the relative height of the work surface, which can cause your client to scrunch their shoulders or keep their arms raised to work, but this can be addressed with a height-adjustable desk (see Section 13.4.2.1). A footrest restricts the number of positions the feet can adopt, limiting your client's postural flexibility.

The angle of the thigh to the torso should be open (i.e., greater than 90°) [26, 29]. A 90° thigh-trunk angle causes the pelvis and sacrum to rotate backwards and the lumbar curve to flatten [43]. Leaning back beyond 105° takes pressure off of the lower back [10, 23, 24, 26, 43], returns the lumbar curve to normal [43], and reduces the work done by the lower back muscles, since body weight is held up by the chair's backrest [29]. There are, of course, trade-offs to reclining the backrest. Leaning backward raises the relative height of the work surface and monitor and moves the user farther away. Leaning backward also requires the neck to flex, stretching the muscles at the back of the neck and applying load to the cervical discs at their front edges [43]. Keyboard (see Section 13.4.3.6) and mouse (see Section 13.4.3.7) arms/ drawers can be used to bring the keyboard and mouse closer.

The head and neck should be straight and upright rather than rotated or flexed [24, 26, 40]. Gaze angle from the eyes to the monitor should be 15 to 45° below horizontal [30]. Gaze angle is dictated by the relative positions of the monitor, the work surface, and the user (which is dictated by the seat pan height and the recline angle of the backrest). Neck rotation can be reduced or eliminated by using a monitor arm (see Section 13.4.3.5) to position the monitor and a copy holder (see Section 13.4.3.4) to position documents.

Moving outward to the arms, the upper arms should be relaxed and close to the body [2, 23, 26, 40]. The position of the upper arms is influenced by the availability of support at the elbow and forearm and the position of the keyboard and mouse. Chair armrests (see Section 13.4.1.3) or independent forearm supports (see Section 13.4.3.1) need to be positioned at the right height and width. Keyboard and mouse arms/drawers can be used to position input devices close to your client's body. The height of the work surface and seat pan should also be set to promote appropriate arm positioning [2].

The elbow angle should be at or greater than 90° to avoid nerve compression at the elbow [26]. In addition, support from an armrest or forearm support should be provided between the elbow and the wrist, rather than at the elbow itself. The wrist should be in a neutral position. Pressure in the carpal tunnel is lowest when the hand is in a natural operating zone of up to 15° wrist extension, lower than 20° flexion, and moderate ulnar deviation [9, 24, 26, 29, 58]. Wrist position is dictated by the shape and orientation of the keyboard (see Section 13.4.4), as well as its height and position relative to the body.

13.5.3   EVALUATING OUTCOMES

By their very nature, documenting whether ergonomic interventions worked is extremely difficult. The challenges in evaluating the effectiveness of ergonomics interventions is further increased when

- Working with a single client as opposed to a large group of workers
- Applying ergonomics to prevent the occurrence of new MSDs, rather than assist in recovery from an existing MSD
- A client is entering a new job, instead of returning to a current job

One approach is to measure the incidence and duration of risk factors (e.g., awkward postures) with and without the interventions in place. Another option is to use subjective measures of pain or discomfort. In both cases, measurements will need to occur over several days or weeks, which may not be practical.

13.6 CASE STUDY

13.6.1 BACKGROUND INFORMATION

James Austin is a right-handed male employed as an IT support staff member. His job requires him to speak on the phone, use a computer at his workstation, and occasionally check other computer monitors in his work area.

Mr. Austin uses a scooter for mobility at work. When he is not at work, he typically uses a rollator (i.e., a walker with wheels). He reports that he has experienced an increasing frequency of falls, so he is reluctant to transfer from his scooter to an office chair at work. Hence, he typically spends most of his work shift in his scooter.

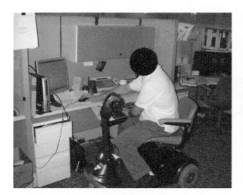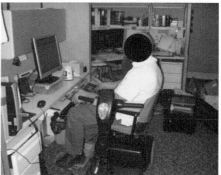

FIGURE 13.21 **(See color insert.)** Case study.

Mr. Austin has no difficulty operating his telephone, a standard 104-key keyboard, or a standard 2-button mouse. His workstation, however, is remarkably poorly configured for his needs. As shown, Mr. Austin must park his scooter parallel to his desk in order to reach the keyboard. His feet are unable to reach the floor when he is seated in his scooter, which forces him to keep his feet on the base of his scooter and rotate his trunk to reach the keyboard. There is a large cabinet in his workstation that forces his monitor to be positioned off to the side, causing him to rotate his neck in the opposite direction from his trunk. His mouse and mouse pad are positioned near the monitor, which requires him to reach forward from the waist and extend his arm to use the mouse.

13.6.2 ASSESSMENT

A complete redesign of Mr. Austin's workstation was discussed during the evaluation. The goal of a new workstation design would be to:

- Create a balanced alignment of Mr. Austin's neck, shoulders, trunk, and legs
- Provide support for Mr. Austin's feet and arms
- Bring the keyboard and mouse closer to Mr. Austin's body to eliminate the need to bend at the waist
- Center the monitor on his desk to reduce neck rotation

These changes were simulated using plastic tubs to give Mr. Austin an idea of the changes that were proposed. Mr. Austin felt that the proposed arrangement would be more comfortable and reduce strain on his muscles and joints.

13.6.3   Recommendations

The following equipment was recommended for Mr. Austin:

A height-adjustable desk. A height-adjustable desk allows the keyboard and monitor to be positioned at appropriate heights to foster an appropriate sitting posture.

Keyboard tray. A low-profile leverless arm that fits both straight or corner desks. Tray tilt can be adjusted ±15° and the adjustable mouse tray tilts and swivels independent of the keyboard tray. A ball-bearing track allows the unit to push underneath the desk or pull out.

ISE flat-panel monitor arm. Adjusts the screen to most comfortable viewing angle—vertically horizontally, and front to back. Includes pivot and tilting capability. Meets Video Electronics Standards Association (VESA) standards.

Height- and angle-adjustable footrest. A footrest sits beneath the user's desk and provides support for the feet. This reduces pressure on the back of the thighs from the seat pan, and improves circulation to the feet.

Alternative seating. Mr. Austin's scooter is not intended to be sat in for extended periods of time, and is poorly suited to replace an office chair. Mr. Austin should schedule a seating and mobility evaluation to consider alternatives to his current scooter.

REFERENCES

1. What is ergonomics. 2010. Available from http://iea.cc/browse.php?contID=what_is_ergonomics (accessed May 26, 2010).
2. Musculoskeletal disorders in the U.S. office workforce. 2001. Zeeland, MI: Herman Miller.
3. Kroemer, K.H.E. 2001. Keyboards and keying: An annotated bibliography of the literature from 1878 to 1999. *Universal Access in the Information Society* 1(2): 98–160.
4. Cohen, A.L. et al. 1997. *Elements of ergonomics programs: A primer based on workplace evaluations of musculoskeletal disorders. DHHS (NIOSH) Publication 97-117*. Cincinnati, OH: National Institute for Occupational Safety and Health.
5. Bernard, B.P., ed. 1997. *Muscuoskeletal disorders and workplace factors: A critical review of epidemiologic evidence for work-related musculoskeletal disorders of the neck, upper extremity, and low back*. DHHS (NIOSH) Publication 97-141, vol. 97-141. Cincinnati, OH: National Institute for Occupational Safety and Health.
6. Buckle, P.W., and J.J. Devereux. 2002. The nature of work-related neck and upper limb musculoskeletal disorders. *Applied Ergonomics* 33(3): 207–217.
7. Waters, T.R., and L.A. MacDonald. 2001. Ergonomic job design to accommodate and prevent musculoskeletal disabilities. *Assistive Technology* 13(2): 88–93.
8. Muggleton, J.M., R. Allen, and P.H. Chappell. 1999. Hand and arm injuries associated with repetitive manual work in industry: A review of disorders, risk factors and preventive measures. *Ergonomics* 42(5): 714–739.

9. Grant, C. 2009. Ergonomics of alternative keyboards. Available from http://office-ergo.com/ergonomic_seating.htm (accessed April 27, 2009).

10. Body support in the office: Sitting, seating, and low back pain. 2002. Zeeland, MI: Herman Miller.

11. Baker, N.A., and M.S. Redfern. 2005. Developing an observational instrument to evaluate personal computer keyboarding style. *Applied Ergonomics* 36(3): 345–354.

12. Grant, C. 2009. Hand and arm basics. Available from http://office-ergo.com/alternat.htm (accessed April 27, 2009).

13. Bufton, M.J. et al. 2006. Effect of keyswitch design of desktop and notebook keyboards related to key stiffness and typing force. *Ergonomics* 49(10): 996–1012.

14. Keir, P.J., J.M. Bach, and D. Rempel. 1999. Effects of computer mouse design and task on carpal tunnel pressure. *Ergonomics* 42(10): 1350–1360.

15. Mital, A., and A. Pennathur. 1999. Musculoskeletal overexertion injuries in the United States: Mitigating the problem through ergonomics and engineering interventions. *Journal of Occupational Rehabilitation* 9(2): 115–149.

16. Cook, C.J., R. Burgess-Limerick, and S. Papalia. 2004. The effect of upper extremity support on upper extremity posture and muscle activity during keyboard use. *Applied Ergonomics* 35(3): 285–292.

17. Pascarelli, E.F., and Y.-P. Hsu. 2001. Understanding work-related upper extremity disorders: Clinical findings in 485 computer users, musicians, and others. *Journal of Occupational Rehabilitation* 11(1): 1–21.

18. Wahlstrom, J. 2005. Ergonomics, musculoskeletal disorders and computer work. *Occupational Medicine* 55(3): 168–176.

19. van den Heuvel, S.G. et al. 2006. Do work-related physical factors predict neck and upper limb symptoms in office workers? *International Archives of Occupational and Environmental Health* 79(7): 585–592.

20. Gerr, F., M. Marcus, and C. Monteilh. 2004. Epidemiology of musculoskeletal disorders among computer users: Lesson learned from the role of posture and keyboard use. *Journal of Electromyography and Kinesiology* 14(1): 25–31.

21. Balci, R., and F. Aghazadeh. 2003. The effect of work-rest schedules and type of task on the discomfort and performance of VDT users. *Ergonomics* 46(5): 455–465.

22. Performance oriented ergonomic checklist for computer (VDT) workstations. 2009. Available from http://ergo.human.cornell.edu/CUVDTChecklist.html.

23. Baker, N.A. 1999. Anthropometry. In *Ergonomics for therapists*, K. Jacobs, ed. Boston: Butterworth Heinemann, pp. 49–84.

24. Hedge, A. 2009. What is the "best" sitting posture? Available from http://www.healthycomputing.com/articles/publish/news/What_is_the_Best_Sitting_Posture.shtml.

25. Grant, C. 2009. Pros and cons of ergonomic office equipment. Available from http://office-ergo.com/pros-cons.htm (accessed April 27, 2009).

26. Ergonomic guidelines for arranging a computer workstation—10 steps for users. 2009. Available from http://ergo.human.cornell.edu/ergoguide.html.

27. Grant, C. 2009. Visual ergonomics in the workplace. Available from http://www.office-ergo.com/setting.htm (accessed April 27, 2009).

28. AbilityNet. 2005. *Ergonomic workstations*. Warwick, UK: AbilityNet.

29. Grant, C. 2009. Conventional wisdom vs. current economics. Available from http://office-ergo.com/conventi.htm (accessed April 27, 2009).

30. Delleman, N.J., and M.B. Berndsen. 2002. Touch-typing VDU operation: Workstation adjustment, working posture and workers' perceptions. *Ergonomics* 45(7): 514–535.

31. Tips for using a computer mouse. 2009. Available from http://ergo.human.cornell.edu/cumousetips.html.

32. Stumpf, B., D. Chadwick, and B. Dowell. 2001. *The kinematics of sitting: Ergonomic criteria for the design of a new work chair*. Zeeland, MI: Herman Miller, p. 3.

33. How to sit in a chair. 1998. Available from http://www.officeorganix.com/Chairsit.htm (accessed August 24, 2006).

34. Grant, C. 2009. A dozen things you should know about eyestrain. Available from http://office-ergo.com/12things1.htm (accessed April 27, 2009).

35. Westgaard, R.H. 2000. Work-related musculoskeletal complaints: Some ergonomics challenges upon the start of a new century. *Applied Ergonomics* 31(6): 569–580.

36. Faucett, J. 2005. Integrating 'psychosocial' factors into a theoretical model for work-related musculoskeletal disorders. *Theoretical Issues in Ergonomics Science* 6(6): 531–550.

37. Karsh, B.-T., F.B.P. Moro, and M.J. Smith. 2001. The efficacy of workplace ergonomic interventions to control musculoskeletal disorders: A critical analysis of the peer-reviewed literature. *Theoretical Issues in Ergonomics Science* 2(1): 23–96.

38. How to choose an ergonomic chair. 2009. Available from http://ergo.human.cornell.edu/AHTutorials/chairch.html.

39. Stumpf, B., D. Chadwick, and B. Dowell. 2001. *The anthropometrics of fit: Ergonomic criteria for the design of a new work chair.* Zeeland, MI: Herman Miller, p. 3.

40. The importance of good seating. 2006. Available from http://www.ace-north.org.uk/pages/resources/documents/ImportanceofGoodSeating.pdf (accessed July 31, 2006).

41. Grant, C. 2009. Demystifying all those chair adjustability options. Available from http://office-ergo.com/ergonomic_seating.htm (accessed April 27, 2009).

42. Everybody deserves a good chair. 2001. Zeeland, MI: Herman Miller.

43. Corlett, E.N. 2006. Background to sitting at work: Research-based requirements for the design of work seats. *Ergonomics* 49(14): 1538–1546.

44. About seat mechanisms. 1998. Available from http://www.officeorganix.com/ChairMechanism.htm (accessed May 5, 2010).

45. HealthyComputing. 2009. The truth about "ergonomic" products. Available from http://www.healthycomputing.com/articles/publish/news/The_Truth_about_Ergonomic_Products.shtml (accessed 2009).

46. Aaras, A. et al. 1997. Postural load during VDU work: A comparison between various work postures. *Ergonomics* 40(11): 1255–1268.

47. Helander, M.G. 2003. Forget about ergonomics in chair design? Focus on aesthetics and comfort! *Ergonomics* 46(13/14): 1306–1319.

48. Computer workstations. 2001. Available from http://www.catea.gatech.edu/quickref-guides/guides/Workstations.php (accessed April 27, 2009).

49. Hedge, A. 2009. Tips for a less-than-ideal workstation. Available from http://www.healthycomputing.com/articles/publish/news/Tips_for_a_Less-Than-Ideal_Workstation.shtml

50. Psihogios, J.P. et al. 2001. A field evaluation of monitor placement effects in VDT users. *Applied Ergonomics* 32(4): 313–325.

51. Ankrum, D.R. 1996, September/October. Viewing distance at computer workstations. *Workplace Ergonomics*, pp. 10–12.

52. Hedge, A., S. Morimoto, and D. McCrobie. 1999. Effects of keyboard tray geometry on upper body posture and comfort. *Ergonomics* 42(10): 1333–1349.

53. Computer keyboard design. 2009. Available from http://ergo.human.cornell.edu/AHTutorials/ckd.htm.

54. Kelaher, D. et al. 2001. An investigation of the effects of touchpad location within a notebook computer. *Applied Ergonomics* 32(1): 101–110.

55. Cook, C.J., and K. Kothiyal. 1998. Influence of mouse position on muscular activity in the neck, shoulder and arm in computer users. *Applied Ergonomics* 29(6): 439–443.

56. Litterick, J. 1981. QWERTYUIOP—Dinosaur in a computer age. *New Scientist* 8(1): 66–68.

57. NIOSH, ed. 1997. Alternative keyboards. Washington, DC: NIOSH.

58. Gilad, I., and S. Harel. 2000. Muscular effort in four keyboard designs. *International Journal of Industrial Ergonomics* 26(1): 1–7.
59. Dvorak, A. 1943. There is a better typewriter keyboard. *National Business Education Quarterly* 12(2): 51–58, 66.
60. Rea, M. 1991. Solving the problem of VDT reflections. In *Progressive architecture* (pp. 35–40). New York: Penton Media.
61. Czerwinski, M. et al. 2006. Large display research overview. In *CHI '06 extended abstracts on human factors in computing systems*. G. Olson, ed. Montreal, Quebec: ACM Press, pp. 69–74.
62. 5 tips for using a laptop computer. 2009. Available from http://ergo.human.cornell.edu/culaptoptips.html.
63. Berkhout, A.L., K. Hendriksson-Larsen, and P. Bongers. 2004. The effect of using a laptop station compared to using a standard laptop PC on the cervical spine torque, perceived strain and productivity. *Applied Ergonomics* 35(2): 147–152.
64. McLean, L. et al. 2001. Computer terminal work and the benefit of microbreaks. *Applied Ergonomics* 32(3): 225–237.
65. Armstrong, T.J. et al. 2001. Developing ergonomic solutions for prevention of musculo-skeletal disorder disability. *Assistive Technology* 13(2): 78–87.
66. Neutral posture typing. 2009. Available from http://ergo.human.cornell.edu/AHTutorials/typingposture.html.

14 Assessment

14.1 INTRODUCTION

Optimizing the fit between the client and his or her computer access technology is critical [1–16]. An inadequate assessment resulting in a poor computer access solution can be costly on a number of levels [1, 5]. At best, an inappropriate computer access solution may merely make someone less efficient. At worst, the wrong computer access solution may actively interfere with an individual's ability to compete in the classroom or workplace [17, 18]. A poor computer access solution is also likely to be abandoned [1], representing a waste of time and resources for all involved.

Doing a good computer access assessment is hard [5]. During the assessment, therapists and consumers must be active problem solvers as they identify purposeful, compensatory strategies and discard less useful or inefficient strategies [19]. The solution must be fitted to the client. No single text entry or pointing device has been shown to be best for all users and tasks [10]. It seems clear that every person and task has a most appropriate device, but no device is most appropriate for every person and task.

14.2 ASSESSMENT PROCESS

A client-centered approach to computer access means understanding the client's needs and abilities first, and working from those toward an appropriate computer access solution [1, 20–22].

14.2.1 CLIENT-CENTERED TEAM-BASED APPROACH

An effective evaluation needs both a goal and a plan [1, 23]. The goal needs to be more specific than to determine whether the client will benefit from computer access technology. Computer access technology is a means to an end, defined by performing specific tasks or participating in specific activities [23]. When planning an evaluation, the clinician needs to consider how many sessions will be needed, where each session will be conducted, which computer access technology will be used during the evaluation, who will participate in each session, who will implement the computer access solution, and what training and follow-up will be provided [23–26]. Involving all stakeholders, including family members, teachers, therapists, and counselors, will lead to better outcomes [2, 27]. Having other team members present can be especially useful if the clinician performing the computer access evaluation is unfamiliar with the client. Other team members can provide important information and help motivate the client during the assessment [23].

14.2.2 SERVICE DELIVERY PROTOCOLS

Several models have been proposed to provide a formal systematic process for conducting assistive technology (AT) assessments. Most models explicitly encourage consideration of the consumer and the consumer's environment, but each differs in which factors are emphasized. Models also differ in whether or not they are specifically designed to be integrated into the special education and individual education plan (IEP) process.

Education Tech Points (ETP) [28] is intended for use with individual students within a special education program and as a means of evaluating the program itself. ETP splits the assessment process into six activities: referral, evaluation, extended assessment, plan development, implementation, and review. Within each activity, the ETP process provides specific questions that should be addressed and decision goals that should be met. Forms and protocols are freely available to implement ETP.

Matching Person and Technology (MPT) [29] is an assessment process that was derived from analyses of AT users and nonusers. MPT focuses on three areas: the consumer's needs and preferences, the environment(s) in which the AT will be used, and the desired functions and features for the AT. MPT is operationalized as a set of forms that are commercially available.

The Human Activity Assistive Technology (HAAT) model [30] examines the consumer, the activities in which the consumer engages, and the environment (including AT) in which the activities take place. In the HAAT model, activities and environment define what abilities the consumer needs. The role of the clinical team is to identify the right modifications to activity and environment to allow the consumer to achieve his or her goals.

AT assessment models provide a framework for organizing the AT assessment process, and many even provide specific procedures or even forms to further formalize the assessment process. In general, the models specify what information should be collected, what factors should be considered, and what decisions should be made. However, these assessment models typically provide little or no assistance with integrating the information that is collected or making decisions. Unfortunately, there are no data available on the effectiveness of these models, making it difficult to compare them [20, 31].

There is no widely accepted protocol for performing a computer access assessment [5, 32, 33]. Most clinicians are on their own in performing an assessment [31, 34, 35]. This often leads to an inefficient trial and error approach [6, 33, 35, 36]. The Physical Characteristics Assessment (PCA) was designed for individuals with CP [35]. The PCA focuses on physical access to the computer (both direct and indirect selection methods) but does not consider cognitive or perceptual impairments. Hwang developed a matrix for identifying appropriate access devices for clients with upper-limb impairments [93]. Denis Anson developed a flowchart for matching clients to the appropriate technology [32, 37]. Advantages of using a structured protocol include:

- Structured protocols help with planning an assessment.
- A clinician is less likely to forget or skip a step.
- Structured protocols are (presumably) based on someone's best practices.

Problems with these models include

- If they are specific, they become outdated by technology. None of the existing models anticipated brain–computer interfaces, multitouch trackpads, or tablet computers.
- They often focus exclusively on physical access and ignore cognitive and perceptual issues. None of them address the interaction between impairments.

14.2.3 What You Need to Learn about the Client

A thorough computer access assessment can feel remarkably invasive. Clinicians and investigators have identified a wide range of factors that can influence the success of a computer access intervention. Not every factor is relevant to every client, of course, but it is up to the clinician to identify which factors are relevant and what weight should be given to each factor. Some factors (like motivation) are not easy to measure objectively and quantitatively and are likely to require multiple interactions with the client [1].

The clinician must get to know the client. It is critical to identify the client's goals and priorities [1, 22, 38–40]. Questions to ask include

- What tasks does the client *need* to perform on a computer?
- What else does the client want to do with a computer?
- Are there any critical performance constraints?

The clinician needs to know about all aspects of the client's life and environment that will impact his or her computer use [1, 6, 22, 38, 40–43]:

- Does the client currently use a computer? What for? What access methods are currently used?
- What other assistive technology does the client already use?
- How old is the client?
- Where does the client live and who does the client live with?
- How active is the client?
- What is the client's socioeconomic status?
- What roles does the client play at home, school, or work?
- How much caregiver assistance does the client receive?
- Who supports the technology (assistive or otherwise) that the client already owns?
- Where will the client use a computer?
- Does the client need to use more than one computer?

The clinician also needs to understand the client's background, including the client's prior experiences with computers and computer access technology, educational and vocational history, and any other relevant prior experiences with technology [22, 40]. Cultural influences can also be important [1, 22, 36, 40, 41]. A client's culture can affect his or her degree of exposure to technology, past experiences, and satisfaction with technology use, all of which influences a client's predisposition to the use of assistive technology [36].

Parette and Angelo found that clinicians often underestimate the influence of families on the success or failure of assistive technology [94]. Cultural values placed on functional support from assistive technologies, as opposed to personal assistance from family members, and the value a client's family places on enhanced independence can also affect an individual's predisposition to use assistive technology [22, 36, 40, 41]. Families are often the first line of defense when a client needs technical or moral support [1, 41].

The client's diagnosis and medical history is obviously important [22, 40, 41], as is the likelihood of change in the client's medical status. A client's diagnosis alone often provides limited information about what computer access technology is most appropriate. Medical assessments often emphasize gross motor functions rather than the fine motor functions needed for computer access. Functional capabilities can vary dramatically across individuals with the same diagnosis, and can be remarkably similar across individuals with very different diagnoses.

Evaluating a client's psychological and emotional state is both important and challenging [6, 22, 40, 41, 43]. The clinician needs to assess the client's motivation, acceptance of assistive technology, and willingness to learn new things [1, 36, 40, 41]. Successfully using computer access technology often requires a willingness to change how the client does things [1].

An accurate assessment of the client's cognitive skills is critical for a successful computer access assessment [6, 22, 26, 41, 43]. Using a computer with computer access technology touches on a range of cognitive skills, including reading, problem solving, memorization, and multitasking. Many computer access technologies decrease the perceptual or motor requirements of operating a computer at the expense of increasing the cognitive load. A clinician should choose interventions with a client's cognitive skills in mind.

A client's sensory impairments must also be understood [6, 22, 40–43], even if a sensory impairment is not the primary reason the client sought a computer access assessment. Computer use is extremely visual in nature, but the growing use of the Internet for distributing audio and video has increased the importance of hearing.

The clinician must examine all of a client's physical skills that are relevant to computer use [6, 22, 38, 40, 42, 43]. For individuals with severe disabilities, the clinician should begin by identifying the physical movements the client can control in a conscious, consistent manner [1, 26, 41]. Once these purposeful movements have been identified, the client needs to assess each movement's accuracy, range, repeatability, strength, and speed [26].

In addition to the client's previous history and current condition, the clinician must consider the client's future needs and abilities [26, 38, 40, 42]. Things to consider include the future course of the client's medical condition, living environment, and amount of personal assistance. Understanding how likely a client's circumstances are to change, and what those changes are likely to be, will help the clinician build in the needed adaptability to the client's computer access solution.

14.2.4 WHAT TO CONSIDER ABOUT EACH COMPUTER ACCESS TECHNOLOGY

Once the client's needs, abilities, and context have been established, the clinician can begin identifying appropriate computer access technologies for the client to evaluate.

Some important questions to consider when examining products include [1, 3, 39]

- Will this device soon be outdated? Is something better on the horizon?
- Does it fit the individual?
- Is it convenient to use in the client's environment(s)?
- Does this device represent the simplest, most efficient way to accomplish the task or is this device too complicated?
- Does it work efficiently and effectively?
- Is it easy to learn to use this device?
- Are all of the technologies compatible with each other and the computer access technologies the client already uses?
- Is the manufacturer willing to provide a loaner for an extended trial before purchase?
- Does the manufacturer provide training in using the device?
- Does the manufacturer have a local sales representative? Do company sales people seem knowledgeable and helpful?
- Is it safe to use?
- Does the device fit well into the user's lifestyle?
- Can the user operate the device independently or with a minimum of assistance?
- Does the device "stick out" too much and advertise the disability of the user?
- Does the device have the potential to increase the quantity and quality of time spent with nondisabled peers or does the device separate the user from others?
- Do the benefits the device provides justify the cost?
- Are there less expensive devices or models that serve the purpose as well?
- Is this device the user's own choice?
- Does the client like this device and want to use it?
- Would the user have preferred some other device or means to perform the task?
- Will using the device always be a chore or can using it become a habit?

Questions specific to hardware (e.g., keyboards, pointing devices) include [1, 3]

- What is the manufacturer's repair policy?
- Does the manufacturer provide a warranty, or a replacement when a device is being repaired?
- Are the company's service people knowledgeable and helpful?
- How long is the device guaranteed to function?
- Are repair services available? At what cost?
- How portable is the product? This includes size and weight, along with the need to install drivers or other supporting software.
- How durable is the product?
- Is the product aesthetically pleasing?
- How easy is it to modify, update, or repair the product?

Questions specific to software include [3]

- Is the software designed to run off of an external disk or thumb drive or does it need to be installed on the computer in order to run?
- What is the company's update policy? How often are updates released? Are updates installed automatically? How often does the company charge for updates?

14.2.5 PERFORMANCE MEASUREMENT

14.2.5.1 Importance of Measuring Performance

Hands-on trials are critical [5, 23, 39]. Finding the best device(s) and optimal configuration requires consideration of multiple aspects of the device. A single measure of performance is rarely enough [21]. Potential computer access solutions should be evaluated across a wide variety of tasks that cover all of the types of activities the client might engage in [24, 41, 44, 45]. On the other hand, while numerous sources emphasize the need to collect performance data, there is limited guidance regarding what data to collect, how to combine the data with subjective observations and other information collected by the clinician, or how to balance conflicting data [21].

14.2.5.2 Objective Performance Measurement

The act of planning and obtaining objective, quantitative measures of performance can improve the quality of service a clinician provides [24, 46, 47]. Quantitative data can be used to make comparisons across potential solutions within a single client during the assessment process [47]. However, quantitative data are also potentially valuable when used to examine a client's performance over time (to determine the effectiveness of training) [24, 25]. Quantitative data can also be used to compare performance across clients [24]. There isn't a standard battery of tests that all computer access clients complete, which makes sense given the variety of people who need computer access technology and the potential interactions between multiple technologies. That being said, individual clinicians (or even multiple clinicians within the same clinic) would still benefit from aggregating outcomes data across their similar clients.

14.2.5.3 Importance of Subjective/Qualitative Data

A clinician should not focus exclusively on quantitative measures. The computer should record the quantitative measures and the clinician should focus on observing the client. Things to look for include posture, compensation for deficits, presence of pain, tremor, spasticity, and signs of fatigue [24]. The client's subjective impressions are also important [2, 48], and will be most accurate when obtained after real tasks. Things to discuss with the client include personal preference, independence, and perceived performance [42].

14.2.5.4 Performance Measurement Tools

Before an alternative input device for a person with a motor impairment can be selected, and evaluated by a therapist working with such an individual, it is necessary to have an objective measure of performance [47]. To determine which strategy of a number of potential interventions is most appropriate for a specific individual, it is necessary to have a quantitative metric for comparing performance using these devices [47]. Furthermore, determining the optimum settings for a particular individual requires an objective measure that is reliable and should also have predictive properties [47]. There are no widely accepted quantitative computer access assessment instruments, service models, or protocols [20, 49]. As a result, computer access assessment is often *ad hoc*, unplanned, and entirely subjective [49].

A performance measurement tool provides one or more skill tests that result in quantitative measures of performance. The tool itself may be software that runs on the computer or it may be a paper-based system. Not many performance measurement tools are available for computer access, and none of the tools that are available have been widely accepted [5, 22, 32, 34, 46].

Manual assessment tools often rely on the subjective judgment of the clinician [50]. Computers are better than people at collecting and aggregating data [46, 50]. Computers can also perform calculations and present data in a meaningful form [50].

One approach to performance measurement is to break computer access down to its component pieces. The other approach is to evaluate specific tasks, perhaps in combination, that the client expects to perform in real life. The advantage of the component pieces approach is that it's more efficient and provides very specific information. A disadvantage of the component pieces approach is that measurement error in a shorter task is more significant than the same error in a much longer task [24]. In other words, being 1 second off when measuring a 10-second task is a bigger deal than being 1 second off when measuring a 100-second task. Another disadvantage of this approach is that the results might not generalize to real life [45].

The advantage of the real tasks approach is that it incorporates the cognitive load involved in task execution, which can be lost when focusing on individual component actions. I recommend using the component pieces approach to narrow the field; then use specific tasks for making the final decision.

14.2.6 TRIAL PERIODS

A client really needs to try out a computer access solution across all of the environments, contexts, and tasks in which it will be used [1, 21–23, 38]. The client should use the technology at different times of day, in different locations, and for different activities. This typically requires renting or borrowing technology for several weeks. A lot of software has trial versions that can be downloaded from the developer's website. Hardware that is sold by an assistive technology company that caters specifically to people with disabilities may be available for loan or rent.

The greatest challenge to the clinician is getting good information from the client during the loan period. It's important to know how often the client actually used the technology and how well it actually worked, but the clinician typically has to rely on the client's self-report.

14.2.7 DOCUMENTATION

The primary output of most assessments is a report documenting the clinician's findings. The report should contain [3, 23]:

- What equipment was used, how the equipment was configured, and the resulting quantitative and qualitative observations
- Measurement instruments employed in the evaluation
- The client's responses and preferences to the equipment tried
- Training needed by team members on the suggested equipment
- How to obtain the equipment as well as what equipment is available for loan or rental
- The recommended system, including settings to use and when or where it might be appropriate to use the equipment
- Recommended environmental and instructional modifications

The International Classification of Functioning, Disability and Health (ICF) provides a systematic scheme for documenting a client's needs and abilities. The ICF model represents a holistic view of functioning, disability, and contextual factors [20]. Unfortunately, most clinicians have little training in the ICF and there are few tools to help use the ICF. The ICF is also not without its limitations. The ICF records whether a person can perform a task with AT, but does not record any information about that performance, such as user satisfaction [20]. This doesn't mean the ICF isn't useful, but it does mean the ICF alone is not sufficient to describe a person's needs and abilities.

14.3   DESIGNING SOLUTIONS

An effective computer access solution is rarely just a device or piece of software. The total solution often involves a combination of technology, appropriate configuration of the technology, modifications to the environment, and training for the client and others around the client [38]. Any sufficiently complex computer access solution will involve trade-offs [9, 21, 51, 52]:

- Easy to use for novices or fast and efficient for expert users
- Most appropriate for right now or able to grow/change to meet future needs
- Limited motor demands or limited cognitive/perceptual demands
- Cost
- Compatibility with existing hardware/software
- Ability to share computer with others

14.3.1   WHEN TO GET SOMETHING NEW

The march of progress within the computer industry is relentless. It often feels as if computer technology becomes obsolete the same day it is purchased. Eventually, all computer hardware and software becomes outdated and must be replaced. As newer versions of software and operating systems are released, the manufacturer may stop supporting older versions. Older computer equipment may not be powerful enough to support new AT or computer software. Older AT may not work with the latest release of a program or operating system.

If the client already has a successful computer access solution in place, the decision to change that solution should not be taken lightly [39, 52]. The clinician and the client should consider whether the reasons for changing the system are sufficient to justify abandoning the effort already spent to develop and learn the old system and investing additional effort in designing and learning a new system [52]. If change is unavoidable, however, then consider which skills developed in using the old system can be transferred to the new system [52].

14.3.2 Integrated vs. Distributed

A client's computer access solution may or may not be integrated with other assistive technology the client owns (e.g., using a wheelchair joystick for mouse control, using an augmentative communication device for text entry). Individuals with limited movement/dexterity or a single access site are good candidates for an integrated computer access solution [3, 38, 42]. Reasons for considering an integrated control system include [42]

- Provides a single, reliable access site
- Reduces training
- Builds on existing skills
- Speed, accuracy, or ease of use improved or long-term endurance increased
- Client or family's personal preference
- Reduced clutter, fewer devices at access site
- Less need for help in transitioning between activities

Reasons to use a distributed control system include [3, 38, 42]

- You can use the most appropriate/efficient input device for each task/device.
- Avoid the increased cognitive demands of learning a more complicated control method.
- Cost: Wheelchair electronics that provide computer access and AAC devices with built-in computers are more expensive.
- If an integrated system breaks, everything goes. If a distributed system breaks, only one component is gone.
- The client may want to access devices separately (e.g., from off of wheelchair, away from AAC device).
- User may already have learned to do some tasks in a specific way or with a specific interface.
- Cognitive or perceptual demands of integrated control may be too great.

14.3.3 Design Guidelines

When designing a computer access solution for a client, consider the types of interventions available [53]:

- Settings and configuration options built in to the computer's operating system
- Software that can be installed on the computer
- Hardware (perhaps in combination with software) that can be attached to the computer

Configuration options that are included in a computer's operating system are the most portable, since they will be available on any computer the client uses. Software (like screen readers) can be carried around on a jump drive. Hardware, particularly devices that are large, complicated, or requires the installation of drivers, is the least portable.

Also keep in mind that people with disabilities often prefer to use standard equipment wherever possible [54]. Relying on configuration options built in to the operating system leaves the computer looking normal. Built-in options are also the least expensive.

Build on the user's existing skills [52]. AT devices are most effective when consumers use their own unique motor abilities instead of trying to move in a manner that looks normal [19]. Don't be seduced by the most expensive high-technology products available. Effective low-tech solutions are often less expensive and more robust [23]. Always include a backup access method, even if it is as simple as a mouthstick.

14.3.3.1 Design for Automaticity

Computer access technology is most efficient, and imposes the least cognitive load, when its use is automatic [52, 55]. Characteristics of tasks that are performed automatically include [52]

- Economy of effort (less energy and attention are required)
- Consistency of performance
- Adaptability (performance can automatically adjust to compensate for task conditions)
- Increased speed
- Dependence on internalized feedback rather than prompts from the environment
- Ability to anticipate the actions of the system
- Ability to multitask

Tasks that are automatic consume far less attention, long-term memory, working memory, executive control, or other cognitive resources than tasks that must be performed deliberately [55]. The design of a computer access solution should promote automaticity [52]. Aspects of a system that promote automaticity include [52]

- Making the system's behavior predictable
- Limiting the amount of visual or auditory feedback needed to operate the system
- Minimizing the number of decisions that need to be made
- Eliminating the need for external prompts or cues during task performance

14.3.3.2 Designing for Initial Ease of Use vs. Expert Use

There is a tension between designing systems that are easy for novices to use and systems that are efficient for experienced users. Systems that provide lots of cues to the user about the current situation and what step to perform next help users to learn the system, but once the system has been mastered, those same cues may be more of a hindrance than a help [52]. Similarly, novices can benefit from frequent requests for confirmation, to reduce errors and provide additional time for planning subsequent actions [21, 52]. More experienced users are more likely to find frequent confirmation requests annoying.

14.4 TRAINING

Service delivery doesn't end after the technology has been selected and configured. Training is a crucial component [1, 2, 36, 38, 52] for both the client and any caregivers who will help the client use the system [2]. Unfortunately, there is often little support for training [52, 56].

Training should consist of more than just stepping the client through isolated tasks. The clinician needs to help the client develop a mental model of how the technology works [52]. A successful mental model will help the user deal with novel situations, correct errors, and predict the actions of the system accurately [52]. An accurate model helps build the user's trust of the system. A clear mental model that allows the user to predict the system's actions makes it less likely that the system will behave in ways the user does not expect [52]. A mental model also helps the user avoid unrealistic expectations of the system and can help the user to avoid transferring old habits from previous computer access solutions [52].

The *task simplification* approach redesigns a task into gradations of complexity. The user begins with a less complex task that incorporates all of the component skills and informational concepts of the full task. As simpler versions of the task are mastered, additional complexity is introduced. This approach is also called the "training wheels" approach, in that the user immediately attains the goal of the task but through a simpler method. Task simplification is appropriate for young children who require the incentive of acquiring the goal. Task simplification is also a useful approach for tasks where the relationship between task components is an important skill component in itself [52].

In the *skill decomposition* method the task is broken down into separate skills or concepts that are practiced individually before being recombined and practiced as a complete task. This approach allows the clinician to determine which task components have been mastered and which haven't. Skill decomposition is well suited for tasks in which one skill is more critical or difficult than others [52].

14.5 FOLLOW-UP

After the equipment is purchased, delivered, and installed, regular follow-up and outcomes evaluation allow the clinician to modify (and hopefully improve) all stages of the decision-making process [2, 44]. Assistive technology in general, and computer access in particular, has very little evidence about what interventions are successful [27]. In part, that is because the definition of *success*, while simple in theory, turns out to be quite elusive in practice. Given the lack of an evidence base, clinicians who provide computer access services are almost required to learn from experience. The problem with learning by experience is that it takes time. New clinicians are less effective because they do not have outcomes to learn from. Computer access decisions are thus often made without the assistance of clinical evidence or quantitative data [44].

Challenges in measuring outcomes include [57]

- Defining/measuring what a good outcome is in the provision of AT
- Separating environmental effects from effects of the AT
- Potential uncertainty in outcomes (good luck vs. bad luck)
- Identifying what factors/circumstances are relevant to the outcome (e.g., environment, support)
- Aggregating individual clients into meaningful groups for analysis and generalization

Another challenge to evaluating outcomes is determining what the goals of the clinician and client are:

- Some AT is chosen to maximize the potential gain (increased mobility, increased independence, increased productivity).
- Other AT is chosen to minimize the potential loss (increased safety, decreased cost, decreased injury).

The outcome of an intervention is just as unique as each individual client. The outcome measure needs to reflect that individuality, which implies a need for one very flexible instrument or a variety of more tailored instruments [27, 57].

The challenges to learning from outcomes include

- Averaging outcomes over multiple (individual) cases.
- Mapping outcomes to specific elements within the decision-making process.
- We may revise our memory of the situation to fit the feedback, rather than the decision-making process.
- Some choices constrain what outcomes are possible.
- Most studies of outcomes are cross-sectional rather than longitudinal, and are not conducted by the clinicians who made the decisions in the first place.

Potential measures/indicators of goodness include

- Abandonment: This is an all-or-nothing measure (no in-between); it may not happen for months or years after the decision is made.
- Agreement with experts: There is no guarantee that experts will agree or even be right; it's hard to measure the distance between two AT solutions.
- Vocational success: Job placement is a binary measure; difficult to compare jobs.
- Educational success: It's possible to increase someone's capabilities, get them in a more advanced class, and have their grades go down even though they are learning more.
- Increased independence: Defining and measuring independence is difficult.
- Increased health: Not all AT directly impacts health (e.g., computer access).
- Frequency and duration of use: Some AT is only intended to be used rarely (e.g., backup access methods).

The term *abandonment* covers a variety of different behaviors [2] and care must be taken when reading the literature to determine how abandonment is defined. Potential reasons a client might abandon a device include [2] (1) exchanging one device with another, (2) no longer needing the device, (3) no longer using the device even though the need persists, (4) partial, reluctant use of the device, and (5) rejection of the notion of using a device before any system is attempted.

One of the most frequently cited studies of AT abandonment was performed by Phillips and Zhao in 1993 [95]. The study encompassed all forms of AT and found that 33% of all assistive technology was abandoned by the user. Other studies of AT abandonment have reported rates as low as 8% and as high as 75% [2, 27, 40, 58]. To date, the evidence regarding abandonment of computer access technology specifically is scant, inconclusive, and often contradictory. In Watson's study, 2 out of 13 participants (students) received a computer access intervention (IntelliKeys keyboard). Neither student abandoned the intervention [27].

14.6   OBSTACLES TO GOOD ASSESSMENT

14.6.1   LACK OF EQUIPMENT

No clinic can have every computer access device and software available on the market. What is important is to have a representative sample of devices for use in the clinic that covers the different options [23] and to encourage clients to do more extended trials of devices at home before purchase.

14.6.2   COMPUTER ACCESS CAN BE ISOLATED FROM OTHER SERVICES

Depending on the facility and the client, computer access services may be provided in isolation from other services (like wheeled seating and mobility, augmentative communication, audiology, vision services, counseling, electronic aids to daily living, home modifications, etc.) [38]. It's not always (or even usually) possible to include all stakeholders (e.g., caregivers, teachers, attendants, family members, employers, vocational rehabilitation counselors) in a single visit to a clinic [58]. In a school or hospital setting, it may be easier to coordinate services. In other environments, this may be impossible. Unless you are working with a client immediately postinjury or postdiagnosis, some services are likely to have already been provided. There is also limited funding to include other clinicians in a computer access evaluation. Even if there was funding, the other clinicians may not have time to participate. One approach to including far-flung team members is to use video conferencing. Several different solutions exist (e.g., Skype, iChat) that include desktop sharing, video, audio, and text messaging.

14.6.3   PROBLEMS WITH A SINGLE SESSION IN A CLINIC

Computer access evaluations are typically conducted in a single session, often in an environment that is unfamiliar to the client [3, 23, 59]. Data collected in a single session in the clinic are unlikely to be representative of the variation in real-world computer use [59]. An assessment that does not include the actual home, school, work, and community environments where a computer and computer access technology will be used is incomplete [58]. Clients, particularly small children, may be nervous or uncomfortable in an unfamiliar clinical environment [58]. Clients can also be fatigued by travel or may have to get up early to make it to a clinic on time [58]. Video conferencing can be used to extend the assessment to the client's environment, but this will only work if the client already has a computer and can borrow or rent the computer access technology under consideration.

14.6.4   LACK OF TIME FOR ASSESSMENT

Time pressure can be a particularly limiting factor in AT assessments. It's hard enough to optimize the configuration of a single device [59, 60]. Optimizing the combination of multiple devices for multiple tasks takes a lot of time. Clinicians rarely have enough time to conduct a completely thorough assessment that compares all potential technologies, configurations, tasks, situations, and environments [21, 24, 49, 56]. The time that a clinician can spend with a client in the clinic can be constrained by factors such as scheduling or fatigue. The time available to the client and clinician to conduct clinic visits, test equipment, and produce a final decision can be constrained by deadlines like the beginning of the school year.

It is critical, then, to make the most efficient use possible of the client's and clinician's time. This begins by planning as much of the assessment as possible prior to the client's arrival. Assessment software that records performance data can also make the assessment process more efficient.

14.6.5   LACK OF TECHNICAL SUPPORT

Clients may not have competent local technical support for their computer access technology [58]. A lack of on-site technical support is especially important for very sophisticated technologies (e.g., eye gaze) and solutions that involve the integration of multiple components (e.g., speech recognition and a screen reader, on-screen keyboard, word prediction, mouse emulator). If on-site technical support is likely to be an issue, then priority should be given to technology from traditional assistive technology manufacturers, who are more likely to provide comprehensive technical support. On-demand technical support services from "big box stores" (e.g., Best Buy's Geek Squad) can also fill in some gaps. Clinicians can also use desktop sharing and video conferencing technology to provide remote technical support.

14.6.6   "ALL THUMBS" PROBLEM

A long-standing challenge in comparing different computer access technologies is that some are easier for novices to use than others, but initial performance may not be indicative of long-term performance after skills are acquired [21, 46, 61, 62]. Clients have a hard time envisioning how a device will work when they are expert at it and it can be hard to convince a client to invest a lot of time learning to use a technology that *may* prove to be more efficient over time. It is hard to predict a client's future performance based on available evidence, because limited evidence is available that is applicable to a specific user/task/technology/environment [21, 52]. Data from expert able-bodied computer users may not be applicable to users with disabilities [21].

A client may favor a device that's easy to use initially over a device with a steeper learning curve that will ultimately be more effective [52, 62–65]. A classic example of this phenomenon is the client who chooses single-switch scanning over Morse code [52]. Extended home trials is one solution, but some technologies (e.g., automatic speech recognition [ASR] or Morse code) can take months to truly master. Another option is to simulate expertise, by focusing on a subset of the functionality or ignoring errors when measuring performance.

14.6.7 LACK OF EVIDENCE BASE

Evidence-based practice means integrating empirical evidence with clinical/educational expertise and stakeholder input, to make decisions that are deemed effective and efficient for a client [31]. There is a tension between real-world data collected as people perform actual tasks in their normal environment and laboratory data. Real-world data may be more representative of a user's actual behavior, and can also capture interactions between multiple tasks and technologies that a controlled study is likely to miss. Real-world data collection also allows participants to work at their own (natural) pace, which may reduce fatigue and stress [59].

On the other hand, real-world data collection lacks the experimental control of data collected in the laboratory. In the real world, when the user has not been given a specific task to accomplish, the goal behind a user's actions may be unclear (or the user may be performing multiple tasks simultaneously) [59]. If an experimenter doesn't tell the subject what to do, it can be hard to tell what he or she is doing. And if the experimenter doesn't know what the subject is doing, it's hard to tell how well he or she is doing it.

It's hard to draw conclusions about an entire class of input devices (i.e., all mice, all trackballs, all joysticks) based on a comparison between a small number of specific instances of each device [60]. There are a huge number of configuration options, with complex interactions [60]. The variety within each device category makes it difficult to identify a representative sample of products and configurations [60]. It's hard to cover all potential combinations. For example, how many different trackballs would be needed to adequately represent all trackballs?

Even carefully performed comparisons become outdated quickly as new devices emerge [24]. It's unclear how empirical results obtained with computer mice that used a ball apply to computer mice that use optical technology. Are results obtained with a traditional trackpad relevant to more modern multitouch trackpads? How do we compare results obtained under Windows 95 and Windows 7?

14.6.8 COGNITIVE/MOTOR/SENSORY TRADE-OFF

Computer access technologies that reduce the motor or sensory requirements of operating a computer typically do so at the expense of increasing the user's cognitive load [10, 21, 33, 66]. For example:

- Screen readers impose significant memory requirements since the contents of the screen aren't visible and must be memorized.
- Screen magnifiers impose similar types of loads because only a portion of the screen is visible, so the rest must be remembered.
- Word prediction and abbreviation expansion impose memory and decision loads.
- ASR requires learning complex commands and processes.

Since AT is the means to operate the computer to perform tasks, rather than an end in itself, AT is almost always used in a multitasking environment [52]. The end result is that computer access technologies that are intended to help the user perform tasks more quickly may actually slow the user down by imposing additional mental operations [67, 68]. AT that imposes less cognitive load on the user is likely to produce better performance [21].

14.6.9 NEED FOR ADAPTATION OVER TIME

A device that is well configured for a novice is likely to be poorly configured for an expert [52, 61]. User's needs change over time. A user's needs may change slowly (due to practice or a degenerative medical condition) or may change quickly (due to fatigue or medicine) [38, 52, 59]. Information technology is constantly changing: new programs are released, old programs are updated. Computer access technology must adapt in response [69].

The computer access solution must therefore be adjusted over time. One implication is that we need computer access technology to automatically adapt [70]. Another implication is that we need lots of people with enough computer access training to feel comfortable making these adaptations, because we can't rely on a small number of rehab engineers to make these frequent modifications.

14.6.10 COMPUTER ACCESS TECHNOLOGY CAN BE EXPENSIVE

In the United States, medical insurance does not reimburse individuals for the cost of computer access technology. School districts and vocational rehabilitation programs will pay for computer access technology, but they have limited budgets and do not provide services to everyone. Without external funding, the cost of some computer access technology can be prohibitive for some clients [36, 71].

14.7 DECISION MAKING

14.7.1 HOW DO PEOPLE MAKE DECISIONS?

A key aspect of the assessment process is choosing between alternative solutions. This section examines what is known about how people (1) collect and integrate information, (2) identify alternatives, and (3) select from among the alternatives they have identified.

14.7.1.1   Collecting and Integrating Information

Collecting and interpreting information accurately is critical to good decision making. However, there are several practical limitations to how much information a decision maker can consider at one time and how accurate that information can be [72]. Constraints on data quantity result from the limited storage capacity of short-term memory. Constraints on the accuracy of information result from imperfect long-term memory and the limited accuracy of "mental arithmetic."

Working memory serves as the "cognitive workbench" for data comparison and manipulation. The amount of information that can be held in working memory at one time is limited [72], and this limit represents the upper bound on the number of facts that can be simultaneously processed. Hence, merely increasing the number of data sources or quantity of information does not necessarily lead to improved decision making.

Long-term memory, on the other hand, serves as the library for background knowledge and experiences. Retrieving, or *recalling*, a specific item from long-term memory depends on how often that item is accessed, and how well connected the item is with other items stored in memory. Knowledge that is older, used less frequently, or is less connected, or *elaborated*, is more difficult to recall [72].

The imperfect nature of long-term memory presents a challenge to clinicians, in that the AT assessment process relies, in part, on recall by the client and caregivers. People tend to be overconfident in their recall of facts, events, and frequency, even for personally witnessed events [73]. Clinicians often ask people to recall specific events that occurred with their current AT, or during an in-home trial of new AT, and people may report greater confidence in their recall than is warranted. Clinicians also have to recall events, and their recall could be similarly overconfident. For example, a clinician might try to recall how a similar client performed with an AT device to determine whether the device might be appropriate for a current client.

People also have difficulty estimating proportions, probabilities, and frequencies [74]. People can generally provide accurate estimates of frequency of occurrence for events that occur 5 to 95% of the time, but have difficulty estimating the frequency of events that happen almost never (less than 5% of the time) or almost always (more than 95% of the time). Another consistent observation is that people's estimates of probabilities and frequencies are "sluggish" and tend to respond slowly to new evidence [72]. Clinicians often ask clients to estimate how frequently things occur (e.g., "How often do you use your tilt feature?" "How often do you experience spasticity?"), and frequency estimates near the extremes could be inaccurate [75].

14.7.1.2   Identifying Alternatives

An important aspect of many decision-making tasks is generating the options from which a choice will be made [76]. If there are many possible options, one can winnow the choices by either starting with an empty set and *including* (adding in) potential choices or starting with all options and *excluding* some. Research has shown that people are more likely to use inclusion when asked for personal judgments, and more likely to use exclusion when there is a single correct answer (e.g., multiple choice tests) [77]. People are also more likely to use exclusion when choosing among items for which it is difficult to provide a single score reflecting the quality of each choice [77]. The exclusion strategy typically leads to larger set sizes [77].

The AT assessment process is driven in large part by the options that a clinician generates and presents to the client. Hence, clinicians need tools and strategies that they can use to generate a small number of the most appropriate options. The AT assessment process has many of the characteristics of tasks that typically favor exclusion (a single correct answer, items that are difficult to score), so it is likely that many clinicians start with a set of all possible options and remove those that are clearly inappropriate. However, since inclusion produces smaller set sizes [76], clinicians might make more efficient use of their time by adopting a strategy based on inclusion to decide which devices to test with a client.

14.7.1.3   Choosing from Multiple Alternatives

Once a set of alternatives has been identified, the decision maker must then choose a single alternative from the set. Decision science has identified several approaches that people use to compare multiple alternatives. *Compensatory* decision strategies make use of all available information about each alternative, and directly compare each alternative on an attribute-by-attribute basis. Each attribute, which can be simple objective items like size or weight or more complex items like language encoding strategy, can be weighted based on its importance to the decision maker. Attributes are often given categorical values (e.g., 0 = heavy, 1 = medium weight, 2 = light) rather than using their unscaled numerical values. Examples of compensatory decision-making strategies are [72]

- Choice by majority of confirming dimensions: Choose the alternative with the greatest number of winning attributes.
- Equally weighted comparison: Choose the alternative for which the sum of the value of each attribute is greatest.
- Weighted additive comparison: Choose the alternative for which the sum of the value for each attribute multiplied by the weight of each attribute is greatest.

Noncompensatory decision strategies, on the other hand, make use of heuristics or other simplifying approaches to produce a decision without considering all of the available information. Because they consider less information, noncompensatory strategies are faster to implement but are less accurate than compensatory strategies. Examples of noncompensatory decision-making strategies are [72]

- Elimination by aspects: Eliminate all choices that fail to meet some threshold (for example, remove from consideration all devices that weigh more than a specific amount).
- Lexicographic heuristic: Choose the alternative that has the highest value for the most important attribute (for example, choose the lightest device).
- Conjunctive heuristic: Set threshold values for all attributes at once, then choose the alternative that exceeds all thresholds (for example, choose the device that is both lighter than a specific amount and smaller than a specific size).

Consciously or not, people have to choose what decision strategy they will use, and they make this choice based on the perceived accuracy and effort of each method [78]. Unfortunately, people are not very good at estimating the effort or accuracy of different decision strategies [79]. When a choice must be made quickly, a noncompensatory decision strategy may be chosen to save time, at the cost of decision quality.

Time pressure can be a particularly limiting factor in AT assessments. The time that a clinician can spend with a client in the clinic can be constrained by factors such as scheduling or fatigue. The time available to the client and clinician to conduct clinic visits, test equipment, and produce a final decision can be constrained by deadlines like the beginning of the school year. It is critical, then, to make the most efficient use possible of the client's and clinician's time.

Additional factors that can influence which strategy and representation are adopted include [80]

- Personal importance of the task to the decision maker
- Familiarity with, or background knowledge of, the task domain
- Temporal duration of possible outcomes
- Moral relevance
- Likelihood of possible outcomes

Clients, clinicians, and third-party payers will all clearly differ according to these factors. For a client, AT has high personal importance and great temporal duration, but the client may have limited familiarity with the AT in question. For a clinician, personal importance may be at a medium level since he or she interacts directly with the client, and familiarity is (hopefully) high. For the third-party payer, there is limited personal importance and the possible outcomes may be measured in monetary terms rather than performance or quality of life. This means that clinicians must take care to present the most relevant information to clients and third-party payers to facilitate their decision making. This also means that clinicians must understand how others are making decisions to be more aware of what each agent's priorities are.

14.7.2   What Limits Decision-Making Accuracy?

Several factors produce suboptimal performance in real-world decision tasks. People making complex decisions are often forced to consider uncertain or ambiguous information. Furthermore, people also have fixed cognitive resources in which to store, analyze, manipulate, and compare information. Finally, people do not always have sufficient time to obtain and make use of all potentially relevant information. These limitations result in several decision-making biases and effects that can lead to inaccurate decisions.

14.7.2.1   Overconfidence

The confidence individuals express in their judgments generally exceeds the accuracy of those judgments for difficult tasks [81]. Even worse, in tasks where repeated judgments are made, but feedback is not given, confidence in the accuracy of judgments can increase while actual accuracy does not [81]. Clinicians often get little or no feedback about the outcomes of their AT recommendations, and any feedback may take a long time to acquire. This implies that clinicians may develop unrealistic confidence in their decisions based on practice without feedback.

14.7.2.2 Sunk Cost Bias

The sunk cost bias refers to a tendency to make decisions based on past investment, rather than future benefits [72]. The sunk cost bias is often observed in stock holders who keep a stock that has lost money, rather than selling. Given the training and cost involved in AT, a sunk cost bias is a real possibility. For example, clinicians may prefer to continue using and recommending older, familiar products in which they have invested much effort to learn rather than newer, more functional devices.

Of course, training and experience are not necessarily bad things, and familiarity is a valid factor in the decision-making process. For example, the effort a consumer has expended learning an encoding scheme like MinSpeak, or a specific interface (JAWS vs. WindowEyes) can have a significant influence on what devices are chosen in the future. Familiarity only becomes sunk cost bias when prior experience is given undue influence over the decision-making process.

14.7.2.3 Optimal Stopping Problem

The problem of *when to stop* seeking information is common in many domains [82, 83]. People typically use a cost-benefit trade-off to decide when to stop seeking information, but people are more sensitive to cost than benefit and often stop seeking information too early [82]. In the AT assessment process, the cost of obtaining more information is often the time and effort needed to test more devices. This time and effort can be significant, particularly if it involves extended home use, and can cause clinicians and clients to stop seeking information too.

14.7.2.4 Predicting Outcomes

An important part of the AT assessment process is predicting, based on a client's novice performance with a device in the clinic, how well a client will perform with a device in the real world once he or she has become expert at that device. This prediction is obviously fraught with uncertainty. When information about the likelihood of outcomes is uncertain or ambiguous, the value of each possible outcome is given more weight in making selections [84]. Since predictions of AT outcomes are uncertain, clients and clinicians are likely to put much more weight on the value of each outcome, rather than its likelihood.

14.7.2.5 Framing Effect

The framing effect is observed when presenting a choice in terms of gains or losses [72]. When a choice is presented in positive terms (e.g., a 100% chance to save 200 lives vs. a 33% chance of saving 600 lives and a 66% chance of saving no lives), then people are more likely to choose the least risky option. However, when a choice is presented in negative terms (e.g., a 100% chance that 400 people will die vs. a 33% chance that no one will die and a 66% chance that 600 people will die), people are more likely to take the more risky option.

Clearly, many AT decisions involve risk. For example, using row/column scanning has a near 100% chance of a low text entry rate, whereas Morse code has a low chance of a high text entry rate and a high chance of no text entry rate (i.e., abandonment). How clinicians present these choices can affect what decisions people make. This is true for both the clinician/client interaction and the clinician/third-party payer interaction.

14.7.2.6 Availability Bias

The availability bias is a cognitive shortcut in which people make exclusive use of information that is readily available in memory [85]. The availability bias can limit the options that a clinician considers to those that are more prominent in memory. Another result of the availability bias is that individuals with more expertise can make poor predictions of the performance of novices, and are resistant to debiasing techniques intended to improve predictions of difficulty. This is in part because experts have trouble recalling their own novice performance [85]. Experts have more ready access to memories of trouble-free task performance than their own novice performance, which can lead them to underestimate the problems that novices will have [85]. Experts are also overconfident in their estimates, which makes it hard to debias them [85]. Clinicians are expert at assistive technology, but must make estimates about the performance of both clients (in using AT) and their families/caregivers (for support, maintenance, and setup). Clinicians should therefore be careful not to underestimate the difficulty that clients and their support network will have.

14.7.2.7 Primacy and Recency

Information is integrated sequentially, over time, and subsequent data force us to update prior beliefs [86]. A *primacy effect* occurs when information encountered early in the sequence is given greater weight, and a *recency effect* occurs when information encountered later in the sequence is given greater weight [86]. People update their belief in a hypothesis by adding/subtracting based on new evidence.

An AT assessment can be a long process, possibly stretched over several sessions, involving complex evidence. This would indicate that a primacy strategy would be favored. Within an evaluation, however, may be several shorter evaluation tasks that involve complex evidence. For example, a client might be asked to choose between three different keyboards or four different pointing devices. As another example, a clinician must choose which subset of devices to present to the client from among many possible keyboards or pointing devices. These shorter, but still complex, decisions would also favor primacy. This implies that the order in which options or evidence is considered will have an effect on what devices are ultimately selected.

14.7.2.8 Anchoring Bias

The anchoring effect is a phenomenon in which an arbitrary number (the anchor) biases subsequent numerical judgments [87]. Anchors are superficially represented in short-term memory as absolute value plus affix (unit) [87]. When numbers are given with high absolute values (e.g., 7,300 m) there is a greater anchor effect than when numbers are given with low absolute values (e.g., 7.3 km) [87]. Clinicians have a variety of scales to choose from (e.g., words per minute vs.

characters per minute). The choice of scale should be made with the anchoring effect in mind. For example, a new keyboard might be justified to a third-party payer in terms of an improvement of 5 characters per minute rather than 1 word per minute.

14.7.2.9   Confirmation Bias

Confirmation bias refers to the tendency of decision makers to pursue evidence that supports their beliefs and ignore evidence that disputes their belief. In the case of an AT assessment, the fixed library of devices available to a clinician can produce confirmation bias. It is unlikely that a clinician will have immediate access to all possible AT devices that might be applicable, and would not have time to try them all even if they were all available. A good example of this is the tongue-touch keypad,* which requires a custom-fit retainer. It's very hard to justify a dental appointment to test something that *might* work and the client *might* like, due to the time and expense involved.

14.7.3   WHAT LIMITS THE USE OF OUTCOMES DATA?

A frequently proposed antidote to poor AT assessments is the use of outcomes data to create a feedback loop. Unfortunately, outcomes in AT are difficult to quantify. Despite numerous efforts to develop a conceptual model with which to evaluate AT outcomes, there is currently no single model that describes and predicts AT outcomes across multiple domains of AT [88]. Second, there are limited opportunities to collect outcomes data (particularly when client and clinician are interacting outside of a school setting). Third, outcomes can take months or years to truly evaluate, which makes it difficult to relate outcomes to what was observed. Even if reliable and accurate AT outcomes are obtained, several obstacles have been identified to integrating feedback into the decision-making process that are particularly relevant to AT.

14.7.3.1   Input Bias

Input bias is the misuse of input information when evaluating outcome quality [89]. Irrelevant input affects judgments of outcome quality even when people realize the input is irrelevant [89]. In particular, inputs that reflect a large quantity (e.g., hours spent at work, cost of the machinery, distance traveled) bias judgments of outcome quality upward [89]. Within the domain of AT, it's possible that a client's or clinician's subjective judgments of AT outcomes may be biased by factors like cost, such that identical functional outcomes are judged differently based on the cost of the underlying system.

14.7.3.2   Hindsight Bias

Hindsight bias makes it difficult to look back at what was known prior to the outcome being observed and assess what should have been foreseen [90]. Often, outcomes seem more inevitable in hindsight than they did in foresight [90]. The hindsight bias differs for people who make decisions (e.g., stock brokers) and people who consume

---

* http://www.newabilities.com/.

decisions (e.g., their clients) [90]. People who evaluate other people's decisions demonstrate hindsight bias for both positive and negative outcomes, whereas people who evaluate their own decisions only demonstrate hindsight bias for positive outcomes [90]. This asymmetric hindsight bias may cause people to be overconfident in their future decisions [90]. Clinicians, clients, and third-party payers all have an interest in analyzing the outcomes of AT interventions. Due to the hindsight bias, clinicians are more likely to focus on positive outcomes when the decisions being evaluated are their own. For this reason, it might be better to train clinicians using the decisions/outcomes from other clinicians.

14.7.3.3 Emotion and Regret

Regret can result from bad decisions (decisions that produce bad outcomes) and from deciding badly (decisions made without sufficient thought) even if the outcome is good [91]. In situations where action is the norm, a decision not to act (inaction) produces greater regret than a wrong action [91].

An emotional reaction to a negative outcome can lead people to switch away from the options they believe are most likely to be successful on the next occasion [92]. Observers are influenced by the outcomes of decisions that others make [92]. Observers rate decision makers as better thinkers, more competent, and having engaged in better decision making when their decisions have a favorable outcome [92]. Similarly, even if the right choice was made but failed due to bad luck, observers rate decision makers more poorly when their decisions result in unfavorable outcomes [92]. When decision makers evaluate their own decisions, regret can cause a change in future behavior when an unfavorable outcome results, even if the choice was correct and subjects believe that option has a greater likelihood of future success [92]. Clients, clinicians, and payers all have to make decisions, and all may experience regret that causes them to change future behavior. For example, a clinician may stop recommending a brand of wheelchair, or a payer may stop approving a class of wheelchairs, because of a single failure.

REFERENCES

1. Beigel, A.R. 2000. Assistive technology assessment: More than the device. *Intervention in School and Clinic* 35(4): 237–243.
2. Johnson, J.M. et al. 2006. Perspectives of speech language pathologists regarding success versus abandonment of AAC. *Augmentative and Alternative Communication* 22(2): 85–99.
3. Kelker, K.A., and R. Holt. 1997. *Family guide to assistive technology*. Billings, MT: Parents, Let's Unite for Kids.
4. Manresa-Yee, C. et al. 2010. User experience to improve the usability of a vision-based interface. *Interacting with Computers* 22(6):594–605.
5. Price, K.J., and A. Sears. 2009. The development and evaluation of performance-based functional assessment: A methodology for the measurement of physical capabilities. *ACM Transactions on Accessible Computing* 2(2).
6. Randolph, A.B., and M.M.M. Jackson. 2010. Assessing fit of nontraditional assistive technologies. *ACM Transactions on Accessible Computing* 2(4).
7. Tanimoto, Y. et al. 2006. Imaging of computer input ability for patient with tetraplegia. *IEEE Transactions on Instrumentation and Measurement* 55(6): 1953–1958.

8. Trewin, S., and H. Pain. 1999. A model of keyboard configuration requirements. *Behaviour and Information Technology* 18(1): 27–35.
9. Trnka, K. et al. 2009. User interaction with word prediction: The effects of prediction quality. *ACM Transactions on Accessible Computing* 1(3).
10. Wood, E. et al. 2005. Use of computer input devices by older adults. *Journal of Applied Gerontology* 24(5): 419–438.
11. Baeker, R., and W. Buxton, eds. 1987. *Readings in human-computer interaction: A multidisciplinary approach.* Los Altos, CA: Morgan Kaufmann.
12. Hansen, P.K., and J. Wanner. 1993. Software drivers for pointers used by persons with disabilities. In *RESNA 1993 Annual Conference.* Las Vegas, NV: RESNA, pp. 443–445.
13. Olson, D.A., and F. DeRuyter, eds. 2002. *Clinician's guide to assistive technology.* St. Louis, MO: Mosby.
14. Poulson, D. 1996. Telematics applications for the integration of the disabled and elderly. In *User fit: A practical handbook on user-centred design for assistive technology.* DG XIII. Brussels-Luxembourg: European Commission.
15. Shein, F. et al. 1989. Guidelines for alternate access system developers. In *RESNA '89: Proceedings of the 12th Annual Conference*, J.J. Presperin, ed. New Orleans: RESNA, pp. 19–20.
16. Shein, F. et al. 1989. A model for alternate access systems. In *RESNA '89: Proceedings of the 12th Annual Conference*, J.J. Presperin, ed. New Orleans: RESNA, pp. 17–18.
17. Fitzgerald, M.M. et al. 2009. Comparison of three head-controlled mouse emulators in three light conditions. *Augmentative and Alternative Communication* 25(1): 32–41.
18. Anson, D.K. et al. 2004. Long-term speed and accuracy of Morse code vs. head-pointer interface for text generation. In *RESNA 27th International Annual Conference*, S.G. Fitzgerald, ed. Orlando, FL: RESNA.
19. Angelo, J. 2000. Factors affecting the use of a single switch with assistive technology devices. *Journal of Rehabilitation Research and Development* 37(5): 591–598.
20. Bernd, T., D. van der Pijl, and L. de Witte. 2009. Existing models and instruments for the selection of assistive technology in rehabilitation practice. *Scandanavian Journal of Occupational Therapy* 16: 146–158.
21. Cress, C.J., and G.J. French. 1994. The relationship between cognitive load measurements and estimates of computer input control skills. *Assistive Technology* 6(1): 54–66.
22. Hoppestad, B.S. 2006. Essential elements for assessment of persons with severe neurological impairments for computer access utilizing assistive technology devices: A Delphi study. *Disability and Rehabilitation: Assistive Technology* 1(1): 3–16.
23. Cormier, C. 2006. Points to consider for an assistive technology evaluation. Available from http://www.connsensebulletin.com/cormiernov2.html (accessed May 4, 2006).
24. Dumont, C., C. Vincent, and B. Mazer. 2002. Development of a standardized instrument to assess computer task performance. *American Journal of Occupational Therapy* 56(1): 60–68.
25. Dumont, C., and B. Mazer. 2006. *Assessment of computer task performance.* Institute de Readaptation en Deficience Physique de Quebec.
26. Access and assessment issues. 2010. Available from http://www.ace-north.org.uk/pages/resources/AssessmentIssues_000.pdf.pdf (accessed July 31, 2006).
27. Watson, A.H. et al. 2010. Effect of assistive technology in a public school setting. *American Journal of Occupational Therapy* 64(1): 17–28.
28. Reed, P., and G. Bowser. 1999. Education Tech Points: A framework for assistive technology planning and systems change in schools. In *Technology and Persons with Disabilities Conference (CSUN).* Los Angeles: California State University, Northridge.
29. Scherer, M.J. et al. 2005. Predictors of assistive technology use: The importance of personal and psychosocial factors. *Disability and Rehabilitation* 27(21): 1321–1331.

30. Cook, A.M., and S. Hussey. 2001. *Assistive technologies: Principles and practice*. 2nd ed. Philadelphia: Mosby, p. 523.
31. Schlosser, R., and P. Raghavendra. 2004. Evidence-based practice in augmentative and alternative communication. *Augmentative and Alternative Communication* 20(1): 1–21.
32. Man, D.W., and M.-S.L. Wong. 2007. Evaluation of computer-access solutions for students with quadriplegic athetoid cerebral palsy. *American Journal of Occupational Therapy* 61(3): 355–364.
33. Mckenna, M.C., and S. Walpole. 2007. Assistive technology in the reading clinic: Its emerging potential. *Reading Research Quarterly* 42(1): 140–145.
34. Fischl, C., and A.G. Fisher. 2007. Development and Rasch analysis of the assessment of computer-related skills. *Scandanavian Journal of Occupational Therapy* 14: 126–135.
35. Fraser, B.A., D.N. Bryen, and C.K. Morano. 1995. Development of a Physical Characteristics Assessment (PCA): A checklist for determining appropriate computer access for individuals with cerebral palsy. *Assistive Technology* 7(1): 26–35.
36. Scherer, M.J. et al. 2007. A framework for modelling the selection of assistive technology devices (ATDs). *Disability and Rehabilitation: Assistive Technology* 2(1): 1–8.
37. Anson, D.K. 1997. *Alternative computer access: A guide to selection*. 1st ed. Philadelphia: F.A. Davis Company, p. 280.
38. Ripat, J., and A. Booth. 2005. Characteristics of assistive technology service delivery models: Stakeholder perspectives and preferences. *Disability and Rehabilitation* 27(24): 1461–1470.
39. *Computer and web resources for people with disabilities*. 2002. Jackson, TN: Alliance for Technology Access (accessed September 4, 2002).
40. Gitlin, L., and D. Burgh. 1995. Issuing assistive devices to older patients in rehabilitation: An exploratory study. *American Journal of Occupational Therapy* 49(10): 994–1000.
41. Angelo, J. et al. 1997. Identifying best practice in the occupational therapy assistive technology evaluation: An analysis of three focus groups. *American Journal of Occupational Therapy* 51(10): 916–920.
42. Guerette, P., and E. Sumi. 1994. Integrating control of multiple assistive devices: A retrospective review. *Assistive Technology* 6(1): 67–76.
43. Jameson, A. 2001. Modeling both the context and the user. *Personal and Ubiquitous Computing* 5(1): 29–33.
44. Hill, K., and B. Romich. 2002. A rate index for augmentative and alternative communication. *International Journal of Speech Technology* 5(1): 57–64.
45. Mahmud, M. 2006. A mixed method for evaluating input devices with older persons. In *8th International ACM SIGACCESS Conference on Computers and Accessibility*, S. Keates, ed. Portland, OR: ACM Press, pp. 295–296.
46. Jenko, M. et al. 2010. A method for selection of appropriate assistive technology for computer access. *International Journal of Rehabilitation Research* 33(4): 298–305.
47. Radwin, R.G., G.C. Vanderheiden, and M.-L. Lin. 1990. A method for evaluating head-controlled computer input devices using Fitts' law. *Human Factors* 32(4): 423–438.
48. Simpson, T. et al. 2008. Tooth-click control of a hands-free computer interface. *IEEE Transactions on Biomedical Engineering* 55(8): 2050–2056.
49. Mazer, B., C. Dumont, and C. Vincen. 2003. Validation of the assessment of computer task performance for children. *Technology and Disability* 15(1): 35–43.
50. Smith, R.O. 1993. Computer-assisted functional assessment and documentation. *American Journal of Occupational Therapy* 11(47): 988–992.
51. Hourcade, J.P. et al. 2010. PointAssist for older adults: Analyzing sub-movement characteristics to aid in pointing tasks. In *28th International Conference on Human Factors in Computing Systems*, E. Mynatt, ed. Atlanta, GA: ACM Press, pp. 1115–1124.

52. Treviranus, J. 1994. Mastering alternative computer access: The role of understanding, trust, and automaticity. *Assistive Technology* 6(1): 26–41.

53. Trewin, S., and H. Pain. 1999. Keyboard and mouse errors due to motor disabilities. *International Journal of Human-Computer Studies* 50(2): 109–144.

54. Trewin, S. 2002. Extending keyboard adaptability: An investigation. *Universal Access in the Information Society* 2(1): 44–55.

55. Fairweather, P.G. 2008. How older and younger adults differ in their approach to problem solving on a complex website. In *10th International ACM SIGACCESS Conference on Computers and Accessibility (ASSETS '08)*, S. Harper, ed. Halifax, Canada: ACM Press, pp. 67–72.

56. Johansen, A.S., and J.P. Hansen. 2006. Augmentative and alternative communication: The future of text on the move. *Universal Access in the Information Society* 5(2): 125–149.

57. Johnson, B.B. et al. 2007. *Multiattribute utility theory: Summarizing a methodology and an evolving instrument for AT outcomes.* Milwaukee: ATOMS Project.

58. Craddock, G., and McCormack, L. 2002. Delivering an AT service: A client-focused, social and participatory service delivery model in assistive technology in Ireland. *Disability and Rehabilitation* 24(1/2/3): 160–170.

59. Hurst, A. et al. 2008. Automatically detecting pointing performance. In Proceedings of the 13th International Conference on Intelligent User Interfaces, S. Staab, ed. Gran Canaria, Spain: ACM, pp. 11–19.

60. Accot, J., and S. Zhai. 1999. Performance evaluation of input devices in trajectory-based tasks: An application of the steering law. In *Proceedings of the SIGCHI Conference on Human Factors in Computing Systems: The CHI Is the Limit.* ACM Press: Pittsburgh, PA.

61. Romich, B., K. Hill, and B.W. Liffick. 2005. Free software for measuring single switch user performance. In *Technology and Persons with Disabilities Conference (CSUN).* Los Angeles: California State University, Northridge.

62. Taveira, A.D., and S.D. Choi. 2009. Review study of computer input devices and older users. *International Journal of Human-Computer Interaction* 25(5): 455–474.

63. Anson, D.K. et al. 2001. Efficiency of the Chubon versus the QWERTY keyboard. *Assistive Technology* 13(1): 40–45.

64. Garcia, F.P., and K.-P.L. Vu. 2011. Effectiveness of hand- and foot-operated secondary input devices for word-processing tasks before and after training. *Computers in Human Behavior* 27(1): 285–295.

65. Zhai, S., P.-O. Kristensson, and B.A. Smith. 2005. In search of effective text input interfaces for off the desktop computing. *Interacting with Computers* 17(3): 229–250.

66. Koester, H., and S.P. Levine. 1994. Modeling the speed of text entry with a word prediction interface. *IEEE Transactions on Rehabilitation Engineering* 2(3): 177–187.

67. Felzer, T., and R. Nordmann. 2006. Alternative text entry using different input methods. In *Eighth International ACM SIGACCESS Conference on Computers and Accessibility.* Portland, OR: ACM Press.

68. Koester, H.H., and S.P. Levine. 1996. Effect of a word prediction feature on user performance. *Augmentative and Alternative Communication* 12(3): 155–168.

69. Schroeder, P. 1998. *Access to multimedia technology by people with sensory disabilities.* Washington, DC: National Council on Disability.

70. Kehoe, A., F. Neff, and I. Pitt. 2009. Use of voice input to enhance cursor control in mainstream gaming applications. *Universal Access in the Information Society* 8(1): 89–96.

71. Shih, C.-T., C.-H. Shih, and C.-H. Luo. 2011. Development of a computer assistive input device through a commercial numerical keyboard by position coding technology for people with disabilities. *Disability and Rehabilitation: Assistive Technology* 6(2): 169–175.

72. Wickens, C.D., and J.G. Hollands. 2000. *Engineering psychology and human performance*. 3rd ed. Upper Saddle River, NJ: Prentice Hall, p. 573.
73. Bornstein, B.H., and D.J. Zickafoose. 1999. "I know I know it, I know I saw it": The stability of the confidence-accuracy relationship across domains. *Journal of Experimental Psychology: Applied* 5(1): 76–88.
74. Varey, C.A., B.A. Mellers, and M.H. Birnbaum. 1990. Judgment of proportions. *Journal of Experimental Psychology: Human Perception and Performance* 16(3): 613–625.
75. Brenner, L.A., and D.J. Koehler. 1996. Overconfidence in probability and frequency judgments: A critical examination. *Organizational Behavior and Human Decision Processes* 65(3): 212–219.
76. Johnson, J.G., and M. Raab. 2003. Take the first: Option-generation and resulting choices. *Organizational Behavior and Human Decision Processes* 91: 215–229.
77. Heller, D., I.P. Levin, and M. Goransson. 2002. Selection of strategies for narrowing choice options: Antecedents and consequences. *Organizational Behavior and Human Decision Processes* 89: 1194–1213.
78. Chu, P.C., and E.E. Spires. 2003. Perceptions of accuracy and effort of decision strategies. *Organizational Behavior and Human Decision Processes* 91: 203–214.
79. Fennema, M.G., and D.N. Kleinmuntz. 1995. Anticipations of effort and accuracy in multiattribute choice. *Organizational Behavior and Human Decision Processes* 63(1): 21–32.
80. Rettinger, D.A., and R. Hasti. 2001. Content effects on decision making. *Organizational Behavior and Human Decision Processes* 85(2): 336–359.
81. Paese, P.W., and J.A. Sniezek. 1991. Influences on the appropriateness of confidence in judgment: Practice, effort, information, and decision-making. *Organizational Behavior and Human Decision Processes* 48: 100–130.
82. Fu, W.-T., and W.D. Gray. 2006. Suboptimal tradeoffs in information seeking. *Cognitive Psychology* 52: 195–242.
83. Lee, M.D. 2006. A hierarchical Bayesian model of human decision-making on an optimal stopping problem. *Cognitive Science* 30(1): 1–26.
84. Honekopp, J. 2003. Precision of probability information and prominence of outcomes: A description and evaluation of decisions under uncertainty. *Organizational Behavior and Human Decision Processes* 90: 124–138.
85. Hinds, P.J. 1999. The curse of expertise: The effects of expertise and debiasing methods on predictions of novice performance. *Journal of Experimental Psychology: Applied* 5(2): 205–221.
86. Hogarth, R.M., and H.J. Einhorn. 1992. Order effects in belief updating: The belief-adjustment model. *Cognitive Psychology* 24(1): 1–55.
87. Wong, K.F.E., and J.Y.Y. Kwong. 2000. Is 7300 m equal to 7.3 km? Same semantics but different anchoring effects. *Organizational Behavior and Human Decision Processes* 82(2): 314–333.
88. Lenker, J.A., and V.L. Paquet. 2003. A review of conceptual models for assistive technology outcomes research and practice. *Assistive Technology* 15(1): 1–15.
89. Chinander, K.R., and M.E. Schweitzer. 2003. The input bias: The misuse of input information in judgments of outcomes. *Organizational Behavior and Human Decision Processes* 91: 243–253.
90. Louie, T.A. 2005. Hindsight bias and outcome-consistent thoughts when observing and making service provider decisions. *Organizational Behavior and Human Decision Processes* 98(1): 88–95.
91. Pieters, R., and M. Zeelenberg. 2005. On bad decisions and deciding badly: When intention-behavior inconsistency is regrettable. *Organizational Behavior and Human Decision Processes* 97(1): 18–30.

92. Ratner, R.K., and K.C. Herbst. 2005. When good decisions have bad outcomes: The impact of affect on switching behavior. *Organizational Behavior and Human Decision Processes* 96(1): 25–37.
93. Hwang, B.-C. 2001. Methodology for the selection and evaluation of computer input devices for people with functional limitations. Doctoral dissertation. Norman, OK: University of Oklahoma.
94. Parette, H., and D.H. Angelo. 1996. Augmentative and alternative communication impact on families: Trends and future directions. *The Journal of Special Education* 30(1): 77–98.
95. Phillips, B., and H. Zhao. 1993. Predictors of assistive technology abandonment. *Assistive Technology* 5(1): 36.

15 Legislation Relevant to Computer Access

Timeline

1973 Rehabilitation Act passed
1981 MS-DOS 1.0 released
1985 MS Windows 1.0 released
1986 Rehabilitation Act amended to include Section 508
1990 Americans with Disabilities Act passed
1992 MS Windows 3.1 released
1994 MS-DOS 6.22 released
1995 Windows 95 released
1996 Telecommunications Act passed
1997 Individuals with Disabilities Education (IDEA) Act passed
1998 Congress strengthens Section 508 of the Rehabilitation Act as part of the Workforce Investment Act
1998 Access Board establishes guidelines for Telecommunications Act
1998 Assistive Technology Act passed
1999 Electronic and Information Technology Access Advisory Committee (EITAAC) establishes guidelines for Section 508
1999 Windows 98 SE released
2001 EITAAC guidelines officially published

15.1 AMERICANS WITH DISABILITIES ACT

The Americans with Disabilities Act of 1990 (ADA) prohibits discrimination on the basis of disability. The law applies to employment, government services, and public spaces. While there is broad agreement that the aspects of the ADA regulating employment and government services apply to computer access and the Internet, the question of whether a website constitutes a public space that falls under the ADA is still under debate.

In the area of employment, the law requires that employers make "reasonable accommodations" in the workplace to allow a qualified person with a disability to be gainfully employed [1], including computer access if an employee needs to use a computer or the Internet to perform his or her job. This does not mean, however, that an employer is obligated to pay any amount of money or an employee is guaranteed to get whatever accommodations he or she wants. An alternative available to an employer is to restructure an employee's duties so that computer access is not required.

The ADA also requires that programs, services, and activities of state and local governments (but not the federal government) be accessible to people with disabilities. There are several ways a government body can meet these requirements [1]:

- Reasonable modifications to rules or practices
- Removal of architectural, communication, or transportation barriers
- Provision of auxiliary aids and services

15.2   TELECOMMUNICATIONS ACT OF 1996

Section 255 of the Telecommunications Act of 1996 requires telecommunications products and services to be directly accessible to people with disabilities or compatible with assistive technology to the extent access is "readily achievable" based on the cost of making products accessible or compatible and the manufacturer's resources [1, 2]. Telecommunications products that are covered by Section 255 include [2]

- Wired and wireless telecommunication devices, such as telephones (including pay phones and cellular phones), pagers, and fax machines
- Other products that have a telecommunication service capability, such as computers with modems

Section 255 only applies to the portion of a product that provides telecommunication services. For example, if a television set-top box enables email communication or Internet access, then the set-top box (but not the television) is covered by Section 255 [2].

15.3   REHABILITATION ACT OF 1973 (AS AMENDED IN 1992 AND 1998)

Several sections of the Rehabilitation Act of 1973 apply to computer access technology. Section 501 of the act requires federal agencies to provide reasonable accommodations for employees, including computer access technology if computer use is a job requirement. Section 504 requires entities that receive federal funds (including universities and state and local governments) to provide access for people with disabilities. Section 508, however, has had the most impact on computer access technology.

15.3.1   Section 508 of the Rehabilitation Act

Section 508 of the Rehabilitation Act (first passed in 1986, then amended in 1992 and 1998) requires that all federal employees and members of the public (with or without disabilities) have access to the same information and data. When federal agencies develop, procure, maintain, or use electronic and information technology (E&IT), they must ensure that [2, 3]

- Federal employees with disabilities have access to information and data that are comparable to those of federal employees who do not have disabilities, unless an undue burden would be imposed on the agency.
- Members of the public with disabilities who are seeking information or services from a federal agency have access to information and data that are comparable to those provided to members of the public who do not have disabilities.

Electronic and information technology (E&IT) includes any product (hardware or software) used to acquire, store, manipulate, or transmit information, including [3, 4]

- Software applications and operating systems
- Web-based information and applications such as distance learning
- Video equipment and multimedia products that may be distributed on the World Wide Web
- Computer hardware

E&IT also includes services and documentation, as well as products [4]. For example, technical support service providers must accommodate the communications needs of persons with disabilities [4].

Section 508 applies to all federal departments and agencies but does not apply to the private sector or entities that receive federal funds (http://www.ittatc.org). Section 508 dictates standards for E&IT that federal agencies purchase but not how or from whom they acquire it [4]. Companies interested in selling E&IT to the federal government are responsible for designing and manufacturing products that comply with Section 508 [4].

Federal agencies can also use Section 508 standards as a yardstick to measure compliance with the ADA and Sections 501 and 504 of the Rehabilitation Act [3]. The ADA and Sections 501 and 504 do not explicitly require accommodations to conform with Section 508 accessibility standards, but the Section 508 requirements can be used as a way of demonstrating that accessibility obligations have been met [3].

15.3.2 Why Do Programmers Violate These Rules?

Before discussing allowable exceptions to the Section 508 requirements, it is worth pausing to consider *why* a company's software might violate the requirements. Modern software is typically constructed out of components (e.g., windows, buttons, sliders) provided by the operating system. In general, when developing software, it is easier to stick with the components that the operating system provides (which typically conform to the 508 requirements) than to develop custom components (that may violate Section 508 requirements), so why do people do it? There are three common reasons:

- Speed. Mediating input and output through the operating system takes time. Video games and media players may write their own software that talks directly with the screen, keyboard, or mouse to increase their responsiveness.

- Looks. Companies have a lot of incentive to make their software look the same on different platforms. Keeping the look of software similar makes it easier for a customer to switch between platforms and simplifies documentation and support for the company.
- Effect. Companies want their software to stand out, so they implement controls that other programs don't have, like volume "knobs" instead of sliders.

15.3.3 EXCEPTIONS TO SECTION 508 REGULATIONS

A federal agency's obligations under Section 508 can be satisfied by acquiring E&IT that meets the applicable technical provisions directly or through "equivalent facilitation" [4]. For example, the Section 508 requirements for software applications and operating systems establish accessibility features that must be available to the user. A product can either build these accessibility features in or be compatible with assistive technology that provides these features [2].

There are several exceptions to the Section 508 regulations, however. All Section 508 requirements are subject to commercial availability [3]. If an accessibility product does not exist (for example, photo editing software that can be operated with a screen reader), then there is no obligation to provide that type of accessibility. Section 508 also exempts E&IT used for military command, weaponry, intelligence, and cryptologic activities and E&IT located in spaces used by service personnel for maintenance, repair, or occasional monitoring of equipment [3].

Federal entities are not required to fundamentally alter products to satisfy Section 508 standards, nor do they have to comply with Section 508 standards if it would impose an undue burden to do so [3]. This is consistent with the ADA and other civil rights legislation, where *undue burden* has been defined as "significant difficulty or expense." However, the federal entity must still provide people with disabilities access to the information or data that are affected [2].

15.3.4 EQUIVALENT FACILITATION

Section 508 also allows agencies to accept EIT offered by vendors that uses designs or technologies that do not meet the applicable technical provisions but provide substantially equivalent or greater access to and use of a product for people with disabilities. This is referred to as equivalent facilitation [4]. Equivalent facilitation does not exempt an agency from providing comparable access. Instead, it is a recognition that technologies may be either developed or used in ways not originally envisioned to provide the same or better functional access. Functional outcome is the key criterion when evaluating whether a technology results in "substantially equivalent or greater access" [4].

15.4 TECHNOLOGY-RELATED ASSISTANCE ACT FOR INDIVIDUALS WITH DISABILITIES OF 1988 (THE TECH ACT)

The Tech Act was the first piece of legislation that defined *AT devices* and *AT services*, terms that were later integrated into IDEA, the Rehabilitation Act, and many state laws. It is also the only piece of legislation intended to cut across all agencies, all ages, all disabilities, and all environments [1]. The Tech Act also requires states receiving funds under the act to comply with Section 508 [3].

15.5 TWENTY-FIRST CENTURY COMMUNICATIONS AND VIDEO ACCESSIBILITY ACT

The Twenty-First-Century Communications and Video Accessibility Act (CVAA) updated the Telecommunications Act of 1996 and established new requirements to ensure that people with disabilities have access to technologies developed since 1996 [5]. The CVAA requires Internet-based communications technologies (equipment, services, and networks) to be accessible by people with disabilities, unless doing so would result in an undue burden. The term *undue burden* has the same meaning given in the ADA [5]. For example, smart phones are required to be accessible to people with visual or auditory impairments [5], including advanced functions such as electronic messaging, unless doing so would result in an undue burden [6].

15.6 VOLUNTARY PRODUCT ACCESSIBILITY TEMPLATES

In 2001, the Information Technology Industry Council (ITI) partnered with the U.S. General Services Administration (GSA) to create the Voluntary Product Accessibility Template (VPAT). VPATs are used by federal contracting and procurement officials to evaluate the extent to which products meet applicable Section 508 regulations. Within a VPAT, the summary table (Table 15.1) provides a snapshot of the Section 508 standards. The leftmost column of the summary table lists the subsections of Subparts B and C of the 508 standards. The middle column summarizes whether the product has features that support the accessibility criteria of the corresponding subsection. The rightmost column includes additional remarks and explanations regarding the product [3].

Each subsequent table within the VPAT contains the actual language of a single subsection, divided into its respective subparagraphs. The leftmost column of each table contains the lettered subparagraphs of the respective subsection. The middle column describes whether the product has features that support the accessibility criteria of the corresponding subparagraph. Suggested language has been developed for completing the middle column of a VPAT, but a vendor may choose which, if any, of the terms to adopt [3].

The rightmost column contains clarifying remarks and explanations regarding the product, including (http://www.itic.org)

- Listing accessibility features or features that are accessible
- Detailing where in the product an exception occurs
- Explaining equivalent methods of facilitation

The following sections focus on two of the VPAT tables that are most relevant to computer access technology.

TABLE 15.1
VPAT Summary Table

Criteria	Supporting Features	Remarks and Explanations
Section 1194.21: Software Applications and Operating Systems		
Section 1194.22: Web-Based Internet Information and Applications		
Section 1194.23: Telecommunications Products		
Section 1194.24: Video and Multimedia Products		
Section 1194.25: Self-Contained, Closed Products		
Section 1194.26: Desktop and Portable Computers		
Section 1194.31: Functional Performance Criteria		
Section 1194.41: Information, Documentation, and Support		

TABLE 15.2
Suggested Terms for VPAT Middle Column

Term	Meaning
Supports	Product fully meets the letter and intent of the criteria.
Supports with exceptions	Product does not fully meet the letter and intent of the criteria, but provides some level of access relative to the criteria.
Supports through equivalent facilitation	Product does not fully meet the intent of the criteria, but an alternate means of satisfying the intent of the criteria has been identified.
Supports when combined with compatible AT	Product fully meets the letter and intent of the criteria when used in combination with compatible assistive technology.
Does not support	Product does not meet the letter or intent of the criteria.
Not applicable	Criteria do not apply to the specific product.
Not applicable—fundamental alteration exception applies	A fundamental alteration of the product would be required to meet the criteria.

15.6.1   SECTION 1194.21: SOFTWARE APPLICATIONS AND OPERATING SYSTEMS

This subsection of Section 508 details the requirements that software, such as word processors, spreadsheets, email clients, and web browsers, must meet.

TABLE 15.3
VPAT Table for Section 1194.21

Criteria	Supporting Features	Remarks and Explanations
(a) When software is designed to run on a system that has a keyboard, product functions shall be executable from a keyboard where the function itself or the result of performing a function can be discerned textually.		
(b) Applications shall not disrupt or disable activated features of other products that are identified as accessibility features, where those features are developed and documented according to industry standards. Applications also shall not disrupt or disable activated features of any operating system that are identified as accessibility features where the application programming interface for those accessibility features has been documented by the manufacturer of the operating system and is available to the product developer.		
(c) A well-defined on-screen indication of the current focus shall be provided that moves among interactive interface elements as the input focus changes. The focus shall be programmatically exposed so that assistive technology can track focus and focus changes.		
(d) Sufficient information about a user interface element including the identity, operation, and state of the element shall be available to assistive technology. When an image represents a program element, the information conveyed by the image must also be available in text.		
(e) When bitmap images are used to identify controls, status indicators, or other programmatic elements, the meaning assigned to those images shall be consistent throughout an application's performance.		
(f) Textual information shall be provided through operating system functions for displaying text. The minimum information that shall be made available is text content, text input caret location, and text attributes.		
(g) Applications shall not override user-selected contrast and color selections and other individual display attributes.		
(h) When animation is displayed, the information shall be displayable in at least one nonanimated presentation mode at the option of the user.		

TABLE 15.3 *(Continued)*
VPAT Table for Section 1194.21

(i) Color coding shall not be used as the only means of conveying information, indicating an action, prompting a response, or distinguishing a visual element.		
(j) When a product permits a user to adjust color and contrast settings, a variety of color selections capable of producing a range of contrast levels shall be provided.		
(k) Software shall not use flashing or blinking text, objects, or other elements having a flash or blink frequency greater than 2 Hz and lower than 55 Hz.		
(l) When electronic forms are used, the form shall allow people using assistive technology to access the information, field elements, and functionality required for completion and submission of the form, including all directions and cues.		

(a) When software is designed to run on a system that has a keyboard, product functions shall be executable from a keyboard where the function itself or the result of performing a function can be discerned textually.

Keyboard access to a program's controls and features allows individuals who cannot use a mouse or other pointing device to use the product. This provision does not, however, prohibit the use of mouse-only functions. Only actions that can be identified or labeled with text are required to be executable from a keyboard. In addition, software that display toolbars with buttons do not need to provide keyboard access to all the buttons in the toolbar as long as the feature activated by a control on a toolbar is a duplicate of a menu function that is keyboard accessible. If the control on the toolbar is unique and cannot be accessed in any other way, the control is required to have a keyboard shortcut [2].

Consider this entry from the Microsoft Word for Mac 2010 VPAT:

(a) When software is designed to run on a system that has a keyboard, product functions shall be executable from a keyboard where the function itself or the result of performing a function can be discerned textually.	Supported with exceptions	Microsoft Word for Mac 2011 supports Mac OS 10.5 (Leopard) accessibility features, including Sticky Keys, Slow Keys, and Mouse Keys. Keyboard access is provided in a number of areas throughout Microsoft Word for Mac 2011. Keyboard shortcuts, shortcut keys, and menu commands are available in Microsoft Word for Mac 2011. Documentation for the Microsoft 2011 for Mac system client programs, which includes Microsoft Word for Mac 2011, is provided in digital format with the product. The Microsoft Office for Mac website contains informational material as well. Functionality that is not keyboard accessible includes the standby audio notes control in notebook layout view, the picture placeholder functionality, dragging media objects from the media browser to the document window, and navigation of the media browser window via the toolbar, some links in the product activation wizard, setting focus on a presence icon, the legacy scrapbook, clicking a file on a SharePoint site, viewing a presence card on a SharePoint site, selecting shapes and advanced typography in publishing layout view, and live table resize. The digital image background removal feature requires a mouse.

Microsoft Word for Mac does not completely satisfy this requirement. The third column specifies which features of the software are not keyboard accessible.

To determine whether a program meets this requirement, consider the following questions:

- Can all menu commands be accessed by keyboard?
- Are there any toolbar buttons that can't be accessed from the keyboard?
- Is Sticky Keys supported?

(b) Applications shall not disrupt or disable activated features of other products that are identified as accessibility features, where those features are developed and documented according to industry standards. Applications also shall not disrupt or disable activated features of any operating system that are identified as accessibility features where the application programming interface for those accessibility features has been documented by the manufacturer of the operating system and is available to the product developer.

The application programming interface (API) is how programs communicate with the operating system and with input and output devices. This requirement prohibits software programs from disabling accessibility features when they have been activated prior to running the application [2]. The intent of this requirement is to discourage software from interfering with a user's assistive technology or operating system settings.

Consider this entry from the Microsoft Word for Mac 2010 VPAT:

(b) Applications shall not disrupt or disable activated features of other products that are identified as accessibility features, where those features are developed and documented according to industry standards. Applications also shall not disrupt or disable activated features of any operating system that are identified as accessibility features where the application programming interface for those accessibility features has been documented by the manufacturer of the operating system and is available to the product developer.	Supported	Microsoft Word for Mac 2011 meets these criteria. It may interact with other Microsoft Office 2011 for Mac applications and Mac OS 10.5 (Leopard). It is compatible with Mac OS 10.5 universal access features, including zoom and Mouse Keys. With certain high-contrast settings, the visual aesthetics may not look good, but the chosen setting is not overridden. Microsoft Word for Mac 2011 provides support for Apple's accessibility APIs (with exceptions). This support can be leveraged by other technologies such as the voice-over technology that is provided by Mac OS 10.5.

In this case, the software completely satisfies the requirement. However, the clarifying remarks do warn that the software's look (its visual aesthetics) may be compromised if the user employs a high-contrast color scheme.

To determine whether a program satisfies this requirement, consider the following questions:

- Support for items in accessibility control panel:
    - Is Sticky Keys supported?
    - Is Filter Keys supported?
    - Is Toggle Keys supported?
    - Is Sound Sentry supported?
    - Is high contrast supported?
    - Are cursor blink rate and width supported?
    - Does Mouse Keys work within this application?
- Accessibility software:
    - Do screen magnifiers work?
    - Do screen readers work?
    - Do on-screen keyboards work?

(c) A well-defined on-screen indication of the current [input] focus shall be provided that moves among interactive interface elements as the input focus changes. The [input] focus shall be programmatically exposed so that assistive technology can track [input] focus and [input] focus changes.

Providing a visual indication of input focus helps someone who is viewing the screen to avoid input errors. Assistive technology must also be able to identify which on-screen element has input focus. This provision requires a program to make the identity of the on-screen element with input focus available through its code to assistive technology [2].

Consider this entry from the Microsoft Word for Mac 2010 VPAT:

(c) A well-defined on-screen indication of the current focus shall be provided that moves among interactive interface elements as the input focus changes. The focus shall be programmatically exposed so that assistive technology can track focus and focus changes.	Supported with exceptions	Microsoft Word for Mac 2011 supports keyboard tabbing. Microsoft Word for Mac 2011 also supports the well-defined on-screen outline that represents current focus, as provided by the operating system in conjunction with voice-over. Exceptions include some areas of the media browser and the code window of Visual Basic for Applications.

In this case, the VPAT discloses that there are some interface elements (such as the media browser) that do not clearly specify where input focus resides. The VPAT does not, however, clarify whether the problem is that input focus is not indicated *visually* to the user or *programmatically* to assistive technology.

To determine whether a program complies with this requirement, consider the following questions:

- Can you tell when menus have focus?
- Can you tell when text fields have focus?
- Can you tell when buttons have focus?
- Do screen readers correctly announce what has focus?

(d) Sufficient information about a user interface element, including the identity, operation, and state of the element, shall be available to assistive technology. When an image represents a program element, the information conveyed by the image must also be available in text.

User interface elements include any feature of a program that is intended to allow the user to perform some action, including buttons, checkboxes, menus, toolbars, and scroll bars. This provision requires that text must be associated with each element that identifies [2]:

- What is the element? (Name of element)
- What does the element do? (Type of element)
- What is the element's current value? (State of element)

The text must be available both visually, to the user, and programmatically, to assistive technology.

Consider this entry from the Microsoft Word for Mac 2010 VPAT:

(d) Sufficient information about a user interface element, including the identity, operation, and state of the element, shall be available to assistive technology. When an image represents a program element, the information conveyed by the image must also be available in text.	Supported with exceptions	Microsoft Word for Mac 2011 provides support for Apple's accessibility APIs (with exceptions); this support can be leveraged by other technologies such as the voice-over technology, which is provided by Mac OS 10.5. Microsoft Word for Mac 2011 supports this criterion with exceptions. Exceptions include: Certain dialogs that have images but aren't mapped to titles. A few images do not have associated screen tips. Dynamic screen tips are disabled in print layout view. Certain custom controls in SDM dialogs may not have associated textual information. In the digital image background removal feature, the following options do not provide the appropriate information using the accessibility APIs: foreground rectangle, foreground/background lines/marks. Also, the scrapbook does not provide the appropriate information using the accessibility APIs.

In this case, there are several instances in which the software fails to satisfy the requirements. Some dialog boxes have images and custom controls that do not have explanatory text associated with them. In addition, the scrapbook feature does not make some explanatory text available programmatically to assistive technology.

To determine whether a program complies with this requirement, consider the following question:

- Do screen readers correctly announce the name (and content) of controls?

(e) When bitmap images are used to identify controls, status indicators, or other programmatic elements, the meaning assigned to those images shall be consistent throughout an application's performance.

This provision only applies to images that are used as input elements or to convey information. Images that are strictly for decoration are not covered. Further, each image should only be used for one thing and the meaning of an image should not change [2].

To determine whether a program complies with this requirement, consider the following questions:

- Does the program use images to convey any information that is not available in other ways?
- Does the meaning of any images change over time?

(f) Textual information shall be provided through operating system functions for displaying text. The minimum information that shall be made available is text content, text input caret location, and text attributes.

The operating system coordinates all of the basic functions that all software relies upon, such as receiving information from the keyboard, displaying information on the computer screen, and storing data on the hard disk. When a program avoids the functions for displaying text or graphics made available by the operating system, assistive technology may not be able to interpret the information. This provision does not prohibit software from using alternative display techniques, but it does require that when an alternative method is used, the information should also be displayed through the operating system [2]. When text is displayed, the program must make the following information available to assistive technology:

- What was written?
- How was it formatted?
- Where is new text input going to go?

Consider this entry from the Microsoft Word for Mac 2010 VPAT:

(f) Textual information shall be provided through operating system functions for displaying text. The minimum information that shall be made available is text content, text input caret location, and text attributes.	Not supported	Microsoft Word for Mac 2011 supports these criteria with exceptions. This is supported in text fields (for example, in certain dialog boxes) and in the Rich Text Edit field. This is not supported in the main Word document window (i.e., the content of the document window does not meet this criterion). However, the text-to-speech technology that is provided by Mac OS 10.5 (Leopard) or later can be used for reading the document content.

Although this entry is small, it contains the most significant accessibility flaw in Microsoft Word for Mac 2010. The main document (i.e., the contents of the file the user is creating) is displayed in a window that does not make the text available to assistive technology such as screen readers. This means that a blind individual using Word for Mac cannot access the contents of a document using a screen reader, which is a fatal accessibility flaw.

To determine whether a program complies with this requirement, consider the following question:

- Do screen readers read all text correctly?

(g) Applications shall not override user-selected contrast and color selections and other individual display attributes.

Persons with disabilities may change the values for configuration options within an operating system, such as colors, contrast, keyboard repeat rate, and keyboard sensitivity. This provision is intended to prevent software from disabling or ignoring these choices. A program can provide alternative settings, but there must be an option within the software to use whatever settings are already in place before the program starts [2].

Consider this entry from the Adobe Connect 8 VPAT:

(g) Applications shall not override user-selected contrast and color selections and other individual display attributes.	Does not support	Adobe Connect does not honor user-defined color and contrast settings in Windows.

The VPAT discloses that Adobe® Connect uses its own color and contrast settings, and does not provide any mechanism for the user to specify that the software should use the settings made at the operating system level.

To determine whether a program complies with this requirement, consider the following questions:

- If high-contrast settings are chosen within the accessibility control panel, are they supported within the application?
- Does a screen magnifier work correctly?

(h) When animation is displayed, the information shall be displayable in at least one nonanimated presentation mode at the option of the user.

Animation can pose serious access problems for users of screen readers or other assistive technology applications. If interface elements or text are animated, the user of assistive technology may not be able to access the application reliably. This provision requires that when animation is used, an application must provide an option to turn off animation [2].

Consider this entry from the iTunes® 10 for Windows VPAT:

(h) When animation is displayed, the information shall be displayable in at least one nonanimated presentation mode at the option of the user.	Partially supported	The visualizer feature does not have an alternative, nongraphical representation.

The iTunes visualizer displays random abstract figures on the screen as music plays. There is no nongraphical alternative to the visualizer available within iTunes, although it is hard to imagine what an alternative might be.

To determine whether a program complies with this requirement, consider the following questions:

- Are animations used to convey information?
- Is the information displayed by animations available on the screen in another modality?
- Can animation be turned off?

(i) Color coding shall not be used as the only means of conveying information, indicating an action, prompting a response, or distinguishing a visual element.

Software should not require a user to distinguish between colors. This provision does not prohibit the use of color to enhance identification of important features, but it does require that some other method of identification, such as text labels, be used in addition to color [2].

Consider this entry from the Microsoft Word for Mac 2010 VPAT:

(i) Color coding shall not be used as the only means of conveying information, indicating an action, prompting a response, or distinguishing a visual element.	Supported with exceptions	Microsoft Word for Mac 2011 does not fully meet this criterion. Color is the only indicator of the difference between grammar and spelling errors, as used by AutoCorrect. There is an alternate way to meet this criterion by using the spelling and grammar dialog under Tools > Spelling and Grammar. Compatibility report doesn't completely meet this criterion, although contrast changes and a flashing icons can be used for purposes of distinguishing between colors. In publishing layout view, color schemes are used for text boxes and color is used to distinguish between different chains of text boxes. Users may create documents that contain information that is distinguished only by color. Users are responsible for adhering to this criterion for documents that they create.

The VPAT identifies several instances where Microsoft Word uses color alone to convey information. For example, Microsoft Word indicates spelling errors by underlining text in red and grammar errors in green. The VPAT also notes that a user may create a document that uses color to convey information, but that is not Microsoft Word's responsibility.

To determine whether a program complies with this requirement, consider the following question:

• Is there any information that is only displayed using color?

(j) When a product permits a user to adjust color and contrast settings, a variety of color selections capable of producing a range of contrast levels shall be provided.

This provision requires more than just providing color choices. The available choices must also allow for different levels of contrast. This does not mean, however, that all software must provide color selections. This provision only applies to products that allow a user to adjust screen colors [2].

Consider this entry from the Adobe Illustrator CS5 VPAT:

(j) When a product permits a user to adjust color and contrast settings, a variety of color selections capable of producing a range of contrast levels shall be provided.	Supports with exceptions	Illustrator CS5 allows a user to customize the brightness of the user interface, the background of his or her document, and the selection guide colors to a wide range of colors supported by the system. However, there may not be sufficient options to allow a range of contrast levels.

Adobe Illustrator allows the user to change the color settings, but does not provide enough color choices. If Adobe Illustrator had not provided any color settings at all, however, then it would not have violated the requirement.

To determine whether a program complies with this requirement, consider the following questions:

- Can the user change color settings within the program?
- Are there many (at least eight) color options?
- If color is changed, does a screen magnifier show the correct colors?

(k) Software shall not use flashing or blinking text, objects, or other elements having a flash or blink frequency greater than 2 Hz and lower than 55 Hz.

This requirement is necessary because displays that flicker or flash can trigger seizures in some individuals with photosensitive epilepsy. The 2 Hz limit was chosen to be consistent with proposed revisions to the ADA accessibility guidelines, which in turn are being harmonized with the International Code Council (ICC)/ANSI standard "Accessible and Usable Buildings and Facilities" (ICC/ANSI A117.1-1998), which references a 2 Hz limit [2].

To determine whether a program complies with this requirement, consider the following questions:

- Are there any blinking objects in the interface?
- Can blinking be turned off?

(l) When electronic forms are used, the form shall allow people using assistive technology to access the information, field elements, and functionality required for completion and submission of the form, including all directions and cues.

Electronic forms are difficult for some people with disabilities to access because the interaction between form controls and assistive technology can be unpredictable, depending upon the design of the interface containing these controls. If keyboard alternatives are provided for navigating through a form, and all elements of the form are labeled with text located in close proximity, the form will most likely meet this provision [2].

Consider this entry from the Adobe Acrobat X for Mac VPAT:

(l) When electronic forms are used, the form shall allow people using assistive technology to access the information, field elements, and functionality required for completion and submission of the form, including all directions and cues.	Supports with exceptions	Form controls in PDF documents support full access to elements and functionality required for completion of the form. However, some dialogs and panels in the Acrobat user interface such as the Share panel, the comments list, and the Portfolio Editor do not provide name, role, and state information for controls and are not fully keyboard accessible.

The VPAT discloses that some dialog boxes and panels (which Adobe considers electronic forms) contain controls that do not make information available programmatically to computer access technology and are not keyboard accessible.

To determine whether a program complies with this requirement, consider the following questions:

- Accessibility control panel:
  - Is Sticky Keys supported?
  - Is Filter Keys supported?
  - Is Toggle Keys supported?
  - Is Sound Sentry supported?
  - Is high contrast supported?
  - Does Mouse Keys work?
- Accessibility software:
  - Do screen magnifiers work?
  - Do screen readers work?
  - Do on-screen keyboards work?

15.6.2 Section 1194.26: Desktop and Portable Computers

This subsection of Section 508 details the requirements that hardware, such as laptops, keyboards, and pointing devices, must meet.

TABLE 15.4
VPAT Table for Section for Section 1194.26

Criteria	Supporting Features	Remarks and Explanations
(a) All mechanically operated controls and keys shall comply with §1194.23 (k) (1) through (4).		
(b) If a product utilizes touch screens or touch-operated controls, an input method shall be provided that complies with §1194.23 (k) (1) through (4).		
(c) When biometric forms of user identification or control are used, an alternative form of identification or activation, which does not require the user to possess particular biological characteristics, shall also be provided.		
(d) Where provided, at least one of each type of expansion slots, ports, and connectors shall comply with publicly available industry standards.		

(a) All mechanically operated controls and keys shall comply with §1194.23 (k) (1) through (4).

The first requirement refers to Subsection §1194.23 of the Section 508 requirements, which specifies accessibility requirements for telecommunications products. Within that subsection, item (k) has four subitems that state:

1. Controls and keys shall be tactilely discernible without activating the controls or keys.
2. Controls and keys shall be operable with one hand and shall not require tight grasping, pinching, or twisting of the wrist. The force required to activate controls and keys shall be 5 lb (22.2 N) maximum.
3. If key repeat is supported, the delay before repeat shall be adjustable to at least 2 seconds. Key repeat rate shall be adjustable to 2 seconds per character.
4. The status of all locking or toggle controls or keys shall be visually discernible, and discernible through either touch or sound.

These provisions cover keyboards, keypads, and other text entry devices along with on/off switches, reset buttons, unlocking controls for docking stations, and releases on items such as Personal Computer Memory Card Association (PCMCIA) card slots and drives [2].

Individual keys must be identifiable and distinguishable from adjacent keys by touch. A product can meet this provision by using various shapes, spacing, or tactile markings. Most computer keyboards, for example, meet this provision because the tactile marks on the *j* and *f* keys permit a user to locate all other keys tactilely, and the physical spacing of the function, number pad, and cursor keys make them easy to locate by touch. Because touch is necessary to discern tactile features, this provision requires keyboards to enable touch without automatically activating a function based on mere contact. Keyboards that are designed to react immediately to touch (e.g., keyboards within touch screens or tablet computers) would not meet this provision because they react as soon as they are touched and have no raised marks or actual keys [2]. The second provision is based on Section 4.27.4 of the ADA accessibility guidelines. This provision is also consistent with the Telecommunications Act accessibility guidelines [2]. The key repeat provision does not require systems to provide a key repeat feature. However, if key repeat is provided, this provision requires the repeat to be adjustable up to 2 seconds between repeats [2].

The status of controls provision deals with latching controls. Buttons that remain depressed when activated and switches with distinct positions satisfy this provision. For buttons that latch but do not remain depressed (e.g., caps lock, scroll lock), the status must be identifiable by either touch or sound, in addition to visual means [2].

Consider this entry from the VPAT for the third-generation Apple iPad:

(a) All mechanically operated controls and keys shall comply with §1194.23 (k) (1) through (4).	Supported with exceptions	Refer to §1194.23 (k) (1) through (4).

Referring to the VPAT table for Section 1194.23, one finds the following:

(k)(1) Products which have mechanically operated controls or keys shall comply with the following: Controls and keys shall be tactilely discernible without activating the controls or keys.	Supported with exceptions	The built-in voice-over screen reader provides audio and visual feedback for touch screen controls without requiring the user to activate them. The home, sleep/wake, side switch, and volume rocker switch are also tactilely discernible. The volume rocker switch must be pressed to determine the current volume setting.

The iPad is not completely in compliance with this regulation because there is no visual representation of the volume level on the iPad. The volume control must be activated (i.e., the user must change the volume) to determine the current volume setting.

(b) If a product utilizes touch screens or touch-operated controls, an input method shall be provided that complies with §1194.23 (k) (1) through (4).

This provision covers desktop, laptop, and tablet computers that use touch screens or other controls that operate by sensing a person's touch. This provision does not prohibit the use of touch screens and contact-sensitive controls. However, if touch-sensitive controls are used, a redundant set of controls must be provided [2].

Consider this entry from the VPAT for the third-generation Apple iPad:

(a) All mechanically operated controls and keys shall comply with §1194.23 (k) (1) through (4).	Supported with exceptions	Refer to §1194.23 (k) (1) through (4).

Referring to the VPAT table for Section 1194.23, one finds the following:

(k)(3) Products that have mechanically operated controls or keys shall comply with the following: If key repeat is supported, the delay before repeat shall be adjustable to at least 2 seconds. Key repeat rate shall be adjustable to 2 seconds per character.	Supported with exceptions	iPad uses a nonmechanical, onscreen keyboard. An external Bluetooth wireless keyboard (available separately) can also be used for text input. Key repeat is only supported on the delete key. The repeat rate and delay before repeat are not adjustable.

Although the iPad uses an on-screen keyboard, a separate wireless keyboard (with mechanical keys) can also be used. The keyboard only allows repeated keystrokes for the delete key, but the repeat rate and delay are not adjustable—in violation of (k)(3).

(d) Where provided, at least one of each type of expansion slots, ports, and connectors shall comply with publicly available industry standards.

This provision requires that any place on a computer system where a user might insert or attach something must comply with an industry standard technical specification that is available to other manufacturers. Examples of items that fall under this requirement include slots for SD cards and DVD ROMs and ports for USB devices. This requirement guarantees that developers of computer access technology will have access to information concerning the design of system connections, and thus be able to produce products that can utilize those connections [2].

Consider this entry from the VPAT for the Apple MacBook Air:

(d) Where provided, at least one of each type of expansion slots, ports, and connectors shall comply with publicly available industry standards.	Supported with exceptions	The MacBook Air has a USB and headphone port on the left side of the unit and Mini DisplayPort and USB on the right side of the unit. USB and headphones are compliant with publicly available industry standards. The Mini DisplayPort provides industry standard output via adapters.

The MacBook Air has a proprietary port (the Mini DisplayPort) for connecting to external displays. The user must buy an adapter that allows the computer to connect to a display using industry standards such as video graphics array (VGA) or high-definition multimedia interface (HDMI).

REFERENCES

1. National Task Force on Technology and Disability. 2007. *Within our reach: Findings and recommendations of the National Task Force on Technology and Disability.* Flint, MI.
2. U.S. Access Board. 2012. Available from http://www.access-board.gov (accessed 2012).
3. Information Technology Technical Assistance and Training Center. 2012. Available from http://www.ittatc.org (accessed 2012).
4. Section508.gov. 2012. Available from http://www.section508.gov (accessed 2012).
5. 21st Century Communications and Video Accessibility Act. 2012. Available from http://www.nad.org/issues/civil-rights/communications-act/21st-century-act (accessed 2012).
6. Richert, M. 2012. The twenty-first century communications and video accessibility act: Highlights of a new landmark communications law. Available from http://www.afb.org/afbpress/pub.asp?DocID=aw130104 (accessed 2012).

Index